# SLEEP, CIRCADIAN RHYTHMS, AND METABOLISM
## THE RHYTHM OF LIFE

# SLEEP, CIRCADIAN RHYTHMS, AND METABOLISM
## THE RHYTHM OF LIFE

*Edited by*
**William Olds**

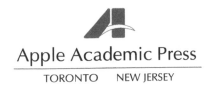

Apple Academic Press

TORONTO    NEW JERSEY

Apple Academic Press Inc. | Apple Academic Press Inc.
3333 Mistwell Crescent | 9 Spinnaker Way
Oakville, ON L6L 0A2 | Waretown, NJ 08758
Canada | USA

©2015 by Apple Academic Press, Inc.

First issued in paperback 2021

*Exclusive worldwide distribution by CRC Press, a member of Taylor & Francis Group*

No claim to original U.S. Government works

ISBN 13: 978-1-77463-079-2 (pbk)
ISBN 13: 978-1-77188-062-6 (hbk)

**Library of Congress Control Number: 2014937347**

---

**Library and Archives Canada Cataloguing in Publication**

---

Sleep, circadian rhythms, and metabolism: the rhythm of life/edited by William Olds.

Includes bibliographical references and index.
ISBN 978-1-77188-062-6 (bound)
1. Circadian rhythms. 2. Sleep. 3. Metabolism. I. Olds, William, editor

QH527.S64 2014          612'.022          C2014-902318-9

---

# ABOUT THE EDITOR

**WILLIAM OLDS, MSc**

William Olds has an undergraduate degree from University of Michigan, and is working on his graduate degree at Yale University, New Haven, Connecticut, in the laboratory of Tian Xu. His current research focuses on satiety signals from the gut and how that communication to the brain breaks down in the pathogenesis of obesity.

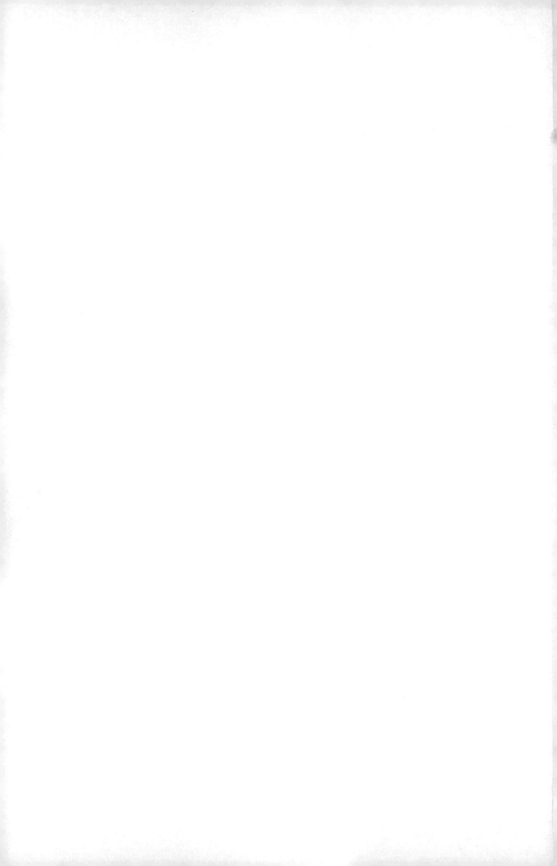

# CONTENTS

# ACKNOWLEDGMENT AND HOW TO CITE

The editor and publisher thank each of the authors who contributed to this book, whether by granting their permission individually or by releasing their research as open source articles or under a license that permits free use, provided that attribution is made. The chapters in this book were previously published in various places in various formats. To cite the work contained in this book and to view the individual permissions, please refer to the citation at the beginning of each chapter. Each chapter was read individually and carefully selected by the editor. The result is a book that provides a nuanced study of the connections between sleep, circadian rhythms, and metabolism.

- Chapter 1 highlights the complexity of our circadian rhythms. Prokineticin 2 is governed by the internal clock, which is malleable and built upon recent history, and, at the same time, the light/dark cycles of our external environment.
- Chapter 2 shows the power of computational biology to uncover new nodes in the network of circadian rhythms.
- Chapter 3 reviews the literature on circadian rhythms as it relates to obesity and acts as a preview to topics that will be explored further in Part 2.
- The work done in Chapter 4 shows how late-night shift conditions impairs our body's ability to keep time and promote metabolic diseases. The authors also show that these effects can be mitigated by strategically planning feeding times, which has potential for therapy for late-night workers suffering from metabolic disease.
- Chapter 5 reviews circadian rhythms with an emphasis on how changing our feeding habits could lead to improved health.
- The previous selections focused on circadian actions of the liver and adipose tissue. Chapter 6 emphasizes circadian rhythms in the brain's neuroendocrine system.
- Chapter 7 investigates the relationship between the suprachiasmatic nuclei and orexin neurons, demonstrating the elegant interplay between our biological clocks and our wakefulness.
- Chapter 8 suggests that the time one eats has as large influence on metabolism as what is consumed.

- Chapter 9 discusses how sleep is an integral part of winding one's metabolic clock. It also serves as a good preview of some of the concepts that will be explored in Part 3.
- Chapter 10 highlights how sleep disorders can result from irregular circadian rhythms and potential ways to diagnose this in individuals.
- Chapter 11 discusses how our globe-trotting and "night-owl" behaviors can disturb the hypothalamic-pituitary-adrenal axis and the repercussions of this disruption on reproduction.
- Unfortunately, our chief model organisms to study circadian rhythms, mice and rats, are nocturnal animals. This makes translational research in this field challenging. Chapter 12 tries to bridge the gap between rats and humans to make our studies easier for comparison across species.
- Thus far, we have focused on how disrupting sleep negatively affects metabolism. However, as discussed in Chapter 13, a high-fat diet can increase sleep duration in rats, revealing an intriguing interplay between diet and sleep.
- After exploring the negative effects of sleep disruption, we conclude with an interesting situation where disruption of sleep is clinically beneficial for depressed patients. Chapter 14 also suggests that our mental state is influenced by circadian rhythms.

# LIST OF CONTRIBUTORS

**Richard R. Almon**
Department of Biological Sciences, State University of New York at Buffalo, Buffalo, NY 14260, USA and Department of Pharmaceutical Sciences, State University of New York at Buffalo, Buffalo, NY 14260, USA

**Roberto Amici**
Department of Biomedical and NeuroMotor Sciences – Physiology, Alma Mater Studiorum – University of Bologna, Piazza di Porta San Donato 2, 40126 Bologna, Italy

**Ioannis P. Androulakis**
Biomedical Engineering Department, Rutgers University Piscataway, NJ 08854, USA

**Johanna L. Barclay**
Max Planck Institute of Biophysical Chemistry, Göttingen, Germany

**Andrew Bierman**
Lighting Research Center, Rensselaer Polytechnic Institute, 21 Union Street, Troy, NY 12180, USA

**Eric L. Bittman**
Department of Biology, University of Massachusetts, Amherst, MA, USA

**Brid Bode**
Max Planck Institute of Biophysical Chemistry, Göttingen, Germany

**Monte S. Buchsbaum**

**John D. Bullough**
Lighting Research Center, Rensselaer Polytechnic Institute, 21 Union Street, Troy, NY 12180, USA

**William E. Bunney, Jr.**

**Maria M. Canal**
Faculty of Life Sciences, University of Manchester, Manchester, UK

**Matteo Cerri**
Department of Biomedical and NeuroMotor Sciences – Physiology, Alma Mater Studiorum – University of Bologna, Piazza di Porta San Donato 2, 40126 Bologna, Italy

**Michelle Y. Cheng**
Department of Pharmacology, University of California, Irvine, CA, USA

**Sehyung Cho**
Department of Neuroscience and Neurodegeneration Control Research Center, Kyung Hee University, Seoul, Korea and Department of Physiology, Kyung Hee University School of Medicine, Seoul, Korea

**Maria Lúcia Corrêa-Giannella**
Laboratory of Cellular and Molecular Endocrinology (LIM/25) - University of São Paulo Medical School, São Paulo, Brazil

**Flavia Del Vecchio**
Department of Biomedical and NeuroMotor Sciences – Physiology, Alma Mater Studiorum – University of Bologna, Piazza di Porta San Donato 2, 40126 Bologna, Italy

**Alessia Di Cristoforo**
Department of Biomedical and NeuroMotor Sciences – Physiology, Alma Mater Studiorum – University of Bologna, Piazza di Porta San Donato 2, 40126 Bologna, Italy

**Debra C. DuBois**
Department of Biological Sciences, State University of New York at Buffalo, Buffalo, NY 14260, USA and Department of Pharmaceutical Sciences, State University of New York at Buffalo, Buffalo, NY 14260, USA

**Mariana G. Figueiro**
Lighting Research Center, Rensselaer Polytechnic Institute, 21 Union Street, Troy, NY 12180, USA

**Oren Froy**
Institute of Biochemistry, Food Science and Nutrition, Robert H. Smith Faculty of Agriculture, Food and Environment, The Hebrew University of Jerusalem, P.O. Box 12, 76100 Rehovot, Israel

**J. Christian Gillin**

**Samer Hattar**
Departments of Biology and Neuroscience, Johns Hopkins University, Baltimore, MD, USA

**Dong-Hee Han**
Department of Neuroscience and Neurodegeneration Control Research Center, Kyung Hee University, Seoul, Korea

**Tamara Hershey**

**Akiko Hida**
Department of Psychophysiology, National Institute of Mental Health, National Center of Neurology & Psychiatry, 4-1-1 Ogawa-Higashi, Kodaira, Tokyo 187-8553, Japan

**Jana Husse**
Max Planck Institute of Biophysical Chemistry, Göttingen, Germany

**J. Chad Johnson**

**William J. Jusko**
Department of Pharmaceutical Sciences, State University of New York at Buffalo, Buffalo, NY 14260, USA

**Chang-Ju Kim**
Department of Physiology, Kyung Hee University School of Medicine, Seoul, Korea

**Kyungjin Kim**
Department of Biological Sciences, Seoul National University, Seoul, Korea

**Mi-Hee Kim**
Department of Neuroscience and Neurodegeneration Control Research Center, Kyung Hee University, Seoul, Korea

**Shingo Kitamura**
Department of Psychophysiology, National Institute of Mental Health, National Center of Neurology & Psychiatry, 4-1-1 Ogawa-Higashi, Kodaira, Tokyo 187-8553, Japan

**A.M.O. Leal**
Divisão de Endocrinologia, Faculdade de Medicina de Ribeirão Preto, Universidade de São Paulo, Ribeirão Preto, SP, Brasil

**Hendrik Lehnert**
Department of Internal Medicine I, University of Lübeck, Lübeck, Germany

**Marco Luppi**
Department of Biomedical and NeuroMotor Sciences – Physiology, Alma Mater Studiorum – University of Bologna, Piazza di Porta San Donato 2, 40126 Bologna, Italy

**Megan M. Mahoney**
Veterinary Biosciences and Neuroscience Program, University of Illinois, 3639 VMBSB MC-002, 2001 S Lincoln Avenue, Urbana, IL 61802, USA

**Oliver J. Marston**
Faculty of Life Sciences, University of Manchester, Manchester, UK

**Davide Martelli**
Department of Biomedical and NeuroMotor Sciences – Physiology, Alma Mater Studiorum – University of Bologna, Piazza di Porta San Donato 2, 40126 Bologna, Italy

**Judit Meyer-Kovac**
Max Planck Institute of Biophysical Chemistry, Göttingen, Germany

**Kazuo Mishima**
Department of Psychophysiology, National Institute of Mental Health, National Center of Neurology & Psychiatry, 4-1-1 Ogawa-Higashi, Kodaira, Tokyo 187-8553, Japan

**Maria Beatriz Monteiro**
Laboratory of Cellular and Molecular Endocrinology (LIM/25) - University of São Paulo Medical School, São Paulo, Brazil

**A.C. Moreira**
Divisão de Endocrinologia, Faculdade de Medicina de Ribeirão Preto, Universidade de São Paulo, Ribeirão Preto, SP, Brasil

**Nadine Naujokat**
Max Planck Institute of Biophysical Chemistry, Göttingen, Germany

**Jong-Yun Noh**
Department of Neuroscience and Neurodegeneration Control Research Center, Kyung Hee University, Seoul, Korea

**Henrik Oster**
Max Planck Institute of Biophysical Chemistry, Göttingen, Germany and Department of Internal Medicine I, University of Lübeck, Lübeck, Germany

**Meric A. Ovacik**
Chemical and Biochemical Engineering Department, Rutgers University Piscataway, NJ 08854, USA

**Youngmi Kim Pak**
Department of Neuroscience and Neurodegeneration Control Research Center, Kyung Hee University, Seoul, Korea and Department of Physiology, Kyung Hee University School of Medicine, Seoul, Korea

**Emanuele Perez**
Department of Biomedical and NeuroMotor Sciences – Physiology, Alma Mater Studiorum – University of Bologna, Piazza di Porta San Donato 2, 40126 Bologna, Italy

**Hugh D. Piggins**
Faculty of Life Sciences, University of Manchester, Manchester, UK

**Mark S. Rea**
Lighting Research Center, Rensselaer Polytechnic Institute, 21 Union Street, Troy, NY 12180, USA

**Rayna E. Samuels**
Faculty of Life Sciences, University of Manchester, Manchester, UK

**Sebastian M. Schmid**
Department of Internal Medicine I, University of Lübeck, Lübeck, Germany

**Gi Hoon Son**
Department of Legal Medicine, Korea University College of Medicine, Seoul, Korea

**Siddharth Sukumaran**
Department of Biological Sciences, State University of New York at Buffalo, Buffalo, NY 14260, USA

**Domenico Tupone**
Department of Biomedical and NeuroMotor Sciences – Physiology, Alma Mater Studiorum – University of Bologna, Piazza di Porta San Donato 2, 40126 Bologna, Italy

**Neil Upton**
Neurology & GI-CEDD, GlaxoSmithKline Pharmaceuticals, New Frontiers Science Park, Third Avenue, Harlow, Essex ,CM19 5AW, UK

**Sandra M.F. Villares**
Laboratory of Cellular and Molecular Endocrinology (LIM/25) - University of São Paulo Medical School, São Paulo, Brazil

**Rhîannan H. Williams**
Faculty of Life Sciences, University of Manchester, Manchester, UK

**Jonathan P. Wisor**
WWAMI Medical Education Program and Department Of Veterinary Comparative Anatomy, Pharmacology and Physiology, Washington State University, Spokane, WA, USA

**Joseph C. Wu**
Department of Psychiatry and Human Behavior, College of Medicine, University of California, Irvine 92717.

**Ji-Ae Yoon**
Department of Neuroscience and Neurodegeneration Control Research Center, Kyung Hee University, Seoul, Korea

**Giovanni Zamboni**
Department of Biomedical and NeuroMotor Sciences – Physiology, Alma Mater Studiorum – University of Bologna, Piazza di Porta San Donato 2, 40126 Bologna, Italy

**Melissa M. Zanquetta**
Laboratory of Cellular and Molecular Endocrinology (LIM/25) - University of São Paulo Medical School, São Paulo, Brazil

**Qun-Yong Zhou**
Department of Pharmacology, University of California, Irvine, CA, USA

# INTRODUCTION

Imagine what the world would be like without a sense of time. How would people know when to meet? How would one cook things or know when to dash out of the house to get to work at the start of the day? Just as our society is built upon times and dates, our organs and even cellular metabolism run by circadian clocks. When these clocks begin to deviate from normalcy, a variety of metabolic and sleep disorders can result.

The circadian rhythm field is an active, multi-disciplicinary area of research encompassing both basic and translational studies. The goals of this text are:

1. To introduce the reader to circadian rhythms in the body and the external cues which set them.
2. Discuss on a molecular and organ-level how disrupting these clocks results in metabolic and sleep disorders.
3. Look at the clinical applications of circadian rhythms, with a focus on sleep.

To this end, the book is broken into three sections, each of which deals with a different aim.

The suprachiasmatic nucleus (SCN) contains the master circadian clock that regulates daily rhythms of many physiological and behavioural processes in mammals. As light is the principal zeitgeber that entrains the circadian oscillator, and PK2 expression is responsive to nocturnal light pulses, Chapter 1, by Cheng and colleagues, investigated the effects of light on the molecular rhythm of PK2 in the SCN. In particular, the authors examined how PK2 responds to shifts of light/dark cycles and changes in photoperiod. They also investigated which photoreceptors are responsible for the light-induced PK2 expression in the SCN. To determine whether light requires an intact functional circadian pacemaker to regulate PK2, this article examined PK2 expression in cryptochrome1,2-deficient

(*Cry1-/-Cry2-/-*) mice that lack functional circadian clock under normal light/dark cycles and constant darkness. Upon abrupt shifts of the light/dark cycle, PK2 expression exhibits transients in response to phase advances but rapidly entrains to phase delays. Photoperiod studies indicate that PK2 responds differentially to changes in light period. Although the phase of PK2 expression expands as the light period increases, decreasing light period does not further condense the phase of PK2 expression. Genetic knockout studies revealed that functional melanopsin and rod-cone photoreceptive systems are required for the light-inducibility of PK2. In *Cry1-/-Cry2-/-* mice that lack a functional circadian clock, a low amplitude PK2 rhythm is detected under light/dark conditions, but not in constant darkness. This suggests that light can directly regulate PK2 expression in the SCN. These data demonstrate that the molecular rhythm of PK2 in the SCN is regulated by both the circadian clock and light. PK2 is predominantly controlled by the endogenous circadian clock, while light plays a modulatory role. The *Cry1-/-Cry2-/-* mice studies reveal a light-driven PK2 rhythm, indicating that light can induce PK2 expression independent of the circadian oscillator. The light inducibility of PK2 suggests that in addition to its role in clock-driven rhythms of locomotor behaviour, PK2 may also participate in the photic entrainment of circadian locomotor rhythms.

Circadian rhythms are 24 hour oscillations in many behavioral, physiological, cellular and molecular processes that are controlled by an endogenous clock which is entrained to environmental factors including light, food and stress. Transcriptional analyses of circadian patterns demonstrate that genes showing circadian rhythms are part of a wide variety of biological pathways. Pathway activity method can identify the significant pattern of the gene expression levels within a pathway. In this method, the overall gene expression levels are translated to a reduced form, pathway activity levels, via singular value decomposition (SVD). A given pathway represented by pathway activity levels can then be as analyzed using the same approaches used for analyzing gene expression levels. In Chapter 2, Ovacik and colleagues propose to use pathway activity method across time to identify underlying circadian pattern of pathways. The authors used synthetic data to demonstrate that pathway activity analysis can evaluate the underlying circadian pattern within a pathway even when circadian patterns cannot be captured by the individual gene expression levels. In addition, they illustrated that pathway activity formulation should be coupled with a significance analysis to distinguish biologically significant information from random deviations. Next, the authors performed pathway activity level analysis on a rich time series of transcriptional profiling in rat liver. The over-represented five specific patterns of pathway activity levels, which cannot be explained by random event, exhibited circadian rhythms. The identification of the circadian signatures at the pathway level identified 78 pathways related to energy metabolism, amino acid metabolism, lipid metabolism and DNA replication and protein synthesis, which are biologically relevant in rat liver. Further, they observed tight coordination between cholesterol biosynthesis and bile acid biosynthesis as well as between folate biosynthesis, one carbon pool by folate and purine-pyrimidine metabolism. These coupled pathways are parts of a sequential reaction series where the product of one pathway is the substrate of another pathway. Rather than assessing the importance of a single gene beforehand and map these genes onto pathways, the authors instead examined the orchestrated change within a pathway. Pathway activity level analysis could reveal the underlying circadian dynamics in the microarray data with an unsupervised approach and biologically relevant results were obtained.

Biological rhythms are present in the lives of almost all organisms ranging from plants to more evolved creatures. These oscillations allow the anticipation of many physiological and behavioral mechanisms thus enabling coordination of rhythms in a timely manner, adaption to environmental changes and more efficient organization of the cellular processes responsible for survival of both the individual and the species. Many components of energy homeostasis exhibit circadian rhythms, which are regulated by central (suprachiasmatic nucleus) and peripheral (located in other tissues) circadian clocks. Adipocyte plays an important role in the regulation of energy homeostasis, the signaling of satiety and cellular differentiation and proliferation. Also, the adipocyte circadian clock is probably involved in the control of many of these functions. Thus, circadian clocks are implicated in the control of energy balance, feeding behavior and consequently in the regulation of body weight. In this regard, alterations in clock genes and rhythms can interfere with the complex mechanism of metabolic and hormonal anticipation, contributing to multifactorial diseases such as obesity and diabetes. The aim of Chapter 3, by Zanquetta and colleagues, was to define circadian clocks by describing their functioning and role in the whole body and in adipocyte metabolism, as well as their influence on body weight control and the development of obesity.

Shiftwork is associated with adverse metabolic pathophysiology, and the rising incidence of shiftwork in modern societies is thought to contribute to the worldwide increase in obesity and metabolic syndrome. The underlying mechanisms are largely unknown, but may involve direct physiological effects of nocturnal light exposure, or indirect consequences of perturbed endogenous circadian clocks. In Chapter 4, Barclay and colleagues employ a two-week paradigm in mice to model the early molecular and physiological effects of shiftwork. Two weeks of timed sleep restriction has moderate effects on diurnal activity patterns, feeding behavior, and clock gene regulation in the circadian pacemaker of the suprachiasmatic nucleus. In contrast, microarray analyses reveal global disruption of diurnal liver transcriptome rhythms, enriched for pathways involved in glucose and lipid metabolism and correlating with first indications of altered metabolism. Although altered food timing itself is not sufficient to provoke these effects, stabilizing peripheral clocks by timed food access can restore molecular rhythms and metabolic function under sleep restriction conditions. This study suggests that peripheral circadian desynchrony marks an early event in the metabolic disruption associated with chronic shiftwork. Thus, strengthening the peripheral circadian system by minimizing food intake during night shifts may counteract the adverse physiological consequences frequently observed in human shift workers.

Obesity has become a serious public health problem and a major risk factor for the development of illnesses, such as insulin resistance and hypertension. Attempts to understand the causes of obesity and develop new therapeutic strategies have mostly focused on caloric intake and energy expenditure. Recent studies have shown that the circadian clock controls energy homeostasis by regulating the circadian expression and/or activity of enzymes, hormones, and transport systems involved in metabolism. Moreover, disruption of circadian rhythms leads to obesity and metabolic disorders. Therefore, it is plausible that resetting of the circadian clock can be used as a new approach to attenuate obesity. Feeding regimens, such as restricted feeding (RF), calorie restriction (CR), and intermittent fasting (IF), provide a time cue and reset the circadian clock and lead to better health. In contrast, high-fat (HF) diet leads to disrupted circadian expression of metabolic factors and obesity. Chapter 5, by Froy, focuses on circadian rhythms and their link to obesity.

Temporal organization is an important feature of biological systems and its main function is to facilitate adaptation of the organism to the environment. The daily variation of biological variables arises from an internal time-keeping system. The major action of the environment is to synchronize the internal clock to a period of exactly 24 h. The light-dark cycle, food ingestion, barometric pressure, acoustic stimuli, scents and social cues have been mentioned as synchronizers or "zeitgebers." The circadian rhythmicity of plasma corticosteroids has been well characterized in man and in rats and evidence has been accumulated showing daily rhythmicity at every level of the hypothalamic-pituitary-adrenal (HPA) axis. Studies of restricted feeding in rats are of considerable importance because they reveal feeding as a major synchronizer of rhythms in HPA axis activity. The daily variation of the HPA axis stress response appears to be closely related to food intake as well as to basal activity. In humans, the association of feeding and HPA axis activity has been studied under physiological and pathological conditions such as anorexia nervosa, bulimia, malnutrition, obesity, diabetes mellitus and Cushing's syndrome. Complex neuroanatomical pathways and neurochemical circuitry are involved in feeding-associated HPA axis modulation. In Chapter 6, Leal and Moriera focus on the interaction among HPA axis rhythmicity, food ingestion, and different nutritional and endocrine states.

Temporal control of brain and behavioral states emerges as a consequence of the interaction between circadian and homeostatic neural circuits. This interaction permits the daily rhythm of sleep and wake, regulated in parallel by circadian cues originating from the suprachiasmatic nuclei (SCN) and arousal-promoting signals arising from the orexin-containing neurons in the tuberal hypothalamus (TH). Intriguingly, the SCN circadian clock can be reset by arousal-promoting stimuli while activation of orexin/hypocretin neurons is believed to be under circadian control, suggesting the existence of a reciprocal relationship. Unfortunately, since orexin neurons are themselves activated by locomotor promoting cues, it is unclear how these two systems interact to regulate behavioral rhythms. In Chapter 7, Marston and colleagues placed mice in conditions of constant light, which suppressed locomotor activity, but also revealed a highly pronounced circadian pattern in orexin neuronal activation. Significantly, activation of orexin neurons in the medial and lateral TH occurred prior to the onset of sustained wheel-running activity. Moreover, exposure to a 6 h dark pulse during the subjective day, a stimulus that promotes arousal and phase advances behavioral rhythms, activated neurons in the medial and lateral TH including those containing orexin. Concurrently, this stimulus suppressed SCN activity while activating cells in the median raphe. In contrast, dark pulse exposure during the subjective night did not reset SCN-controlled behavioral rhythms and caused a transient suppression of neuronal activation in the TH. Collectively these results demonstrate, for the first time, pronounced circadian control of orexin neuron activation and implicate recruitment of orexin cells in dark pulse resetting of the SCN circadian clock.

In modern society, growing numbers of people are engaged in various forms of shift works or trans-meridian travels. Such circadian misalignment is known to disturb endogenous diurnal rhythms, which may lead to harmful physiological consequences including metabolic syndrome, obesity, cancer, cardiovascular disorders, and gastric disorders as well as other physical and mental disorders. However, the precise mechanism(s) underlying these changes are yet unclear. Chapter 8, by Yoon and colleagues, therefore examined the effects of 6 h advance or delay of usual meal time on diurnal rhythmicities in home cage activity (HCA), body temperature (BT), blood metabolic markers, glucose homeostasis, and expression of genes that are involved in cholesterol homeostasis by feeding young adult male mice in a time-restrictive manner. Delay of meal time caused locomotive hyperactivity in a significant portion (42%) of subjects, while 6 h advance caused a torpor-like symptom during the late scotophase. Accordingly, daily rhythms of blood glucose and triglyceride were differentially affected by time-restrictive feeding regimen with concurrent metabolic alterations. Along with these physiological changes, time-restrictive feeding also influenced the circadian expression patterns of low density lipoprotein receptor (LDLR) as well as most LDLR regulatory factors. Strikingly, chronic advance of meal time induced insulin resistance, while chronic delay significantly elevated blood glucose levels. Taken together, these findings indicate that persistent shifts in usual meal time impact the diurnal rhythms of carbohydrate and lipid metabolisms in addition to HCA and BT, thereby posing critical implications for the health and diseases of shift workers.

In Chapter 9, Wisor proposes a mechanistic link between cellular metabolic status, transcriptional regulatory changes and sleep. Sleep loss is associated with changes in cellular metabolic status in the brain. Metabolic sensors responsive to cellular metabolic status regulate the circadian clock transcriptional network. Modifications of the transcriptional activity of circadian clock genes affect sleep/wake state changes. Changes in sleep state reverse sleep loss-induced changes in cellular metabolic status. It is thus proposed that the regulation of circadian clock genes by cellular metabolic sensors is a critical intermediate step in the link between cellular metabolic status and sleep. Studies of this regulatory relationship may offer insights into the function of sleep at the cellular level.

Metabolic, physiological and behavioral processes exhibit 24-hour rhythms in most organisms, including humans. These rhythms are driven by a system of self-sustained clocks and are entrained by environmental cues such as light-dark cycles as well as food intake. In mammals, the circadian clock system is hierarchically organized such that the master clock in the suprachiasmatic nuclei of the hypothalamus integrates environmental information and synchronizes the phase of oscillators in peripheral tissues. The transcription and translation feedback loops of multiple clock genes are involved in the molecular mechanism of the circadian system. Disturbed circadian rhythms are known to be closely related to many diseases, including sleep disorders. Advanced sleep phase type, delayed sleep phase type and nonentrained type of circadian rhythm sleep disorders (CRSDs) are thought to result from disorganization of the circadian system. Evaluation of circadian phenotypes is indispensable to understanding the pathophysiology of CRSD. It is laborious and costly to assess an individual's circadian properties precisely, however, because the subject is usually required to stay in a laboratory environment free from external cues and masking effects for a minimum of several weeks. More convenient measurements of circadian rhythms are therefore needed to reduce patients' burden. In Chapter 10, Hida and colleagues discuss the pathophysiology and pathogenesis of CRSD as well as surrogate measurements for assessing an individual's circadian phenotype.

Circadian rhythms and "clock gene" expression are involved in successful reproductive cycles, mating, and pregnancy. Chapter 11, by Dr. Mahoney, explores how alterations or disruptions of biological rhythms, as commonly occurs in shift work, jet lag, sleep deprivation, or clock gene knock out models, are linked to significant disruptions in reproductive function. These impairments include altered hormonal secretion patterns, reduced conception rates, increased miscarriage rates and an increased risk of breast cancer. Female health may be particularly susceptible to the impact of desynchronizing work schedules as perturbed hormonal rhythms can further influence the expression patterns of clock genes. Estrogen modifies clock gene expression in the uterus, ovaries, and suprachiasmatic nucleus, the site of the primary circadian clock mechanism. Further work investigating clock genes, light exposure, ovarian hormones, and reproductive function will be critical for indentifying how these factors interact to impact health and susceptibility to disease.

Light and dark patterns are the major synchronizer of circadian rhythms to the 24-hour solar day. Disruption of circadian rhythms has been associated with a variety of maladies. Ecological studies of human exposures to light are virtually nonexistent, however, making it difficult to determine if, in fact, light-induced circadian disruption directly affects human health. In Chapter 12, Rea and colleagues used a newly developed field measurement device to record circadian light exposures and activity from day-shift and rotating-shift nurses. Circadian disruption defined in terms of behavioral entrainment was quantified for these two groups using phasor analyses of the circular cross-correlations between light exposure and activity. Circadian disruption also was determined for rats subjected to a consistent 12-hour light/12-hour dark pattern (12L:12D) and ones subjected to a "jet-lagged" schedule. Day-shift nurses and rats exposed to the consistent light-dark pattern exhibited pronounced similarities in their circular cross-correlation functions and 24-hour phasor representations except for an approximate 12-hour phase difference between species. The phase difference reflects the diurnal versus nocturnal behavior of humans versus rodents. Phase differences within species likely reflect chronotype differences among individuals. Rotating-shift nurses and rats subjected to the "jet-lagged" schedule exhibited significant reductions in phasor magnitudes compared to the day-shift nurses and the 12L:12D rats. The reductions in the 24-hour phasor magnitudes indicate a loss of behavioral entrainment compared to the nurses and the rats with regular light-dark exposure patterns. This paper provides a quantitative foundation for systematically studying the impact of light-induced circadian disruption in humans and in animal models. Ecological light and activity data are needed to develop the essential insights into circadian entrainment/disruption actually experienced by modern people. These data can now be obtained and analyzed to reveal the interrelationship between actual light exposures and markers of circadian rhythm such as rest-activity patterns, core body temperature, and melatonin synthesis. Moreover, it should now be possible to bridge ecological studies of circadian disruption in humans to parametric studies of the relationships between circadian disruption and health outcomes using animal models.

Sleep restriction leads to metabolism dysregulation and to weight gain, which is apparently the consequence of an excessive caloric intake. On the other hand, obesity is associated with excessive daytime sleepiness in humans and promotes sleep in different rodent models of obesity. Since no consistent data on the wake–sleep (WS) pattern in diet-induced obesity rats are available, in Chapter 13, Luppi and colleagues studied the effects on the WS cycle of the prolonged delivery of a high-fat hypercaloric (HC) diet leading to obesity in Sprague-Dawley rats. The main findings are that animals kept under a HC diet for either four or eight weeks showed an overall decrease of time spent in wakefulness (Wake) and a clear Wake fragmentation when compared to animals kept under a normocaloric diet. The development of obesity was also accompanied with the occurrence of a larger daily amount of REM sleep (REMS). However, the capacity of HC animals to respond to a "Continuous darkness" exposure condition (obtained by extending the Dark period of the Light–Dark cycle to the following Light period) with an increase of Sequential REMS was dampened. The results of the present study indicate that if, on one hand, sleep curtailment promotes an excess of energy accumulation; on the other hand an over-exceeding energy accumulation depresses Wake. Thus, processes underlying energy homeostasis possibly interact with those underlying WS behavior, in order to optimize energy storage.

Sleep deprivation is a rapid, nonpharmacologic antidepressant intervention that is effective for a subset of depressed patients. The objective of Chapter 14, by Wu and colleagues, was to identify which brain structures' activity differentiates responders from nonresponders and to study how metabolism in these brain regions changes with mood. Regional cerebral glucose metabolism was assessed by positron emission tomography (PET) with ['8F]deoxyglucose (FDG before and after total sleep deprivation in 15 unmedicated awake patients with unipolar major depression and 15 normal control subjects, who did the continuous performance test during FDG uptake. After sleep deprivation, four patients showed a 40% or more improvement on the Hamilton Rating Scale for Depression. Before sleep deprivation the depressed responders had a significantly higher cingulate cortex metabolic rate than the depressed nonresponders, and this normalized after sleep deprivation. The normal control subjects and nonresponding depressed patients showed no change in cingulate metabolic rate after sleep deprivation. Overactivation of the limbic system as assessed by PET scans may characterize a subset of depressed patients. Normalization of activity with sleep deprivation is associated with a decrease in depression.

# PART I

# INTRODUCTION:
# THE WATCH INSIDE ALL OF US

# CHAPTER 1

# REGULATION OF PROKINETICIN 2 EXPRESSION BY LIGHT AND THE CIRCADIAN CLOCK

MICHELLE Y. CHENG, ERIC L. BITTMAN, SAMER HATTAR, AND QUN-YONG ZHOU

## 1.1 BACKGROUND

Light is the principal zeitgeber that entrains circadian rhythms of physiology and behaviour [1,2]. The major light input pathway to the suprachiasmatic nucleus (SCN) is the retinohypothalamic tract [3], which arises from a population of retinal ganglion cells [4]. Recent studies have demonstrated that melanopsin-containing retinal ganglion cells, rods, and cones all convey photic information to the SCN, and mice lacking these photoreceptive systems cannot be entrained by light [5-11]. Excellent progress has been made in the understanding of circadian photic entrainment [12-15]. This includes light-induced transcriptional activation of core clock genes in the SCN, such as *Per1* and *Per2*, as well as immediate-early gene *c-fos*. Exposure to light pulses at night induces expression of these genes in the

*This chapter was originally published under the Creative Commons Attribution License. Cheng MY, Bittman EL, Hattar S, and Zhou Q-Y. Regulation of Prokineticin 2 Expression by Light and the Circadian Clock. BMC Neuroscience 6,17 (2005). doi:10.1186/1471-2202-6-17.*

SCN, and this light induction mechanism has been suggested as a critical pathway for the resetting of circadian clock in response to changes in light/dark conditions [16-19]. Intercellular signalling mechanisms between SCN neurons are also important in circadian photic entrainment, as mice with mutation in a neuropeptide receptor for VIP (Vasoactive Intestinal Peptide) and PACAP (Pituitary Adenylate Cyclase Activating Peptide) are unable to sustain normal circadian behaviour and exhibit loss of sensitivity to light [20].

In addition to the effect of light on circadian entrainment, light also has a direct effect on physiology and behaviour, generally termed as "masking" [21,22]. For instance, light pulses given at night acutely suppress the locomotor behaviour of nocturnal rodents [21,22], and this can occur without functional clockwork [23-27]. Masking may account for the maintenance under normal light/dark conditions of wheel-running rhythms in cryptochrome-deficient (*Cry1-/-Cry2-/-*) mice, which are behaviourally arrhythmic under constant darkness. The contribution of masking to normal locomotor activity rhythms is unclear, as is the participation of the SCN in masking effects of light. Vitaterna et al (1999) first observed a light-driven *Per2* rhythm in the SCN in *Cry1-/-Cry2-/-* mice, and have suggested that the light-driven molecular rhythm in the SCN may be related to the preservation of their locomotor rhythm [25].

We previously found that prokineticin 2 (*PK2*) is a first order clock-controlled gene, whose expression in the SCN is regulated by CLOCK and BMAL1 acting on the E-boxes in the gene's promoter [28]. We have also demonstrated that *PK2* may function as a SCN output molecule that transmits circadian locomotor rhythm via activation of a G protein-coupled receptor [28,29]. Interestingly, we also observed that *PK2* expression is rapidly induced by light pulses administered at night [28], a characteristic that is usually seen with core clockwork genes but not clock-controlled genes. Here we further investigated the light regulation of the rhythm of *PK2* expression in the SCN. In particular, we investigated the photoreceptive mechanisms responsible for the light-induced *PK2* expression in the SCN. Utilizing *Cry1-/-Cry2-/-* mice, we also determined whether light can drive *PK2* expression in the SCN independent of a functional circadian clock.

## 1.2 RESULTS

### 1.2.1 PK2 *RESPONDS DIFFERENTIALLY TO THE DELAY AND ADVANCE OF LIGHT/DARK CYCLES*

We first examined the effects of abrupt shifts of light/dark cycles on *PK2* mRNA rhythm in the SCN. Animals were first entrained for two weeks under 12 hour light: 12 hour dark (LD), then subjected to either a 6 hour delay (6hrD) shift or 6 hour advance (6hrA) shift of light/dark cycles. We measured *PK2* mRNA in the SCN of these animals to examine how quickly the *PK2* mRNA rhythm re-entrains to the shifted light/dark cycles. Under LD, *PK2* mRNA peaks during the day and remains low or undetectable during the night. During the first cycle of the delayed shift (6hrD), the *PK2* mRNA rhythm responds quickly: the rising phase of *PK2* expression adjusts rapidly to the delayed light/dark cycles, while the falling phase still resembles that of the unshifted light/dark cycles (Figure 1A). In contrast, the *PK2* mRNA rhythm responds very little to a 6 hour advance shift (6hrA). During the first cycle of the advance shift, the *PK2* oscillation pattern remains similar to that of the unshifted LD (Figure 1B). These changes in *PK2* expression during 6hrD or 6hrA shift indicate that the endogenous circadian clock exerts dominant control over the *PK2* rhythm, as *PK2* expression cannot respond immediately and completely to the shifts of light/dark cycles.

As it normally takes about 1–2 days for locomotor rhythms to stably entrain to phase delays and about 5–6 days to entrain to phase advances [30,31], we next examined the timecourse of shifts of the *PK2* rhythm to 6 hour phase advances and delays. Consistent with the animal's locomotor behaviour, the *PK2* mRNA rhythm reaches stable phase within 2 days of 6hrD shift (Figure 1C). In contrast, only the rise of *PK2* reaches stable phase within 2 days of 6hrA shift, while the fall of *PK2* takes longer (Figure 1D). Thus, we further examined whether the *PK2* rhythm is stably entrained after 6 days of 6hrA shift. As expected, the *PK2* rhythm is completely entrained to 6hrA shift after 6 days (Figure 1D). Together,

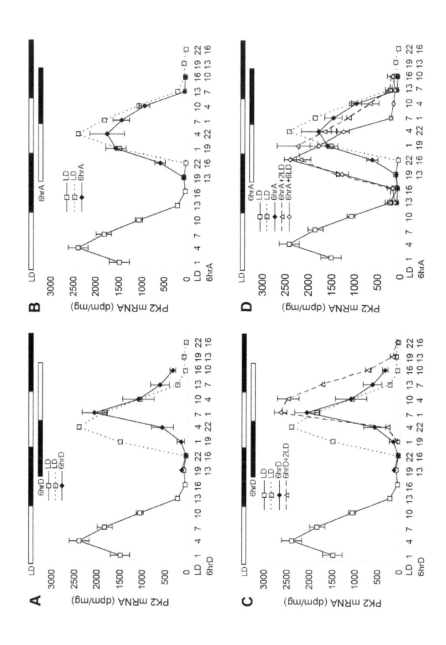

**FIGURE 1:** Temporal profiles of *PK2* mRNA in the SCN in response to abrupt shifts of light/dark cycles. Animals were entrained to 12L:12D (LD) and subjected to either 6-hour delay of light/dark cycles (6hrD), 6-hour advance (6hrA), 6-hour delay followed by adaptation of 2 additional LD (6hrD+2LD), or 6-hour advance followed by adaptation of 2 additional LD (6hrA+2LD) or 6 additional LD (6hrA+6LD). Open and filled horizontal bars indicate light and dark periods, respectively. The LD data is doubled plotted as dashed line (open square) in all graphs. The zeitgeber time (ZT) on the x-axis reflects the timescale for LD, 6hrD or 6hrA. Please note that the additional LD adaptation groups use the same timescale as the 6hrD or 6hrA. (A) Temporal profiles of *PK2* mRNA under 6hrD and LD. Note that *PK2* mRNA responds quickly to the 6hrD shift. (B) Temporal profiles of *PK2* mRNA rhythm under 6hrA and LD. Note that *PK2* mRNA did not adjust to the 6hrA shift. (C) Temporal profiles of *PK2* mRNA rhythm under 6hrD, 6hrD+2LD and LD to indicate adaptation of *PK2* rhythm under 6hrD. Note that *PK2* rhythm is stably entrained to 6hrD after two days. (D) Temporal profiles of *PK2* mRNA rhythm under 6hrA, 6hrA+2LD, 6hrA+6LD and LD to illustrate adaptation of *PK2* rhythm under 6hrA. Note that *PK2* rhythm did not stably entrained to 6hrA until after 6 days. Each value is the mean ± SEM of 3 animals.

the differential responses of *PK2* rhythm to a 6hrD or 6hrA shift indicate that the endogenous circadian clock predominantly controls *PK2* rhythm, as circadian oscillators typically show rapid phase delays but advance with transients [31,32]. The entrainment patterns of *PK2* during phase shifts are consistent with behavioural studies in animals and human subjects [30,31].

## 1.2.2 PK2 RHYTHM IS ENTRAINED BY DIFFERENT PHOTOPERIODS

We next examined the effect of photoperiod on the *PK2* molecular rhythm in the SCN. *PK2* mRNA was measured in the SCN of mice entrained under different photoperiods: 8 hour light: 16 hour dark (8L:16D), 16 hour light: 8 hour dark (16L:8D), or 20 hour light: 4 hour dark (20L:4D). During 12L:12D, *PK2* mRNA is highly expressed during the 12 hour light phase with peak level at ZT4 (Figure 1A, Figure 3A). Under 16L:8D, *PK2* mRNA expands to the entire 16 hour light phase and is essentially undetectable during the 8 hour dark period (Figure 2B). However, the expression of *PK2* mRNA is not confined to the light phase of the shorter photoperiod (8L:16D), as *PK2* mRNA rises before lights on and persists after lights off (Figure 2A). The temporal profile of *PK2* mRNA under this short photoperiod (8L:16D) is very similar to that observed under 12L:12D (Figure 1A, Figure 3A) or constant darkness (2DD) [28]. Thus, although light can induce *PK2* mRNA and expand the duration of *PK2* expression, the phase angle of *PK2* expression is determined by the circadian clock, and its duration cannot be further compressed under shorter photoperiods. Interestingly, the peak of *PK2* mRNA expression was significantly higher in long days (16L:8D) than in shorter days (8L:16D) (Figure 2A–B), further indicate the enhancing effect of light on *PK2* expression. However, a significant reduction in the *PK2* peak level is observed under a very long photoperiod (20L: 4D) (Figure 2C). We also noticed that under 20L:4D, *PK2* mRNA is further expanded and becomes detectable even in dark phase (Figure 2C). Under this long photoperiod (20L:4D), the difference between the peak and basal level of *PK2* is only about 4 fold (Figure 2C). As it has been reported that the rhythms of *mPer1* and *mPer2* mRNAs in the SCN are also entrained with different phase angles under a variety of photoperiods [33-35], we have also examined *Per1* and *Per2* rhythm in our photoperiod studies (see 1). The *Per1* and *Per2* rhythm we observed under these photoperiods are consistent with previous findings [35]. Taken together, these results indicate that changes in photoperiod alter *PK2* rhythm in the SCN, and the amplitudes of *PK2* mRNA oscillation are greatly reduced in very long photoperiods.

### 1.2.3 LIGHT INDUCIBILITY OF PK2 IS ELIMINATED IN MICE THAT LACK MELANOPSIN, ROD AND CONE PHOTOTRANSDUCTION SYSTEM (OPN4-/-, GNAT1-/- CNGA3-/- MICE)

As melanopsin has been implicated in circadian photoreception [5-11], we examined whether the *PK2* molecular rhythm is normally entrained in melanopsin-deficient (*Opn4-/-*) mice. Figure 3 shows that the oscillation profile of *PK2* in the SCN of *Opn4-/-* mice is essentially identical to that observed in the wild type mice under LD. This normal temporal profile of *PK2* mRNA corresponds with the normal locomotor rhythm of

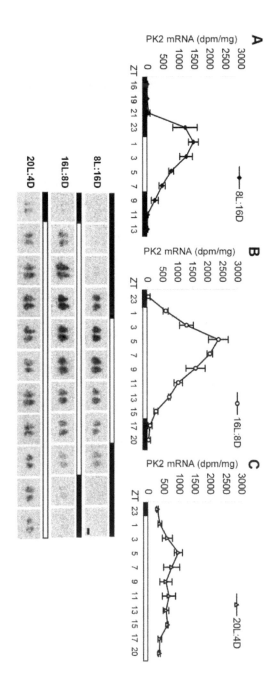

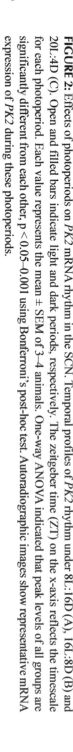

**FIGURE 2:** Effects of photoperiods on *PK2* mRNA rhythm in the SCN. Temporal profiles of *PK2* rhythm under 8L:16D (A), 16L:8D (B) and 20L:4D (C). Open and filled bars indicate light and dark periods, respectively. The *zeitgeber* time (ZT) on the x-axis reflects the timescale for each photoperiod. Each value represents the mean ± SEM of 3–4 animals. One-way ANOVA indicated that peak levels of all groups are significantly different from each other, p < 0.05–0.001 using Bonferroni's post-hoc test. Autoradiographic images show representative mRNA expression of *PK2* during these photoperiods.

*Opn4-/-* mice under light/dark conditions [7,8]. As *Opn4-/-* mice display attenuated phase resetting in response to light pulses and exhibit impaired light masking responses to bright light [36], we also examined whether light inducibility of *PK2* is blunted in *Opn4-/-* mice. Figure 3B shows that light pulse-induced *PK2* in the SCN of *Opn4-/-* mice was significantly reduced by about 50% and 60%, one and two hours after the light pulse, respectively.

The *Opn4-/-* light pulse studies show that a residual *PK2* expression is still present after a light pulse, suggesting that without melanopsin, other phototransduction system can still transmit light information to induce *PK2* expression. Thus, we decided to examine the light inducibility of *PK2* in triple knockout mice lacking melanopsin, rod and cone phototransduction systems (*Opn4-/- Gnat1-/- Cnga3-/-* mice), as these animals free run under light dark conditions (LD) and lack masking responses to light [10]. Figure 3C shows that the light pulse-induced *PK2* in the SCN is completely eliminated in these triple knockout mice, consistent with their malfunctioning photoentrainment systems and their lack of masking responses to light [10]. In addition, we also observed that *PK2* mRNA followed the free-running locomotor rhythms in these triple knockout mice (Figure 3D), with high levels of *PK2* during the inactive phase (CT3) and low levels during active phase (CT15). Together, these results suggest that melanopsin contributes to the light inducibility of *PK2*, and intact melanopsin with functional rod/cone phototransduction systems are required for the light inducibility of *PK2*.

## 1.2.4 A LOW AMPLITUDE PK2 RHYTHM IS PRESERVED IN CRYPTOCHROME-DEFICIENT (CRY1-/-CRY2-/-) MICE UNDER LIGHT/DARK CONDITIONS

Previous studies have shown that the light-regulated Per2 rhythm is maintained in the SCN of cryptochrome-deficient (*Cry1-/-Cry2-/-*) mice that lack functional circadian clock [25,37]. In order to determine whether the regulation of *PK2, Per1, Per2* and *Bmal1* expression by light requires an intact circadian pacemaker, we systematically assessed the temporal mRNA profiles of clockwork genes in *Cry1-/-Cry2-/-* mice under both

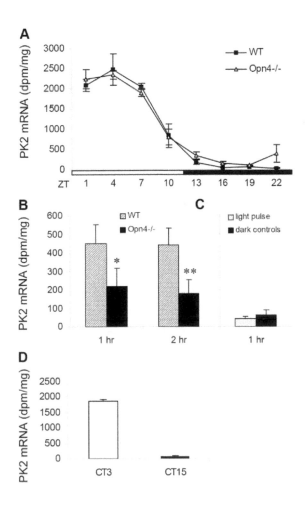

**FIGURE 3:** *PK2* mRNA rhythm in the SCN of melanopsin-deficient (*Opn4-/-*) mice and triple knockout mice (*Opn4-/- Gnat1-/- Cnga3-/-* mice). (A) Temporal profiles of *PK2* mRNA rhythm in wildtype (filled squares) and *Opn4-/-* mice (open triangles) under LD. Open and filled bars indicate light and dark periods, respectively. Each value represents the mean ± SEM of 3–4 animals. Two-way ANOVA indicated that there is no significant difference between genotypes. (B) Light pulse-induced *PK2* mRNA expression in wildtype (shaded bars) and *Opn4-/-* mice (filled bars). *PK2* mRNA was measured one and two hours after brief light pulse at ZT14. Each value represents the mean ± SEM of 6–8 animals. *p < 0.05, **p < 0.01, Student's t-test. (C) Light-pulse induced *PK2* mRNA expression in triple knockout mice that lack melanopsin, rod and cone photoreceptive system (*Opn4-/- Gnat1-/- Cnga3-/-* mice). Dark controls received no light pulse. Each value represents the mean ± SEM of 3 animals. (D) *PK2* mRNA expression in triple knockout mice at circadian time (CT) 3 and 15.

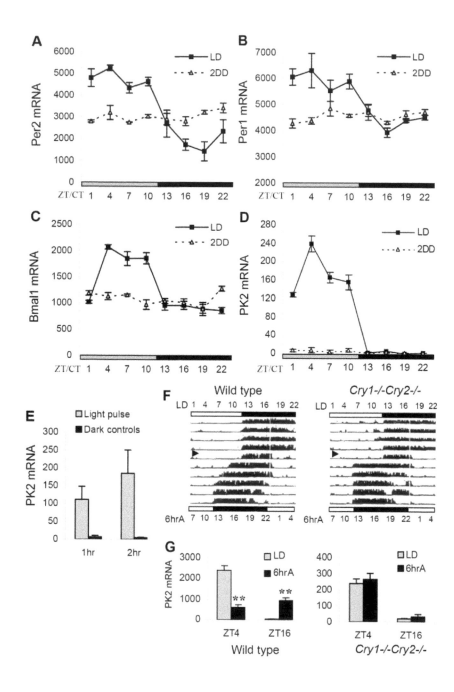

**FIGURE 4:** Light-driven molecular rhythms in the SCN of *Cry1-/-Cry2-/-* mice. Temporal mRNA profiles of *Per2* (A), *Per1* (B), *Bmal1* (C) and *PK2* (D) in *Cry1-/-Cry2-/-* mice under 12L:12D (LD) or two days constant darkness (2DD). Each value represents the mean ± SEM of 3–4 animals. Two-way ANOVA with Bonferroni's posthoc analysis was used to test for significant interactions between expression across time of sampling and under different lighting conditions (LD vs 2DD). $p < 0.0001$ (*Per2*), $p < 0.002$ (*Per1*), $p < 0.0001$ (*Bmal1*) and $p < 0.0001$ (*PK2*). (E) Light pulse-induced *PK2* mRNA in *Cry1-/-Cry2-/-* mice. *PK2* mRNA was measured one and two hours after brief light pulse at ZT14 (shaded bar). Black bar represents dark controls that did not receive light pulse. Each value represents the mean ± SEM of 5–6 animals. Two-way ANOVA indicates a significant difference in *PK2* expression between light and dark treatment ($p < 0.05$), however, the *PK2* induction is not significantly different between the two timepoints (1 hr vs 2 hr). (F) Locomotor behavioural rhythms of wild type (left) and *Cry1-/-Cry2-/-* mice (right) in response to 6 hour advance of light/dark cycle. Open and filled bars indicate light and dark periods, respectively. Black arrow indicates the day of 6 hour advance shift (6hrA). Numbers above and below the actograms represent timescale in zeitgeber time (ZT) for LD and 6hrA. (G) Rapid adjustment of *PK2* rhythm in *Cry1-/-Cry2-/-* mice to 6 hour advance (6hrA). *PK2* mRNA was quantitated in the SCN of wildtype and *Cry1-/-Cry2-/-* mice under LD (shaded) or 6hrA (black). Each value represents the mean ± SEM of 3–4 animals. Three-way ANOVA with Bonferroni's post hoc analysis indicates a significant interaction between light/dark cycle (LD vs 6hrA), timepoint (ZT4 vs ZT16) and genotype (wildtype vs *Cry1-/-Cry2-/-* mice), $p < 0.001$. Two-way ANOVA with Bonferroni's post hoc analysis show that there is significant difference in wildtype *PK2* expression level between LD and 6hrA, (ZT4, ***$p < 0.001$; ZT16, **$p < 0.01$), but not in *Cry1-/-Cry2-/-* mice (ZT4, $p = 1.000$; ZT16, $p = 1.000$).

light/dark (LD) and constant dark (DD) conditions. Figure 4 shows that the molecular rhythm of *Per2* remained largely intact in *Cry1-/-Cry2-/-* mice entrained under 12L:12D, with levels about 4-fold higher during the light phase than the dark phase. This amplitude of the *Per2* oscillation profile was similar to that observed in wild type mice [18,38]. A low amplitude *Per1* rhythm in *Cry1-/-Cry2-/* mice was also apparent under LD, but not DD (Figure 4B). We further detected a light-driven *Bmal1* rhythm in the SCN of *Cry1-/-Cry2-/-* mice under LD, but not DD (Figure 4C). Interestingly, this *Bmal1* rhythm in *Cry1-/-Cry2-/-* mice peaked during light phase, opposite from the *Bmal1* rhythm in wild type mice and in phase with *Per1* [39,40]. As it has been suggested that *PER2* can positively regulate Bmal1 expression via inhibition of the orphan nuclear receptor

REV-ERBα [41,42], it is possible that this *Bmal1* rhythm is secondary to the light-driven *Per2* rhythm. Further studies are required to clarify this observation.

We also examined the molecular rhythm of *PK2* in *Cry1-/-Cry2-/-* mice. Figure 4D shows that *PK2* mRNA rhythm in the SCN of *Cry1-/-Cry2-/-* mice was apparent under LD, with the presence of a low level *PK2* during light phase and absence of *PK2* during dark phase (see 2). Similar to wild type mice, the peak level of this low amplitude *PK2* rhythm was around ZT4, although its peak was only about 8% of that observed in wild type mice (Figure. 4D, Figure 1A, Figure 3A). No *PK2* rhythm was evident when *Cry1-/-Cry2-/-* mice were placed under DD (Figure 4D). Furthermore, the inducibility of *PK2* to nocturnal light pulses is also maintained in *Cry1-/-Cry2-/-* mice. *PK2* mRNA increased one and two hours after a brief light pulse at ZT14 (Figure 4E). Nevertheless, light-induced *PK2* was still detected in *Per1,2,3-/-* mice and *Clk-/-* mice that lack functional circadian clock (Cheng, Weaver & Zhou, unpublished observations). As *PK2* remains responsive to light in these clock mutant mice that lack functional circadian clock, it is likely that the low amplitude *PK2* rhythm in *Cry1-/-Cry2-/-* mice under LD is directly driven by light.

In order to test whether this light-driven *PK2* rhythm may be related to the maintenance of behavioural rhythms observed in *Cry1-/-Cry2-/-* mice under LD, we studied the responses of *Cry1-/-Cry2-/-* mice to a 6 hour advance of lighting schedule. In contrast to the transients of entrainment of locomotor rhythms in wild type mice (which takes about 4-5 days to re-entrain to phase advance), the locomotor activity of *Cry1-/-Cry2-/-* mice adjusted rapidly to 6 hr advance (Figure 4F). Such a rapid response is characteristic of masking. A correlative rapid adjustment of *PK2* was also observed in the SCN of *Cry1-/-Cry2-/-* mice (Figure 4G). As *Cry1-/-Cry2-/-* mice lack functional circadian clock and their locomotor behaviour and *PK2* expression patterns are completely light driven, our results suggest that this low amplitude, light-driven rhythm of *PK2* may contribute to or underlie the masking of locomotor behaviour in these animals.

## 1.3 DISCUSSION

Our studies indicate that the molecular rhythm of *PK2* in the SCN is predominantly controlled by the circadian clock, with light playing a modulatory role. Abrupt shifts of light/dark cycles significantly altered the phase of the *PK2* rhythm. While *PK2* expression re-entrained rapidly to phase delays, it takes several cycles of transients for *PK2* to be stably entrained to phase advances (Figure 1). The rate of re-entrainment of *PK2* molecular rhythms to these shifts is consistent with that of behavioural adaptation of animals and human subjects [30,31]. Our photoperiod studies indicate that *PK2* expression in the SCN responds differentially to changes in photoperiod length (Figure 2). Although increasing light period can induce *PK2* expression and expand the duration of *PK2* rhythm (Figure 2B), shortening of the light period does not lead to corresponding reduction of the duration of *PK2* expression (Figure 2A). It appears that a minimal duration of *PK2* expression is maintained under short photoperiod (Figure 2A) and constant darkness [28], which further indicate the dominant control of *PK2* expression by the circadian clock. Interestingly, the amplitude of the *PK2* oscillation was greatly reduced under very long photoperiod (20L:4D) (Figure 2C). As the amplitude of both *Per1* and *Per2* rhythms were also reduced during 20L:4D (see 1), it is likely that these depressed rhythms of clockwork genes may contribute to the depressed *PK2* rhythm observed. Whether reduction in the amplitude of expression in any of these genes is related to arrhythmicity in LL deserves further examination.

Our studies with *Cry1-/-Cry2-/-* mice revealed the presence of a light-driven *PK2* molecular rhythm in the SCN under LD, indicating that light can drive *PK2* rhythm independent of functional circadian clock. Interestingly, the molecular rhythms of some clockwork genes such as *Per2, Per1,* and *Bmal1* were also partially maintained in the SCN of *Cry1-/-Cry2-/-* mice under LD (Figure 4). Thus, light-driven molecular oscillations of clockwork or clock-controlled output genes exist in the absence of functional circadian clock. Vitaterna et al (1999) first noticed such light-regulated *Per2* molecular rhythm in the SCN of *Cry1-/-Cry2-/-* mice, and suggested the term of "light-driving" effect [25]. As *Cry1-/-Cry2-/-* mice lack functional circadian clocks and their locomotor behaviour remains rhythmic under LD, but not under DD conditions [24,25], it is likely that these light-driven molecular rhythms may drive the locomotor rhythms in these animals. As we have previously shown that *PK2* may be a critical output molecule responsible for circadian locomotor rhythms, the presence of this light-driven *PK2* rhythm in *Cry1-/-Cry2-/-* mice may thus contribute to or underlie masking as well as the free running behavioural rhythms in these animals. It is well established that an intact SCN is necessary for the preservation of free running locomotor rhythms [43]. The role of the SCN in masking of locomotor activity by light is controversial, with similar studies having produced contradictory results [23,44]. Thus, it is possible that there might be common signal molecule(s) that mediate(s) the light-masking and the circadian clock-controlled locomotor behaviour. Construction of *PK2*-deficient mice will be necessary to resolve the exact role of *PK2* in the light-driven locomotor rhythms.

The light inducibility of *PK2* in the SCN is an unusual characteristic for a clock-controlled gene. Our results demonstrate that melanopsin-positive retinal ganglion cells, in conjunction with rods and cones, are responsible for the light-inducibility of *PK2* (Figure 3). The same photoreceptive system has been shown responsible for the entrainment of locomotor rhythm [5-11]. The light inducibility of *PK2* may be related to the presence of a putative cyclic AMP response element (CRE) in the promoter of the *PK2* gene [28]. CRE-dependent activation is critical for light-induced gene expression in the SCN [45-48]. The reduced light inducibility of *PK2* in mutant mice that lack functional clock may indicate that CRE-dependent pathway and CLK/BMAL1 transcriptional factors may interact in the light-induced *PK2* expression in the SCN. Accumulative data have implicated the photic regulation of the transcription of clock genes such as *Per1* and *Per2* in the entrainment of behavioural rhythms [30,34]. The phase of the core SCN clock gene expression determines the timing of clock-controlled SCN output signals that ultimately regulate physiology and behaviour. Unlike the *Per1* promoter, whose activation in the SCN shifts rapidly when the LD cycle is advanced [31], *PK2* exhibits transients during phase advance, more similar to those of *Cry1* and *Cry2* [30,31]. This is consistent with the role for *PK2* as a clock-controlled gene and thus is downstream from the light-regulated expression of *Per1* or

*Per2*. The presence of E box motifs in the *PK2* promoter suggests that light-regulated *Per1* (and perhaps *Per2*) expression can influence *PK2* expression. However, the light inducibility of *PK2* indicates that *PK2* may have a more direct and central role in entrainment in addition to its putative role as an SCN output signal. In other words, whether *PK2* functions completely outside the central circadian loops or partly within them has yet to be determined. It is well established that the activation of glutamate receptor and its downstream actions are critical for the retinohypothalamic inputs of light to the SCN [49]. As receptor for *PK2* is highly expressed in the SCN [28] and activation of the *PK2* receptor triggers similar signalling pathways as that of glutamate receptors [29], it is possible that the circadian clock and/or light-driven *PK2* may feed back to the core circadian loops in the SCN. In addition, *PK2* has recently been shown to excite neurons that express *PK2* receptor [50], further suggesting that *PK2* may activate the firing of SCN neurons, and thus possibly participate in the synchronization of the circadian clock. Thus, the light inducibility of *PK2* may be relevant to both the phase resetting of the core circadian loops and critical SCN output signals.

## 1.4 CONCLUSION

Our studies demonstrate that *PK2* is predominantly driven by the circadian clock, as *PK2* expression exhibits circadian transients in response to phase advances. Furthermore, shortening of the light period does not result in corresponding reduction of the phase of *PK2* rhythm, also consistent with the dominant control from the circadian clock on *PK2* expression. However, light also modulates *PK2* rhythm. Nocturnal light pulses can directly induce *PK2* expression in the SCN. Studies with *Cry1-/-Cry2-/-* mice revealed that light can drive a low amplitude *PK2* molecular rhythm in the SCN in the absence of functional circadian oscillators. These studies demonstrate that *PK2* molecular rhythm in the SCN is controlled by dual mechanisms: dominantly by the circadian transcriptional loops but also directly by light. The light inducibility of *PK2* in the SCN suggest that in addition to *PK2*'s role as a SCN output signal, *PK2* may also participate in the photic entrainment of circadian clock and perhaps in masking.

## 1.5 METHODS

### 1.5.1 EXPERIMENTS OF LIGHT/DARK CYCLE SHIFTS

Male adult C57BL/6 mice (Taconic Farms, New York) were entrained under 12 hour light: 12 hour dark (12L:12D, lights on at 0700 h) cycle for two weeks with food and water available ad libitum. Light phase was either delayed by 6 hours (lights on at 1300 h) or advanced by 6 hours (lights on at 0100 h) and samples were taken every three hours for the 24 hour period (Zeitgeber time, ZT, ZT1-22). To examine *PK2* expression two days after the shift, animals were placed in two additional light/dark cycles and brain samples were collected. All animal procedures were approved by the Institutional Animal Care and Use Committee and consistent with Federal guidelines. In situ hybridization was used in all studies to examine *PK2* mRNA expression in the SCN [28]. Antisense and sense riboprobes containing the coding region of mouse *PK2* (accession number AF487280 1-528 nt), mouse *Per1* (accession number AF022992 340-761nt), mouse *Per2* (accession number AF035830 9-489 nt) and mouse *Bmal1* (accession number AB015203 864-1362 nt) were generated.

### 1.5.2 PHOTOPERIOD STUDIES

Animals were initially entrained under 12L:12D for one week, followed by placement in different photoperiods (light intensity ~400 lux) for three to four weeks: 8 hour light:16 hour dark (8L:16D, lights on at 0900 h, lights off at 1700 h), 16 hour light: 8 hour dark (16L:8D, lights on at 0500 h, lights off at 2100 h). For the 20 hour light: 4 hour dark (20L:4D, lights on at 0300 h, lights off at 2300 h), animals were first placed in 14L:10D for one week, transferred to 16L:8D for another week, followed by two weeks in 20L:4D. All brain samples were taken every two hours throughout the 24 hour cycle, except the first and the last two time points which were sampled every three hours.

## 1.5.3 STUDIES OF MELANOPSIN-DEFICIENT MICE AND MICE THAT LACK MELANOPSIN, RODS AND CONES

Wild type and melanopsin-deficient (*Opn4-/-*) mice (on C57BL/6:129 hybrid background) [5] were entrained to 12L:12D and sampled every three hours for the 24 hour period (ZT1-22). For light pulse studies, wild type, *Opn4-/-* mice and triple knockouts (*Opn4-/- Gnat1-/- Cnga3-/-* mice) that lack melanopsin, rod and cone phototransduction systems were used [10]. Animals received a 15 min light pulse (~200 lux) at ZT14 and brains were sampled one or two hours after light pulse. Dark control animals did not receive a light pulse.

## 1.5.4 STUDIES OF CRYPTOCHROME-DEFICIENT (CRY1-/-CRY2-/-) MICE

Cryptochrome-deficient (*Cry1-/-Cry2-/-*) mice on a C57BL/6:129 hybrid background were kindly provided by Dr. Aziz Sancar (University of North Carolina at Chapel Hill). Wild type and *Cry1-/-Cry2-/-* mice were entrained to 12L:12D and sampled every three hours for the 24 hour period (ZT1-22). A second group of *Cry1-/-Cry2-/-* mice were placed into two days of constant darkness (2DD) (Circadian time, CT, CT1-22). The mRNA levels of *PK2, Per2, Per1* and *Bmal1* were measured in the SCN. For light pulse experiments, *Cry1-/-Cry2-/-* mice received a 15 min light pulse (~400 lux) at ZT14, and sampled one or two hours after light pulse. Dark control *Cry1-/-Cry2-/-* mice did not receive a light pulse. For the shifting experiments, wildtype and *Cry1-/-Cry2-/-* mice were initially entrained under 12L:12D, then subjected to an acute 6 hour advance of lighting schedule. Running-wheel activities of these mice were monitored 10 days before and 10 days after the 6 hour advance shift. The 6 hour phase advance was then repeated and brains were collected at ZT4 and ZT16 on the day of the shift.

## REFERENCES

1.    Reppert SM, Weaver DR: Molecular analysis of mammalian circadian rhythms. Annu Rev Physiol 2001, 63:647-676.

2.   Reppert SM, Weaver DR: Coordination of circadian timing in mammals. Nature 2002, 418(6901):935-941.
3.   Moore RY: Entrainment pathways and the functional organization of the circadian system. Prog Brain Res 1996, 111:103-119.
4.   Ebling FJ: The role of glutamate in the photic regulation of the suprachiasmatic nucleus. Prog Neurobiol 1996, 50(2–3):109-132.
5.   Hattar S, Liao HW, Takao M, Berson DM, Yau KW: Melanopsin-containing retinal ganglion cells: architecture, projections, and intrinsic photosensitivity. Science 2002, 295(5557):1065-1070.
6.   Berson DM, Dunn FA, Takao M: Phototransduction by retinal ganglion cells that set the circadian clock. Science 2002, 295(5557):1070-1073.
7.   Panda S, Sato TK, Castrucci AM, Rollag MD, DeGrip WJ, Hogenesch JB, Provencio I, Kay SA: Melanopsin (Opn4) requirement for normal light-induced circadian phase shifting. Science 2002, 298(5601):2213-2216.
8.   Ruby NF, Brennan TJ, Xie X, Cao V, Franken P, Heller HC, O'Hara BF: Role of melanopsin in circadian responses to light. Science 2002, 298(5601):2211-2213.
9.   Lucas RJ, Hattar S, Takao M, Berson DM, Foster RG, Yau KW: Diminished pupillary light reflex at high irradiances in melanopsin-knockout mice. Science 2003, 299(5604):245-247.
10.  Hattar S, Lucas RJ, Mrosovsky N, Thompson S, Douglas RH, Hankins MW, Lem J, Biel M, Hofmann F, Foster RG, Yau KW: Melanopsin and rod-cone photoreceptive systems account for all major accessory visual functions in mice. Nature 2003, 424(6944):76-81.
11.  Panda S, Provencio I, Tu DC, Pires SS, Rollag MD, Castrucci AM, Pletcher MT, Sato TK, Wiltshire T, Andahazy M, Kay SA, Van Gelder RN, Hogenesch JB: Melanopsin is required for non-image-forming photic responses in blind mice. Science 2003, 301(5632):525-527.
12.  Dunlap JC: Genetics and molecular analysis of circadian rhythms. Annu Rev Genet 1996, 30:579-601.
13.  Lowrey PL, Takahashi JS: Genetics of the mammalian circadian system: Photic entrainment, circadian pacemaker mechanisms, and posttranslational regulation. Annu Rev Genet 2000, 34:533-562.
14.  Hastings M, Maywood ES: Circadian clocks in the mammalian brain. Bioessays 2000, 22(1):23-31.
15.  Cermakian N, Sassone-Corsi P: Environmental stimulus perception and control of circadian clocks. Curr Opin Neurobiol 2002, 12(4):359-365.
16.  Rusak B, Robertson HA, Wisden W, Hunt SP: Light pulses that shift rhythms induce gene expression in the suprachiasmatic nucleus. Science 1990, 248(4960):1237-1240.
17.  Kornhauser JM, Nelson DE, Mayo KE, Takahashi JS: Photic and circadian regulation of c-fos gene expression in the hamster suprachiasmatic nucleus. Neuron 1990, 5(2):127-134.
18.  Albrecht U, Sun ZS, Eichele G, Lee CC: A differential response of two putative mammalian circadian regulators, mper1 and mper2, to light. Cell 1997, 91(7):1055-1064.

19. Shigeyoshi Y, Taguchi K, Yamamoto S, Takekida S, Yan L, Tei H, Moriya T, Shibata S, Loros JJ, Dunlap JC, Okamura H: Light-induced resetting of a mammalian circadian clock is associated with rapid induction of the mPer1 transcript. Cell 1997, 91(7):1043-1053.

20. Harmar AJ, Marston HM, Shen S, Spratt C, West KM, Sheward WJ, Morrison CF, Dorin JR, Piggins HD, Reubi JC, Kelly JS, Maywood ES, Hastings MH: The VPAC(2) receptor is essential for circadian function in the mouse suprachiasmatic nuclei. Cell 2002, 109(4):497-508.

21. Mrosovsky N: Masking: history, definitions, and measurement. Chronobiol Int 1999, 16(4):415-429.

22. Redlin U: Neural basis and biological function of masking by light in mammals: suppression of melatonin and locomotor activity. Chronobiol Int 2001, 18(5):737-758.

23. Redlin U, Mrosovsky N: Masking by light in hamsters with SCN lesions. J Comp Physiol [A] 1999, 184(4):439-448.

24. van der Horst GT, Muijtjens M, Kobayashi K, Takano R, Kanno S, Takao M, de Wit J, Verkerk A, Eker AP, van Leenen D, Buijs R, Bootsma D, Hoeijmakers JH, Yasui A: Mammalian Cry1 and Cry2 are essential for maintenance of circadian rhythms. Nature 1999, 398(6728):627-630.

25. Vitaterna MH, Selby CP, Todo T, Niwa H, Thompson C, Fruechte EM, Hitomi K, Thresher RJ, Ishikawa T, Miyazaki J, Takahashi JS, Sancar A: Differential regulation of mammalian period genes and circadian rhythmicity by cryptochromes 1 and 2. Proc Natl Acad Sci U S A 1999, 96(21):12114-12119.

26. Bae K, Jin X, Maywood ES, Hastings MH, Reppert SM, Weaver DR: Differential functions of mPer1, mPer2, and mPer3 in the SCN circadian clock. Neuron 2001, 30(2):525-536.

27. Bunger MK, Wilsbacher LD, Moran SM, Clendenin C, Radcliffe LA, Hogenesch JB, Simon MC, Takahashi JS, Bradfield CA: Mop3 is an essential component of the master circadian pacemaker in mammals. Cell 2000, 103(7):1009-1017.

28. Cheng MY, Bullock CM, Li C, Lee AG, Bermak JC, Belluzzi J, Weaver DR, Leslie FM, Zhou QY: Prokineticin 2 transmits the behavioural circadian rhythm of the suprachiasmatic nucleus. Nature 2002, 417(6887):405-410.

29. Lin DC, Bullock CM, Ehlert FJ, Chen JL, Tian H, Zhou QY: Identification and molecular characterization of two closely related G protein-coupled receptors activated by prokineticins/endocrine gland vascular endothelial growth factor. J Biol Chem 2002, 277(22):19276-19280.

30. Reddy AB, Field MD, Maywood ES, Hastings MH: Differential resynchronisation of circadian clock gene expression within the suprachiasmatic nuclei of mice subjected to experimental jet lag. J Neurosci 2002, 22(17):7326-7330.

31. Yamazaki S, Numano R, Abe M, Hida A, Takahashi R, Ueda M, Block GD, Sakaki Y, Menaker M, Tei H: Resetting central and peripheral circadian oscillators in transgenic rats. Science 2000, 288(5466):682-685.

32. Daan S, Pittendrigh C: A functional analysis of circadian pacemakers in nocturnal rodents. IV. Entrainment: pacemaker as clock. J Comp Physiol A Neuroethol Sens Neural Behav Physiol 1976, 106:291-331.

33. Messager S, Ross AW, Barrett P, Morgan PJ: Decoding photoperiodic time through Per1 and ICER gene amplitude. Proc Natl Acad Sci U S A 1999, 96(17):9938-9943.

34. Albrecht U, Zheng B, Larkin D, Sun ZS, Lee CC: MPer1 and mper2 are essential for normal resetting of the circadian clock. J Biol Rhythms 2001, 16(2):100-104.

35. Steinlechner S, Jacobmeier B, Scherbarth F, Dernbach H, Kruse F, Albrecht U: Robust circadian rhythmicity of Per1 and Per2 mutant mice in constant light, and dynamics of Per1 and Per2 gene expression under long and short photoperiods. J Biol Rhythms 2002, 17(3):202-209.

36. Mrosovsky N, Hattar S: Impaired masking responses to light in melanopsin-knockout mice. Chronobiol Int 2003, 20(6):989-999.

37. Okamura H, Miyake S, Sumi Y, Yamaguchi S, Yasui A, Muijtjens M, Hoeijmakers JH, van der Horst GT: Photic induction of mPer1 and mPer2 in cry-deficient mice lacking a biological clock. Science 1999, 286(5449):2531-2534.

38. Shearman LP, Zylka MJ, Weaver DR, Kolakowski LF Jr, Reppert SM: Two period homologs: circadian expression and photic regulation in the suprachiasmatic nuclei. Neuron 1997, 19(6):1261-1269.

39. Gekakis N, Staknis D, Nguyen HB, Davis FC, Wilsbacher LD, King DP, Takahashi JS, Weitz CJ: Role of the CLOCK protein in the mammalian circadian mechanism. Science 1998, 280(5369):1564-1569.

40. Hogenesch JB, Gu YZ, Jain S, Bradfield CA: The basic-helix-loop-helix-PAS orphan MOP3 forms transcriptionally active complexes with circadian and hypoxia factors. Proc Natl Acad Sci U S A 1998, 95(10):5474-5479.

41. Preitner N, Damiola F, Lopez-Molina L, Zakany J, Duboule D, Albrecht U, Schibler U: The orphan nuclear receptor REV-ERBalpha controls circadian transcription within the positive limb of the mammalian circadian oscillator. Cell 2002, 110(2):251-260.

42. Ueda HR, Chen W, Adachi A, Wakamatsu H, Hayashi S, Takasugi T, Nagano M, Nakahama K, Suzuki Y, Sugano S, Iino M, Shigeyoshi Y, Hashimoto S: A transcription factor response element for gene expression during circadian night. Nature 2002, 418(6897):534-539.

43. Stephan FK, Zucker I: Circadian rhythms in drinking behavior and locomotor activity of rats are eliminated by hypothalamic lesions. Proc Natl Acad Sci U S A 1972, 69(6):1583-1586.

44. Li X, Gilbert J, Davis FC: Disruption of masking by hypothalamic lesions in Syrian hamsters. J Comp Physiol A Neuroethol Sens Neural Behav Physiol 2004.

45. Gau D, Lemberger T, von Gall C, Kretz O, Le Minh N, Gass P, Schmid W, Schibler U, Korf HW, Schutz G: Phosphorylation of CREB Ser142 regulates light-induced phase shifts of the circadian clock. Neuron 2002, 34(2):245-253.

46. Obrietan K, Impey S, Smith D, Athos J, Storm DR: Circadian regulation of cAMP response element-mediated gene expression in the suprachiasmatic nuclei. J Biol Chem 1999, 274(25):17748-17756.

47. Tischkau SA, Mitchell JW, Tyan SH, Buchanan GF, Gillette MU: Ca2+/cAMP response element-binding protein (CREB)-dependent activation of Per1 is required for light-induced signaling in the suprachiasmatic nucleus circadian clock. J Biol Chem 2003, 278(2):718-723.

48. Yokota S, Yamamoto M, Moriya T, Akiyama M, Fukunaga K, Miyamoto E, Shibata S: Involvement of calcium-calmodulin protein kinase but not mitogen-activated protein kinase in light-induced phase delays and Per gene expression in the suprachiasmatic nucleus of the hamster. J Neurochem 2001, 77(2):618-627.
49. Ding JM, Chen D, Weber ET, Faiman LE, Rea MA, Gillette MU: Resetting the biological clock: mediation of nocturnal circadian shifts by glutamate and NO. Science 1994, 266(5191):1713-1717.
50. Cottrell GT, Zhou QY, Ferguson AV: Prokineticin 2 modulates the excitability of subfornical organ neurons. J Neurosci 2004, 24(10):2375-2379.

*There are several supplemental files that are not available in this version of the article. To view this additional information, please use the citation information cited on the first page of this chapter.*

# CHAPTER 2

# CIRCADIAN SIGNATURES IN RAT LIVER: FROM GENE EXPRESSION TO PATHWAYS

MERIC A. OVACIK, SIDDHARTH SUKUMARAN,
RICHARD R. ALMON, DEBRA C. DUBOIS, WILLIAM J. JUSKO, AND
IOANNIS P. ANDROULAKIS

## 2.1 BACKGROUND

Circadian rhythms are 24 hour oscillations in many behavioural, physiological, cellular and molecular processes that are controlled by an endogenous clock which is entrained to environmental factors including light, food and stress [1]. These oscillations synchronize biological processes with changes in environmental factors thus allowing the organism to adapt, anticipate, and respond to changes effectively.

Some examples of the biological processes and parameters that show circadian oscillations include body temperature, sleep-wake cycles, endocrine functions, hepatic metabolism and cell cycle progression [2]. Furthermore, disruption of circadian oscillations is linked to many diseases and disorders including cancer, metabolic syndrome, obesity, diabetes, and cardiovascular diseases. In mammals, the central (sometimes referred

This chapter was originally published under the Creative Commons Attribution License. Ovacik MA, Sukumaran S, Almon RR, DuBois DC, Jusko WJ, and Androulakis IP. Circadian Signatures in Rat Liver: From Gene Expression to Pathways. BMC Bioinformatics 11,540 (2010). doi:10.1186/1471-2105-11-540.

to as the master) clock is present in the suprachiasmatic nucleus (SCN) in the anterior part of the hypothalamus. Circadian oscillators that are present in other parts of the brain and in other organs are referred to as "peripheral clocks" and are controlled by the central master clock. At the molecular level the clock mechanism involves a transcriptional and post-transcriptional auto-regulatory negative feedback loop consisting of BMAL1 and CLOCK transcription factors which form the positive arm and the PERIOD and CRYPTOCHROME transcription factors which form the negative arm of the feedback loop [3,4]. In addition to these core transcription factors, many other transcription factors which are directly regulated by the core factors including REV-ERBs, RORs and PAR-bZip transcription factors are also involved in the regulation of the circadian expression of the transcriptome which in turn regulates various biological processes [5-7].

Transcriptional analyses of circadian patterns [1,8-10], performed in both drosophila and mammalian systems, demonstrate that genes showing circadian rhythms are part of a wide variety of biological pathways. The expression of several circadian rhythms in a single pathway may ensure a tighter circadian regulation of a pathway or be parts of the circadian clock taking place in other biological functions. The issue of this type of analysis, however, is that moderate but steady changes in the gene expression levels within a pathway could be missed if relatively few individual genes appear significant. Consequently, the identification of biological pathways related to circadian phenomenon could be missed.

We propose to analyze the gene expression data at the pathway level. The starting point of such an analysis is that moderate but steady circadian patterns in the gene expression levels within a pathway could be missed if relatively few individual genes appear circadian. The effectiveness of this approach was illustrated in a study comparing gene expression profiles in muscle of type 2 diabetics (DM2) relative to non-diabetics by [11]. Gene-set enrichment analysis (GSEA) revealed a subset of genes involved in oxidative phosphorylation as being differentially expressed, even though no single gene appeared as differentially expressed between samples. The relationship between oxidative phosphorylation and DM2 is richly supported by the literature [11]. To address the time course gene expression data, Rahnenfuhrer et al. identified the degree of co-expression of genes within a pathway over time [12]. First, the average correlation between gene expression levels within a pathway is computed. Then, the significance of the average correlation of within a pathway is evaluated by a randomization procedure based on the entire microarray. This method, however, can only evaluate whether there is a significant gene expression pattern within a pathway but cannot illustrate the significant pattern itself. Therefore, this method is not able to identify the circadian pattern of a pathway. Alternatively, pathway activity method [13] can identify the significant pattern of the gene expression levels within a pathway. In this method, the overall gene expression levels are translated to a reduced form, pathway activity levels, via singular value decomposition (SVD). A given pathway represented by pathway activity levels can then be as analyzed using the same approaches used for analyzing gene expression levels [13]. Yet, pathway activity method is applied only to evaluate the differentiation between two treatment groups [13,14], i.e. control and treated samples. We propose to use pathway activity method across time to identify underlying circadian pattern of pathways.

Liver is an important organ that is involved in carrying out a wide variety of critical processes including systemic energy regulation processes, metabolism and detoxification of both endogenous and exogenous compounds and hormonal production [9]. Liver is the only tissue that stores glucose in the form of glycogen that can be released in response to glucagon or epinephrine to maintain systemic concentrations [15]. In addition to glucose storage and release, liver can also synthesize glucose de novo through the process of gluconeogenesis. In addition to carbohydrate metabolism, the liver is central to whole body lipid metabolism. About one-half of the cholesterol in the body is produced in the liver, much of which is used for bile acid synthesis [16]. Furthermore, liver is the most important organ that is involved in the metabolism of many drugs and hence contributes to the disposition of these compounds from the body [2]. Proper timing of these processes is of utmost importance for the maintenance of the homeostasis in the system. Previous studies have shown that circadian rhythms are observed at all levels of organization in liver from molecular to the cellular level such as enzyme activity, gene expression, metabolite concentration, DNA synthesis and morphological changes [17]. One of the important levels of organization in the cell is biochemical pathways, which are the ensemble of biochemical reactions to fulfil a particular function. An appreciation of the circadian characteristics of the biological pathways in liver is essential for understanding both the normal physiological and pathophysiological functioning of liver.

In this paper, we used synthetic data to demonstrate that pathway activity analysis can evaluate the underlying circadian pattern within a pathway even when circadian patterns cannot be captured by the individual gene expression levels. In addition, we illustrated that pathway activity formulation should be coupled with a significance analysis to distinguish biologically significant information from random deviations. Next, we performed pathway activity level analysis on a rich time series of transcriptional profiling in rat liver [9]. The over-represented specific patterns of pathway activity levels exhibited circadian rhythms.

## 2.2 METHODS

### 2.2.1 EXPERIMENTAL DATA

Fifty-four male normal Wistar animals (250-350 g body weight) were housed in a stress free environment with light: dark cycles of 12 hr:12hr. Animals were sacrificed on three successive days at each of 18 selected time points within the 24 hour cycle. The time points were 0.25, 1, 2, 4, 6, 8, 10, 11, 11.75 hr after lights on to capture light period and 12.25, 13, 14, 16, 18, 20, 22, 23, 23.75 h after lights on to capture the dark period. To obtain a clear picture, two 24 hour periods were concatenated to obtain a 48 hour period and are meant only as a visual check that curves do in fact "meet" at the light/dark transitions Our research protocol adheres to the "Principles of Laboratory Animal Care" (NIH publication 85-23, revised in 1985) and was approved by the University at Buffalo Institutional Animal Care and Use Committee. The details of the experiment can be found in [9]. The data is available under the accession number GSE8988 http://www.ncbi.nlm.nih.gov/geo/.

## 2.2.2 CIRCADIAN SIGNATURE OF GENE EXPRESSION LEVELS

The circadian pattern of a gene expression is approximated using the sinusoidal model $A \cdot \sin(B \cdot t + C)$ [9]. The coefficients are amplitude (A), frequency (B), and phase (C) of the model. The frequency of the sinusoidal model identifies the essence of the circadian behaviour, which is characterized by one full period in 24 hour. The multiplication of total time (t, 24 hr) and frequency (B) should be equal to $2 \cdot \pi$ in order to characterize one full period (circadian) by the sinusoidal model.

A non-linear curve fitting algorithm is used to define the parameters of the sinusoidal model that would fit best to the gene expression levels over time. The fitted models that have the coefficient B between 0.24 and 0.28 are kept for further analysis to assure the circadian dynamics. Once a model is built for a given gene expression level, the correlation between the data and the model is the criterion to define the circadian signature. Genes are characterized as exhibiting circadian pattern if the correlation between the gene expression and the fitted sinusoidal model is equal or greater than 0.8.

## 2.2.3 PATHWAY ACTIVITY LEVELS

We adapted the pathway activity level formulation to include an additional statistical analysis to evaluate pathway levels [13]. The pathway activity analysis begins with mapping gene expressions of microarray onto pathways. Pathway annotations of gene expressions are retrieved from the publicly available database The Molecular Signatures Database (MSigDB) [18]. Subsequently, gene expression levels within a given pathway are reduced to the pathway activity levels using singular value decomposition (SVD). It is considered that pathway activity levels express the underlying dynamics of a pathway. Next, the significance of the pathway activity levels is evaluated with respect to a randomly permutated microarray data. Then, pathways are filtered out based on the significance analysis.

The matrix $\Xi_p$ (k,t) is composed of k genes and t different conditions (correspond to time points and samples) for the gene expression matrix of a given pathway P of size k genes and t samples, and is normalized to have a mean of 0 and a standard deviation of 1. The singular value decomposition (SVD) of $\Xi_p(k,t)$ is given as:

$$\Xi_p(k,t) = U_p(k,k) \cdot S_p(k,t) \cdot V_p'(t,t) \tag{1}$$

The columns of the matrix $U_p(k, k)$ are the orthonormal eigenvectors of $\Xi_p(k,t)$. The $S_p(k,t)$ is a diagonal matrix containing the associated eigenvalues, and the columns of the matrix $V'_p(t,t)$ are projections of the associated eigenvectors of $\Xi_p(k,t)$. As the elements of $S_p(k,t)$ are sorted from the highest to the lowest, the first row of $V'_p(t,t)$, represents the most significant correlated gene expression pattern within a pathway across different samples. Pathway activity level, $PAL_p(t)$ is defined as the first eigenvector of the $V'_p(t,t)$

$$PAL_p(t) = V_p'(t,1) \tag{2}$$

The first column of $U_p(k, k)$ is a vector of weights, one weight for each gene within the pathway. The weights can be positive or negative values indicating the direction of the expression levels with respect to the pathway activity levels. A higher absolute weight of a gene specifies a higher contribution to $PAL_p(t)$

The fraction of the overall gene expression $(f_p)$ that is captured by $PAL_p(t)$ is:.

$$f_p = \frac{S_p(1,1)^2}{\sum_{g=1}^{t} S_p(g,g)^2} \tag{3}$$

To evaluate whether $PAL_p(t)$ can represent significant information of the pathway of interest, referred as the significance analysis of $PAL_p(t)$ in this study, we perform an additional analysis. This analysis indicates whether there is significant expression pattern shared by individual genes within a pathway [14]. This is performed by evaluating the significance of the $f_p$ value. First, 10,000 random gene sets of the same size of each pathway are generated from the microarray. Next, the $f_p$ values for the random data sets are evaluated and compared to the actual $f_p$ value. The p-value of $f_p$ is computed as the fraction of the $f_p$ of the randomly generated matrices that exceeded the actual fP . If the fP of the randomly generated matrices exceeds the actual $f_p$ by more than 5%, then the actual $f_p$ is attributed to a random variation in the microarray data (p-value < 0.05). Finally, the pathways are filtered based on the associated p-value of their $f_p$ value.

Subsequently, $PAL_p(t)$ (Eq. (2)) is applied to describe the pathway activity levels over time. Each entry of $PAL_p(t)$ represents the pathway activity level of corresponding experimental condition ($\Xi_p(k,t)$ includes replicate measurements at each time point). However, $PAL_p(t)$ do not indicate any up-or down-regulation in pathway behaviour, instead $PAL_p(t)$ evaluates the relative change across different experimental conditions. The sign $PAL_p(t)$ can be chosen based on the pattern the genes that have the highest contribution to $PAL_p(t)$ ($PAL_p(t) \equiv -PAL_p(t)$) [13].

## 2.2.4 CLUSTERING ANALYSIS OF PATHWAY ACTIVITY LEVELS

To cluster the statistically significant pathway activity levels, we applied an unsupervised clustering approach proposed by Nguyen et al. [19]. This approach was applied to detect the significant clusters of co-expressed genes. In this study, we use pathway activity levels instead of gene expression levels.

First, ANOVA is used as a part of the clustering algorithm of the pathway activity levels, where three replicates of each measurement are averaged [20]. Therefore, we applied ANOVA (p-value < 0.01) to remove the pathway activity levels that are not statistically changing across time points prior to the clustering calculation. ANOVA analysis ensures that the observed changes in pathway activity levels occur over time. Following, repeated measurements are averaged for clustering [20]. Subsequently, the optimum number of clusters are decided after considering several clustering methods (hclust, diana, kmeans, pam, som, mclust), metrics (Euclidian,

Pearson correlation, and Manhattan) and an agreement matrix that quanti-fies the frequency which two pathways belong to the same cluster based on the pathway activity levels. Then a subset of pathways is selected to ensure that no pathway is present with an ambiguous cluster assignment with any other pathway in the analysis with a confidence level δ. The δ is the threshold to say whether the agreement level of two pathways belong to one (δ). or two clusters (1 -δ) is consistent or not. The last step is divid-ing the selected subset into a number of patterns based on the agreement matrix. The details of the algorithm can be found in [19]. In this analysis we use δ = 0.65.

## 2.2.5 SYNTHETIC DATA

A hypothetical pathway that consists of 45 gene expressions across T = 54 samples (3 replicates at 18 time points) is constructed following previ-ously described methods. The gene expression values within the synthetic pathway, $g_i$, are generated based on a widely accepted model of periodic gene expression

$$g_i = \beta \cdot \cos(\omega \cdot t + \varphi) + \varepsilon_t \qquad (4)$$

where β is a positive constant, $\omega \in (0, \pi)$, φ uniformly distributed in $(-\pi, \pi]$ where $\varepsilon_t$ is a sequence of uncorrelated random variables with mean 0 and variance $\sigma^2$, independent of φ. We assume φ = 0 for all simulated profiles. In order to simulate different signal to noise ratios we also assume the amplitude for baseline variation constant, but add different noise compo-nent ε for individual profiles. The ε value for each fraction was taken as a random number $\varepsilon_t \in [0,50 \cdot i]$, i = 0,1,2,...100. When the noise level, i, is zero, all 45 genes have the same circadian pattern. As we increase the noise level, the profiles of the individual gene expressions deviate from the circadian pattern and converge to random variation.

To quantify the effect of the noise level on the individual genes within the synthetic pathway, 1000 replicates of the synthetic pathway are generated at different noise levels. For each generated replicate, the fraction of the circadian genes within the synthetic pathway is evaluated and then compared to a given percentage value, i.e. 50%. If the actual the fraction of the circadian genes within the synthetic pathway is smaller than the 0.5, the event that 50% of the genes within the synthetic pathway are circadian is attributed to a random variable. The ratio of the total number of the event that 50% of the genes within the synthetic pathway are circadian to 1000 identifies the p-value. In addition to p-value for the event that 50% of the genes within the synthetic pathway are circadian, p-values for the event that 10% and 90% of the genes within the synthetic pathway are circadian at different noise level.

We evaluate the $PAL_p(t)$ of the synthetic data as the noise level is increased and a non-linear curve fitting algorithm is used to define the parameters of the sinusoidal model that would fit best to the pathway activity levels over time. The procedure for the determination of circadian pattern of pathway activity levels is similar to the determination of circadian pattern of gene expression levels. The synthetic pathway is identified as exhibiting a circadian pattern if the correlation between $PAL_p(t)$ and the fitted sinusoidal model is equal to or greater than 0.8.

## 2.3 RESULTS

### 2.3.1 SYNTHETIC DATA

To test the hypothesis that pathway activity analysis can identify changes that emerge at the pathway level that cannot be identified at the individual gene expression level, a synthetic pathway consisting of 45 genes was constructed and data representative of circadian pattern is generated at different noise levels. Subsequently we compared the significance of the event when 90, 50 and 10% of the genes within the synthetic pathway are circadian. These results are compared with the significance of the synthetic pathway showing circadian pattern in its pathway activity level in Figure 1. For either method, a significance value close to unity indicates that the event is highly likely. A typical threshold used to consider the significance of an event is 0.95. The purpose of this analysis is to evaluate the effect of noise level on the number of genes showing circadian pattern within the pathway.

From Figure 1, we observe that at low noise levels ($0 < i < 6$) we are confident that at least 90% of the genes within the synthetic pathway are circadian. However, the confidence level of detecting 90% of the genes is circadian decreases sharply as we increase the noise level. At this noise level, the underlying circadian pattern can be identified via both evaluating the circadian genes and pathway activity levels. At a noise level of 17, we can confidently conclude that only 50% of the genes are circadian. At higher noise levels, i.e. $i = 30$, we cannot even conclude that 10% of the genes are circadian (p-value $> 0.05$). Thus gene expression alone will not be able to provide information about the significant circadian pattern at this noise level. However, pathway activity analysis predicts with high confidence level (p-value $< 0.0001$) that there is an underlying circadian pattern within the synthetic pathway at this noise level ($i = 30$). Therefore, pathway activity levels are more robust than the gene expression levels in identifying underlying expression pattern within a pathway.

Nevertheless, a critical issue arises when we consider whether the variation captured by $PAL_p(t)$ can represent the overall gene expression within a pathway. While we can be confident that a circadian pattern does exist, we cannot be confident that this pattern is real or due to random variations. To address this issue of random noise in the data vs. real gene expression changes, we evaluated the significance of the $PAL_p(t)$ (presented in Figure 2 at different noise levels). Even though $PAL_p(t)$ might predict confidently a circadian pattern, that event could be the results of random variability in the data, as quantified by the significance of $PAL_p(t)$. For example, at $\alpha = 10$, the significance of the synthetic pathway being circadian is high; however, the significance of $PAL_p(t)$ is considerably lower. This result indicates that the observed pattern cannot be solely attributed to the underlying structure of the data. Therefore, determining significance level $PAL_p(t)$ is necessary for a reliable representation of circadian pathways.

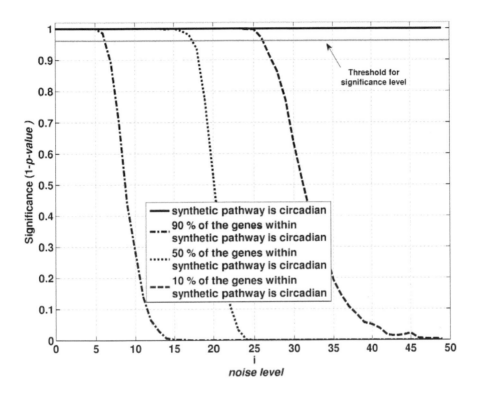

**FIGURE 1:** Effect of noise level on the circadian dynamics of the synthetic pathway. As the noise level is increased, the significance (1-p-value) of the event that synthetic pathway is circadian and the events that 10, 50 and 90% of the genes within the synthetic pathway are circadian are illustrated. The calculations of the p-values are explained in the methods section.

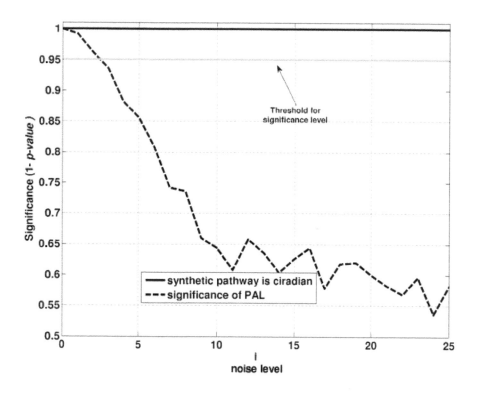

**FIGURE 2:** Effect of noise level on the significance of PAL. As the noise level is increased, the significance (1-p-value) of the event that synthetic pathway is circadian and the significance of PAL are illustrated.

## 2.3.2 CIRCADIAN SIGNATURES OF PATHWAYS IN RAT LIVER

We analyzed a rich time series of transcriptional profiling in rat liver where the rats were maintained in 12:12 hours light/dark cycle and exposed to the least possible environmental disturbances to minimize stress. We evaluated pathway activity level analysis on the microarray data and following applied a clustering analysis of the pathway activity levels.

As a result of the significance analysis $f_p$486 of the 638 defined pathways in MSigDB are considered for further analysis. Having eliminated the pathway activity levels that do not exhibit a significant change over time (ANOVA, p-value < 0.01), the clustering analysis yielded five significant patterns of pathway activity levels (Figure 3). We follow an unsupervised approach and identify the emergent pathway activity level patterns that appeared to have sinusoidal circadian patterns. The significant clusters represent the most populated pathway activity levels patterns within the data, whereas the rest of the data can be associated with random deviations. To quantify the characteristics of the circadian patterns, we perform the approximation of the centroid of each cluster to a sinusoidal function. The correlation between the centroid of each cluster and the associated fitted sinusoidal model exhibit high correlation (correlation = > 0.96, given on top of each graph in Figure 3). The outline of this analysis is depicted in Figure 4.

The peak and nadir points are referred as the turning points. Cluster 1, Cluster 2 have their turning points around the middle of the light period (~6th-8th hours of the 24 hour cycle) and around the middle of the dark period (~18th and 20th hours 24 hour cycle). Cluster3, Cluster 4 and Cluster 5 have their turning points around the transition between the light and the dark period (~10th-13th hours of the 24 hour cycle) and their the turning points around the beginning of the light period and at the end of the dark period (~1st -2nd hours and ~20th and 22nd of the 24 hour cycle).

Evaluating pathway activity levels resulted cases where two pathways have similar fraction of overall gene expression captured by $PAL_p(t)$, $f_p$ values, however the associated p-values, vary significantly. In example, $f_p$ MAPK Pathway, Nicotinate and nicotinamide metabolism and glycine, serine and threonine metabolism pathway are 0.23, 0.21 and 0.22 respectively (top panel of Figure 5).

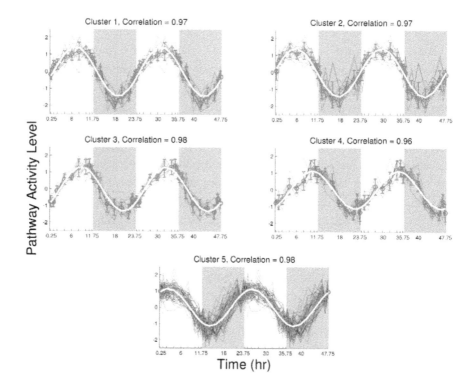

**FIGURE 3:** The five significant clusters identified by a consensus clustering analysis [19] using $\delta = 0.65$. The pathway activity level (PAL) of pathways represents the presented curves and the exact reverse curves; PAL = (-) PAL. The signs of PAL are chosen so that PAL has the similar patterns for a better representation and clustering purposes. The centroids of each cluster is shown with the red error bars, the fitted sinusoidal model to the centroids of each cluster is depicted in white.

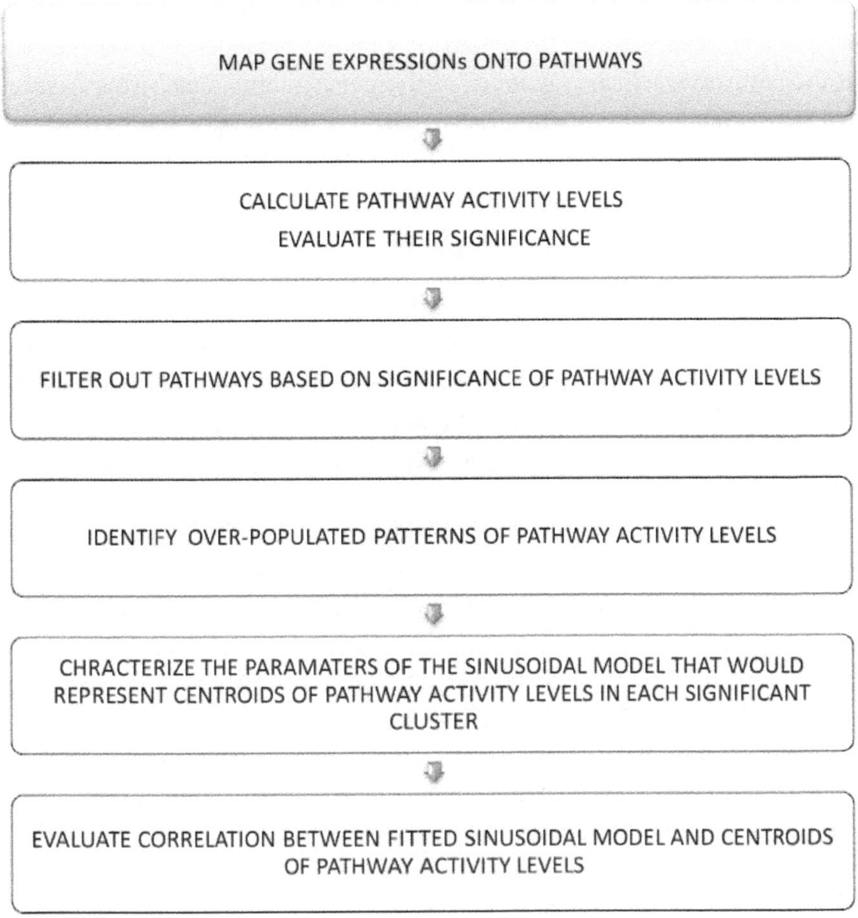

**FIGURE 4:** The outline for clustering analysis of pathway activity levels. Pathway activity analysis begins with mapping gene expression onto known pre-defined groups of genes, pathways. Subsequently, the pathway activity levels are calculated using SVD and the significance of pathway activity levels are evaluated. Pathways are filtered based on the significance of the PALs. Following, the over-populated patterns are identified by using a consensus clustering approach proposed in [19]. Then, the parameters of the sinusoidal model $A \cdot \sin(B \cdot t + C)$ that would best fit the centroids of the pathway activity levels (in each clusters) are characterized. Finally, the correlation between fitted sinusoidal model and the centroids of the pathway activity levels in each cluster is evaluated.

On the other hand, their associated p-values are rather different; 0.66, 0.12 and 0, respectively (top panel of Figure 5). Depending on the size of the pathways, which is number of the genes within a pathway, $f_p$ value can be obtained from random variations. Therefore, $f_p$ value itself is not an objective feature to identify whether the information captured overall gene expression by $PAL_p(t)$ is significant. The significance analysis of $PAL_p(t)$ enables us to filter out pathways that exhibit circadian rhythms by chance. For example, MAPK pathway and Nicotinate and nicotinamide metabolism may be identified as exhibiting circadian pattern without the significance analysis of $PAL_p(t)$ because $PAL_p(t)$ of MAPK Pathway and Nicotinate and nicotinamide metabolism exhibit high correlation with the fitted sinusoidal model (bottom left and bottom middle panels in Figure 5).

Glycine, serine and threonine metabolism exhibit both significant $PAL_p(t)$ and high correlation with the fitted sinusoidal model (top right and bottom right panels in Figure 5). To study the effect of individual gene expression on the pathway activity level, we depict the relationship between the weights and the correlation of the individual genes (the correlation between gene expression levels and the fitted sinusoidal model that represent the circadian pattern) in glycine, serine and threonine metabolism pathway Figure 6. The weight of a gene characterizes its contribution to the pathway activity level compared to the rest of the genes in the pathway.

It can be seen from Figure 6, that Gldc, Cth, Chka, Chkb, Cbs, Bhmt and Shtm1 exhibit circadian patterns (correlation > 0.8) and also their weights are among the highest (weight > | -0.25|). In addition, the genes, which correlation is slightly under the threshold (correlation ~> 0.7) such as Gatm, Shtm2 and Alas1, have comparably higher absolute weights (weight ~> | -0.25|). The positive and negative values of weights indicate the direction of the gene expression when compared to the pathway activity level. In example, the genes that have negative weights have their peak in the early light period and their nadir in the early dark period (e.g. Chka, Cth), whereas the genes that have positive values have their nadir in the early light period and peak in the early dark period (e.g. Shmt1) (Figure 7.). The pathway activity levels of glycine, serine and threonine metabolism (bottom right panel in Figure 5) follow the genes that have the positive weight value (e.g. Chka, Cth) and have its turning point in the early light period. The sign (positive or negative) of the weights can be chosen

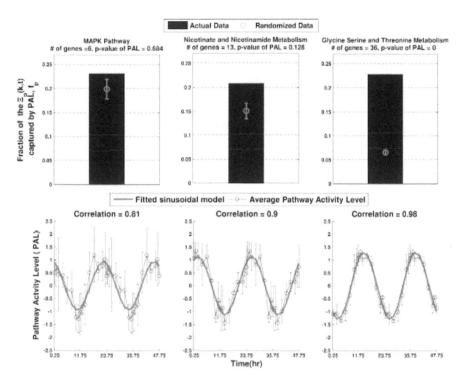

**FIGURE 5:** Pathway activity levels for select pathways. A) The comparison of the $f_p$ to the permutated $f_p$ for MAPK Pathway, nicotinate and nicotinamide metabolism and glycine, serine and threonine metabolism pathway. The mean and the standard deviation interval of permutated $f_p$ is given. The same value of $f_p$ can be obtained by randomly permutated data in MAPK Pathway and nicotinate and nicotinamide metabolism, whereas the $f_p$ captured by randomly permutated data is much lower compared to $f_p$ in glycine, serine and threonine metabolism pathway B) Pathway activity levels and fitted sinusoidal models for the pathways. The mean and the standard deviation interval of the pathway activity levels are given. The correlation between pathways activity level and fitted sinusoidal model is presented for each pathway on top of each graph.

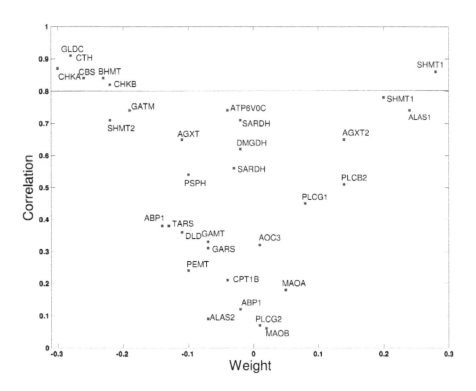

**FIGURE 6:** The relationships between weight and the correlation of the genes within glycine, serine and threonine metabolism. The correlation is between gene expressions and the fitted sinusoidal models and is set to identify circadian genes. The threshold for circadian genes is correlation > 0.8. The weights are evaluated from the SVD analysis. The absolute value of the weights represents the contribution of the individual genes to the pathway activity level. The genes that have higher correlation values have relatively higher absolute weights.

to represent pathway activity level as pathway activity levels indicate the overall orchestrated significant change in the gene expression within a pathway. Furthermore, we observe that there are genes, which correlation is slightly under the threshold (correlation $\sim> 0.7$) but they have low absolute weights (weight $\sim< 0$) such as Atp6voc and Sardh. The expression pattern of these genes, (as an example we depicted the expression pattern of Atp6voc in Figure 7) does not coincide with the rest of the genes that have higher absolute weights, therefore do not contribute to the pathway activity level as much and has low weights.

By applying SVD, a number of possible correlated variables (gene expressions) are mapped onto a smaller number of uncorrelated variables (the rows of $V'_p(t,t)$ in Eq. (1). Pathway activity is denoted as the most significant data pattern which corresponds to the first row of $V'_p(t,t)$ (Eq. (2))as the elements of $S_p(k,t)$ are sorted from the highest to the lowest (Additional File 1). The latter rows correspond to the other patterns which significances are determined with the associated eigenvalues. The matrix $V'_p(t,t)$ is orthonormal matrix; therefore the rows represent different data patterns. The two sets of circadian patterns in glycine, serine and threonine metabolism (Figure 7) are retrieved via the first two rows of $V'_p(t,t)$. $V'_p(t,1)$ and $V'_p(t,2)$ have high correlation with fitted sinusoidal model (Additional File 2.). The p-value of $V'_p(t,1)$ is statistically significant whereas the p-value of $V'_p(t,2)$ is not statistically significant.

Table 1 provides the detailed list of identified pathways in each cluster. In total, there are 78 pathways in five clusters. The list of genes in these pathways, associated gene expressions, the weights, the correlation between fitted sinusoidal model and the individual gene expressions can be found in Additional File 3. The identification of the circadian signatures at the pathway level identified biologically relevant processes. As such, gene expression, metabolite concentration and enzyme activity in energy metabolism (e.g. glycolysis and gluconeogenesis), amino acid metabolism (e.g. lysine degradation, urea cycle) [23,24], lipid metabolism (e.g. fatty acid biosynthesis) [25] and DNA replication and protein synthesis (e.g. DNA replication reactome, Purine metabolism) [26] exhibited having circadian dynamics in mammals liver.

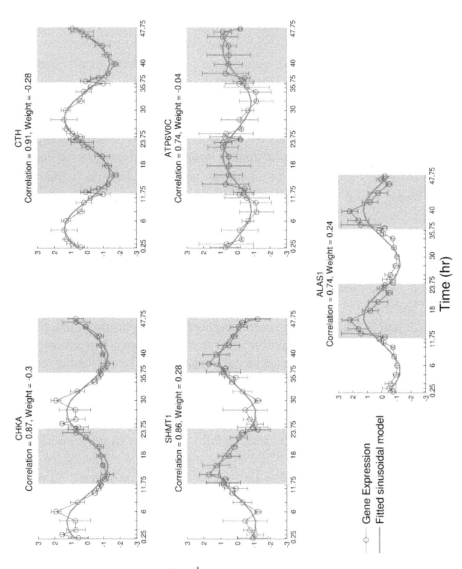

**FIGURE 7:** Selected gene expressions within glycine, serine and threonine metabolism. The correlation between the gene expression levels and the fitted sinusoidal models and the weights, which are evaluated via SVD analysis, of the genes are given on top of each graph. The signs (positive and/or negative) of weights indicate opposite direction in the gene expression.

**TABLE 1:** Circadian pathways and associated cluster numbers.

| Pathway name | Cluster ID |
| --- | --- |
| ASCORBATE AND ALDARATE METABOLISM | 1 |
| BUTANOATE METABOLISM | 1 |
| PURINE METABOLISM | 1 |
| LIMONENE AND PINENE DEGRADATION | 1 |
| DNA POLYMERASE | 1 |
| ATP SYNTHESIS | 1 |
| DNA REPLICATION REACTOME | 1 |
| LYSINE DEGRADATION | 1 |
| HISTIDINE METABOLISM | 1 |
| PHENYLALANINE METABOLISM | 1 |
| 3 CHLOROACRYLIC ACID DEGRADATION | 1 |
| G1 TO S CELL CYCLE REACTOME | 2 |
| FATTY ACID METABOLISM | 2 |
| BILE ACID BIOSYNTHESIS | 2 |
| UREA CYCLE AND METABOLISM OF AMINO GROUPS | 2 |
| VALINE LEUCINE AND ISOLEUCINE DEGRADATION | 2 |
| TRYPTOPHAN METABOLISM | 2 |
| P53 SIGNALING PATHWAY | 2 |
| CELL CYCLE KEGG | 2 |
| G2 PATHWAY | 2 |
| ARGININE AND PROLINE METABOLISM | 2 |
| RNA POLYMERASE | 2 |
| IFNA PATHWAY | 2 |
| ST TYPE I INTERFERON PATHWAY | 2 |
| POLYUNSATURATED FATTY ACID BIOSYNTHESIS | 3 |
| CELL COMMUNICATION | 3 |

**TABLE 1:** *Cont.*

| Pathway name | Cluster ID |
| --- | --- |
| ANTIGEN PROCESSING AND PRESENTATION | 3 |
| MRP PATHWAY | 3 |
| FRUCTOSE AND MANNOSE METABOLISM | 3 |
| TYROSINE METABOLISM | 3 |
| ETC PATHWAY | 4 |
| TYROSINE METABOLISM | 4 |
| MALATEX PATHWAY | 4 |
| PROTEASOME PATHWAY | 4 |
| ALANINE AND ASPARTATE METABOLISM | 4 |
| GLYCOLYSIS AND GLUCONEOGENESIS | 4 |
| SA CASPASE CASCADE | 4 |
| CHOLESTEROL BIOSYNTHESIS | 5 |
| GLYCEROPHOSPHOLIPID METABOLISM | 5 |
| TERPENOID BIOSYNTHESIS | 5 |
| RNA TRANSCRIPTION REACTOME | 5 |
| BIOSYNTHESIS OF STEROIDS | 5 |
| CIRCADIAN EXERCISE | 5 |
| CYANOAMINO ACID METABOLISM | 5 |
| FEEDER PATHWAY | 5 |
| GLYCEROLIPID METABOLISM | 5 |
| GLYCINE SERINE AND THREONINE METABOLISM | 5 |
| METHIONINE METABOLISM | 5 |
| LYSINE BIOSYNTHESIS | 5 |
| NUCLEOTIDE SUGARS METABOLISM | 5 |
| ETHER LIPID METABOLISM | 5 |
| SPHINGOLIPID METABOLISM | 5 |
| ONE CARBON POOL BY FOLATE | 5 |
| BASAL TRANSCRIPTION FACTORS | 5 |
| CIRCADIAN RHYTHM | 5 |
| LYSINE BIOSYNTHESIS | 5 |
| LYSINE DEGRADATION | 5 |
| MEF2 D PATHWAY | 5 |
| METHANE METABOLISM | 5 |
| METHIONINE METABOLISM | 5 |

**TABLE 1:** *Cont.*

| Pathway name | Cluster ID |
|---|---|
| METHIONINE PATHWAY | 5 |
| ONE CARBON POOL BY FOLATE | 5 |
| SA G1 AND S PHASES | 5 |
| SELENOAMINO ACID METABOLISM | 5 |
| TID PATHWAY | 5 |
| TOLL PATHWAY | 5 |
| APOPTOSIS | 5 |
| APOPTOSIS GENMAPP | 5 |
| CARM ER PATHWAY | 5 |
| EPONFKB PATHWAY | 5 |
| FXR PATHWAY | 5 |
| G1 PATHWAY | 5 |
| GSK3 PATHWAY | 5 |
| LEPTIN PATHWAY | 5 |
| P53 PATHWAY | 5 |
| RACCYCD PATHWAY | 5 |
| SA REG CASCADE OF CYCLIN EXPR | 5 |
| TALL1 PATHWAY | 5 |

*) Since gene products can function in multiple pathways, some pathways that may not be active in liver can be identified as circadian. For example small cell lung cancer, SNARE interactions in vesicular transport, prion disease are not defined in liver tissue. For the statistical analysis, we are not biased by the tissue specific pathways; however an additional filtering is performed for the biologically relevant pathways.

In addition, we evaluated the enrichment of the pathways with the genes that exhibited circadian patterns in [9]. MSigDB database [18] offers an annotation tool that explore gene set annotations to gain further insight into the biology behind a gene set in question. The end result is a p-value indicating the significance of the overlap of the genes with a pathway http://www.broadinstitute.org/gsea/msigdb/annotate.jsp.

The genes that exhibit circadian dynamics in [9] have been mapped to 34 pathways (Additional File 4), nine of which have significant p-value < 0.05.

To further explain the biological significance of the pathway activity level analysis, we studied the coordination between different pathways that is another level of organization in cellular processes, especially in cases where the product of one pathway is the substrate of another pathway. One classic example is the production of bile acids and it needs cholesterol as its starting material. Previous studies have shown that the pathways for steroid and bile acid biosynthesis are coordinated and coupled with cholesterol biosynthesis pathway for maximizing the efficiency of these processes. It has been established that bile acid levels are tightly controlled to ensure appropriate cholesterol catabolism, and promote optimal solubilization and absorption of fat and other essential nutrients [25,27]. Figure 8 shows the fitted sinusoidal models of PAL curves for cholesterol and bile acids biosynthesis. From the Figure 8, we could see that both pathways shows circadian rhythmicity with the phase of oscillations for cholesterol biosynthesis with a peak reaching at 15 hours after lights on, but the bile acid biosynthesis pathway shows a slight time lag in its oscillation with the peak occurring at 17 hours after lights on. In the figure, the PAL curves reach its peak during the mid-dark period and nadir during the mid-light period. As mentioned previously, the peak and nadir of PAL curves represent the maximum variation in the temporal gene expression in the pathway and the exact reverse of the PAL curve is mathematically same as the PAL curve itself (PAL-PAL). But from the literature, we know that these pathways peak during the dark period when the animals are actively feeding. Furthermore, the circadian oscillations in expression of many of the genes involved in the pathway (including the rate limiting genes like HMGCR for cholesterol biosynthesis [16] and CYP7A1 for bile acid biosynthesis [28] peaks during the dark/active period in the 24 hours light/dark cycle. So to deduce the biological significance of the PAL curve, along with the PAL curve pattern one should take into account of the oscillation patterns of the individual gene expression (including the rate limiting genes) along with any existing knowledge about the biological function and regulation of a given pathway. Additional file 5 and 6 provides the expression of individual genes in these pathways. Similar coupling of pathways are observed such as folate biosynthesis and one carbon pool by folate are coupled with purine and pyrimidine metabolism [29].

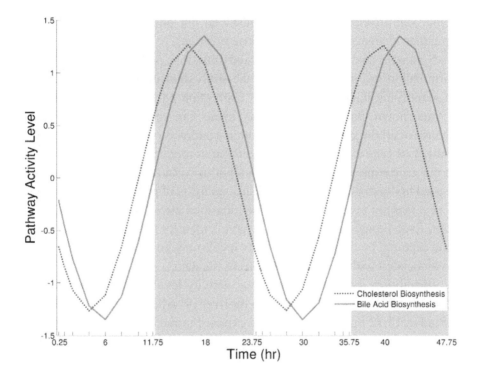

**FIGURE 8:** Fitted sinusoidal models of pathway activity levels for cholesterol biosynthesis and bile acid biosynthesis.

## 2.4 DISCUSSION

The goal of this study is to characterize the dynamic evaluation of pathways based on transcriptional profiling. Pathway activity level formulation enabled us to identify circadian signatures of pathways by reducing the overall gene expression level to a single response. We improved the former formulation of the pathway activity level analysis with an additional significance analysis that enhanced our ability to detect relevant circadian changes and reduce the false positives.

Synthetic data was used to demonstrate that pathway activity levels formulation are more robust than the individual gene expression levels in identifying underlying circadian expression pattern within a pathway. It was shown that pathway activity levels can capture the orchestrated change of all the gene expression within a pathway, whereas analysis at the individual gene expression levels could miss moderate but steady changes in the gene expression levels within a pathway. In addition, synthetic data is used to illustrate that the significance analysis of pathway activity levels is necessary to evaluate whether the identified circadian pattern is significant. Even though pathway activity levels identify a circadian pattern, the data captured by the pathway activity levels may not be significant and can be associated with random variations in the data.

In addition, we evaluated pathway activity levels based on a rich time series of transcriptional profiling in rat liver [9] where the rats were maintained in 12:12 light/dark cycle and exposed to the least possible environmental disturbances to minimize stress. Unlike the synthetic data, we did not know the underlying patterns in the microarray data. As a result of the clustering analysis, the most populated patterns of pathway activity levels exhibited circadian rhythms (Figure 3). The over-representation of specific patterns in the data cannot be explained by random events. Therefore, we can conclude that pathway activity level can identify the underlying circadian pattern in the data.

The five main clusters shown in Figure 3 represent the presented curves and the exact reverse curves; PAL = (-) PAL. The turning points can characterize both the peak and the nadir points in biochemical processes. In Figure 3, the signs of PALs are chosen so that PALs have the similar patterns for a better representation and clustering purposes. The sign of PAL can be chosen based on the pattern the genes that have the highest contribution to PAL. For example, we represent pathway activity levels of cholesterol biosynthesis and bile acid synthesis peaking in dark period (Figure 8). From the literature; we know that these pathways peak during the dark period when the animals are actively feeding.

Moreover, the list of the genes that exhibit circadian dynamics were mapped to 34 pathways. Our unsupervised approach identified the entire 34 mapped pathway, whereas nine of mapped pathway exhibited statistically significant enrichment. Additional biologically relevant pathways were identified by pathway activity level analysis such as pathways related to cell cycle, DNA replication and apoptosis exhibited having circadian dynamics in mammals [26,30]. Similar to synthetic data, analysis of biological data emphasizes studying at the individual gene expression levels could miss changes at the pathway level.

Characterizing the circadian regulation at the pathway level is an important piece of information that may help reveal the complex relationships such as understanding the liver functioning. The biological relevance of pathway activity level formulation to analyze circadian rhythms is well illustrated by analyzing coupled pathways. As shown in Figure 8, PAL analysis suggests that bile acid biosynthesis pathways are intrinsically coupled with cholesterol biosynthesis pathway, which is the case as reported by previous studies. Furthermore, this is physiologically important as cholesterol is an important substrate for the biosynthesis of both bile acids. Bile acids are involved in the digestion of dietary lipids and higher levels of bile acid biosynthesis occur during the dark period which represents the active feeds period in rats.

Moreover, we observe series of pathways related to protein synthesis and degradation having circadian patterns. Studies examining the gene expression and enzyme activities related to amino acid metabolism showed persistent circadian rhythms [17]. These studies indicate that amino acid metabolism components tend to correlate with food intake. Though no conclusive evidence is available, transport and metabolic substrates of amino acids have shown clock-regulated changes.

This current analysis is limited, as any pathway method, by currently available pathway knowledge. For example, there are two genes, SHMT1 and SHMT2, which have exactly opposite circadian oscillations in gene expression and hence opposite weights. SHMT1 is a cytosolic enzyme and SHMT2 is a mitochondrial enzyme. Though they catalyze the same reaction, the cellular purposes of these enzymes are different. In addition, several genes not linked to known pathways are not considered in pathway analysis. As more specific pathway databases such as tissue specific pathway databases or cellular compartment specific pathway databases are created and the pathway knowledge databases are improved, the power of this pathway analysis method will increase. Another limitation of this study is that it looks the dynamics of the pathway only at the mRNA levels. But it is a known fact that many biological processes are also regulated at the levels of translation of proteins (like microRNA regulation), activation state (phosphorylation, functionalization, etc), degradation and interaction with other proteins. But again this is just the limitation of the dataset available and we are confident that the methodology can be applied to any proteomics, microRNA arrays dataset, etc in the same way as we applied for our dataset.

## 2.5 CONCLUSIONS

In summary, rather than assessing the importance of a single gene beforehand and map these genes onto pathways, we instead examined the orchestrated change within a pathway. Pathway activity level analysis could reveal the underlying circadian dynamics in the microarray data with an unsupervised approach and biologically relevant results were obtained. We believe that our analysis of circadian pathways based on transcriptional profiling can contribute to filling the gaps between circadian regulation and biochemical activity. While transcriptional profiling is a valuable tool for unrevealing potential connections between the circadian clock and biochemical activity [31], complementing the transcriptional studies with proteomic and metabolomics analyses will provide new insights to the circadian phenomenon.

## REFERENCES

1.  Panda S, Antoch MP, Miller BH, Su AI, Schook AB, Straume M, Schultz PG, Kay SA, Takahashi JS, Hogenesch JB: Coordinated transcription of key pathways in the mouse by the circadian clock. Cell 2002, 109(3):307-320.
2.  Sukumaran S, Almon RR, DuBois DC, Jusko JJ: Circadian rhythms in gene expression: relationship to physiology, disease, drug disposition and drug action. Advanced drug delivery reviews 2010.
3.  Dunlap JC: Molecular bases for circadian clocks. Cell 1999, 96(2):271-290.
4.  Mirsky HP, Liu AC, Welsh DK, Kay SA, Doyle FJ: A model of the cell-autonomous mammalian circadian clock. Proc Natl Acad Sci USA 2009, 106(27):11107-11112.
5.  Preitner N, Damiola F, Lopez-Molina L, Zakany J, Duboule D, Albrecht U, Schibler U: The orphan nuclear receptor REV-ERBalpha controls circadian transcription within the positive limb of the mammalian circadian oscillator. Cell 2002, 110(2):251-260.
6.  Jetten AM: Retinoid-related orphan receptors (RORs): critical roles in development, immunity, circadian rhythm, and cellular metabolism. Nucl Recept Signal 2009, 7:e003.
7.  Gachon F: Physiological function of PARbZip circadian clock-controlled transcription factors. Ann Med 2007, 39(8):562-571.
8.  Harmer SL, Hogenesch JB, Straume M, Chang HS, Han B, Zhu T, Wang X, Kreps JA, Kay SA: Orchestrated transcription of key pathways in Arabidopsis by the circadian clock. Science 2000, 290(5499):2110-2113.
9.  Almon RR, Yang E, Lai W, Androulakis IP, Dubois DC, Jusko WJ: Circadian Variations in Liver Gene Expression: Relationships to Drug Actions. J Pharmacol Exp Ther 2008. OpenURL
10. Keegan KP, Pradhan S, Wang JP, Allada R: Meta-analysis of Drosophila circadian microarray studies identifies a novel set of rhythmically expressed genes. PLoS Comput Biol 2007, 3(11):e208..
11. Mootha VK, Lindgren CM, Eriksson KF, Subramanian A, Sihag S, Lehar J, Puigserver P, Carlsson E, Ridderstrale M, Laurila E, et al.: PGC-1alpha-responsive genes involved in oxidative phosphorylation are coordinately downregulated in human diabetes. Nat Genet 2003, 34(3):267-273.
12. Rahnenfuhrer J, Domingues FS, Maydt J, Lengauer T: Calculating the statistical significance of changes in pathway activity from gene expression data. Stat Appl Genet Mol Biol 2004, 3:Article16.
13. Tomfohr J, Lu J, Kepler TB: Pathway level analysis of gene expression using singular value decomposition. BMC Bioinformatics 2005, 6:225.
14. Levine DM, Haynor DR, Castle JC, Stepaniants SB, Pellegrini M, Mao M, Johnson JM: Pathway and gene-set activation measurement from mRNA expression data: the tissue distribution of human pathways. Genome Biol 2006, 7(10):R93..
15. Tirone TA, Brunicardi FC: Overview of glucose regulation. World J Surg 2001, 25(4):461-467.

16. Russell DW: Cholesterol biosynthesis and metabolism. Cardiovasc Drugs Ther 1992, 6(2):103-110.

17. Davidson AJ, Castanon-Cervantes O, Stephan FK: Daily oscillations in liver function: diurnal vs circadian rhythmicity. Liver Int 2004, 24(3):179-186.

18. Subramanian A, Tamayo P, Mootha VK, Mukherjee S, Ebert BL, Gillette MA, Paulovich A, Pomeroy SL, Golub TR, Lander ES, et al.: Gene set enrichment analysis: a knowledge-based approach for interpreting genome-wide expression profiles. Proc Natl Acad Sci USA 2005, 102(43):15545-15550.

19. Nguyen TT, Nowakowski RS, Androulakis IP: Unsupervised selection of highly coexpressed and noncoexpressed genes using a consensus clustering approach. OMICS 2009, 13(3):219-237.

20. Yeung KY, Medvedovic M, Bumgarner RE: Clustering gene-expression data with repeated measurements. Genome Biol 2003, 4(5):R34.

21. Ptitsyn AA, Zvonic S, Gimble JM: Permutation test for periodicity in short time series data. BMC Bioinformatics 2006, 7(Suppl 2):S10.

22. Wichert S, Fokianos K, Strimmer K: Identifying periodically expressed transcripts in microarray time series data. Bioinformatics 2004, 20(1):5-20.

23. Robinson JL, Foustock S, Chanez M, Bois-Joyeux B, Peret J: Circadian variation of liver metabolites and amino acids in rats adapted to a high protein, carbohydrate-free diet. J Nutr 1981, 111(10):1711-1720.

24. Froy O: The relationship between nutrition and circadian rhythms in mammals. Front Neuroendocrinol 2007, 28(2-3):61-71.

25. Akhtar RA, Reddy AB, Maywood ES, Clayton JD, King VM, Smith AG, Gant TW, Hastings MH, Kyriacou CP: Circadian cycling of the mouse liver transcriptome, as revealed by cDNA microarray, is driven by the suprachiasmatic nucleus. Curr Biol 2002, 12(7):540-550.

26. Schibler U: Circadian rhythms. Liver regeneration clocks on. Science 2003, 302(5643):234-235.

27. Akhtar MK, Kelly SL, Kaderbhai MA: Cytochrome b(5) modulation of 17{alpha} hydroxylase and 17-20 lyase (CYP17) activities in steroidogenesis. J Endocrinol 2005, 187(2):267-274.

28. Russell DW, Setchell KD: Bile acid biosynthesis. Biochemistry 1992, 31(20):4737-4749.

29. Fox JT, Stover PJ: Folate-mediated one-carbon metabolism. Vitam Horm 2008, 79:1-44.

30. Levi F, Schibler U: Circadian rhythms: mechanisms and therapeutic implications. Annu Rev Pharmacol Toxicol 2007, 47:593-628.

31. Rutter J, Reick M, McKnight SL: Metabolism and the control of circadian rhythms. Annu Rev Biochem 2002, 71:307-331.

*There are several supplemental files that are not available in this version of the article. To view this additional information, please use the citation information cited on the first page of this chapter.*

# CHAPTER 3

# BODY WEIGHT, METABOLISM, AND CLOCK GENES

MELISSA M. ZANQUETTA, MARIA LÚCIA CORRÊA-GIANNELLA, MARIA BEATRIZ MONTEIRO, AND SANDRA M. F. VILLARES

## 3.1 INTRODUCTION

The prevalence of obesity is growing rapidly, affecting all ages and social classes, despite all scientific efforts to clarify its causes. Excess body weight has become one of the biggest health issues today, and is principally due to increased food availability, high caloric diets and sedentary lifestyles. Recent studies have shown the importance of new discoveries regarding the intracellular mechanisms which can trigger obesity and other metabolic disturbances.

Some studies have suggested that altered patterns of sleep/wake cycle and feeding behavior were associated to 24-hour lifestyles and changes in body weight although the mechanisms by which daily rhythms are transformed into increased adiposity remain unclear [1,2].

*This chapter was originally published under the Creative Commons Attribution License. Zanquetta MM, Corrêa-Giannella ML, Monteiro MB, and Villares SMF. Body weight, Metabolism, and Clock Genes. Diabetology & Metabolic Syndrome 2,53 (2010). doi:10.1186/1758-5996-2-53.*

Circadian rhythms are biological events that constantly repeat in a 24-hour period and are generated by an endogenous mechanism. This endogenous mechanism is composed of circadian clocks, including the central clock (located in the suprachiasmatic nucleus- SCN) and peripheral clocks (located in all other cells of the organism), and is defined as the intrinsic molecular mechanisms that allow the organism to adapt to changes in its environment [3]. The clocks are synchronized or adjusted to coincide with periodical environmental events such as the day/night cycle. A well-synchronized clock guarantees that all physiological and behavioral rhythms take place in a coordinated manner over the 24-hour period [4].

Many researchers are investigating the function of the circadian clocks in circadian physiology regulation. Hence, the knowledge regarding the role of peripheral circadian clocks in glucose and lipids metabolism is starting to emerge. The adipocyte has an important role in endocrine system regulations, energy homeostasis, satiety signaling and in cell differentiation and proliferation. The circadian clock of the adipose cell is also probably involved in the control of many of these functions. It is reasonable to deduce that alterations in the peripheral circadian clock of adipose tissue can induce the onset of obesity or intensify its causes and consequences, for example, by generating modifications in adipose tissue metabolism or acting on hunger/satiety and energy balance regulation. The aim of this review was to define the circadian clocks by describing their functioning, their role in the whole body, in adipocyte metabolism, as well as their influence on body weight control and the development of obesity.

## 3.2 CIRCADIAN CLOCKS

It is well known that the life of plants, animals and humans seems to be adapted to their respective environment and that each species' survival depends on the capacity of the organism to adapt in response to periodical changes. Biological rhythms have emerged in an attempt to facilitate evolution by enabling the anticipation of many regulatory, physiological and behavioral mechanisms that improve the chances of survival of both the individual and the species. In other words, due to the physiological anticipation of the stimuli of the environment, the reactions of the organism occur at the right time of day. Alterations in the natural synchrony between cycles of day/night, activity/rest, and hormonal or feeding behavior etc. can induce modifications in this highly complex mechanism of metabolic and hormonal anticipation.

The control of circadian rhythm expression involves regulation at the cellular level through the clock genes [3,5]. The clock genes codify a family of proteins that generate an auto-regulatory mechanism of positive and negative transcriptional feedback loops which occur on a 24-hour basis [3]. In mammals, the clock mechanism is composed of at least 9 main proteins: CLOCK (circadian locomotor output cycles kaput), BMAL1 (brain and muscle ARNT-like protein 1), PER1 (period 1), PER2 (period 2), PER3 (period 3), CRY1 (cryptochrome 1), CRY2 (cryptochrome 2), REVERBα (reverse erythroblastosis virus α) and RORα (retinoid-related orphan receptor- α). Many of these proteins act as transcriptional factors, since they have PAS (Per-ARNT-Sim; involved in protein-protein interactions) and bHLH (basic helix-loop-helix; involved in protein-DNA interaction) domains. With these characteristics, the proteins comprising the clock work together activating and inhibiting their own transcription. CLOCK and BMAL1 form a heterodimer that binds to E-box on the promoter of other clock genes, such as *Per1, Per2, Per3, Cry1, Cry2, Reverba, Rora* and many output genes that are controlled by the clock (CCGs: clock-controlled genes). The heterodimer CLOCK/BMAL1 also stimulates Bmal1 transcription, generating a positive feedback loop. Conversely, a negative feedback loop of the clock takes place through the heterodimerization of CRY and PER. The heterodimer CRY/PER translocates to the nucleus and inhibits the transcriptional activity of the CLOCK/BMAL1 heterodimer [6,7]. Nuclear receptors REVERBα and RORα participate in the regulation of Bmal1 expression, inhibiting or activating the transcription, respectively [8] (Figure 1).

The circadian clock components show distinct characteristics and actions on the clock's functioning. Thus, any alterations that occur in gene expression and/or protein translation may result in impaired functioning of the entire mechanism. High tissue specificity of the circadian clock also guarantees perfect working of this complex intrinsic mechanism, which is primordial for physiological and behavioral circadian responses to be triggered at the optimum time of day.

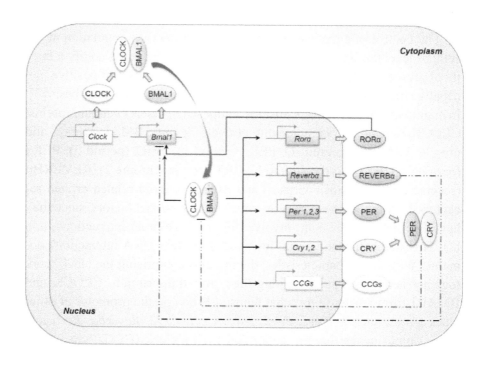

**FIGURE 1:** Molecular machinery of the circadian clock. The core clock components CLOCK and BMAL1 heterodimerize in the cytoplasm, forming a protein complex. The heterodimer is then translocated to the nucleus and binds to E-boxes on the promoter of target genes, controlling their expression. These genes include *Per1*, *Per2*, *Per3*, *Cry1*, *Cry2*, *Reverba*, *Rora* and many clock-controlled genes (CCGs). CLOCK/BMAL1 heterodimer also stimulates transcription of Bmal1 itself, forming the positive feedback loop of the mechanism. Negative feedback loop is mainly regulated by CRY and PER, that heterodimerize in the cytoplasm, translocate to the nucleus and inhibits CLOCK/BMAL1 transcription activity. Gene expression of *Bmal1* is also regulated by REVERBα (inhibition) and RORα (stimulation), that compete for the same ROR elements present in the *Bmal1* promoter. Regulation of CCGs expression by the circadian clock confers rhythmicity to a variety of molecular and physiological processes. Straight lines: stimulation. Dashed lines: inhibition.

The optimization of the organism's responses at the right time of day directly depends on the synchronization between central and peripheral clocks and with regular cycles of the environment. Zeitgebers (from the German word, Zeit = time; geber = give) or synchronizers are the factors responsible for synchronizing the circadian clocks. Sun light determines the precise length of day and night in the 24-hour period, accurately orienting the subject in relation to the point of day. As a consequence, light is one of the most powerful synchronizers of the circadian rhythms.

Environmental light is the zeitgeber for the central circadian clock, being transmitted to the SCN through a neuronal pathway that starts at the retina [9]. The zeitgebers of the peripheral clocks are neuro-humoral factors, some of which have previously been described as glucocorticoids, and in food restriction and melatonin [9-11]. Melatonin is one of the most important neuro-humoral zeitgebers for the synchronization of the internal system, since it is a hormone produced and secreted only during the night by the pineal gland, which receives retino-hypothalamic neural signals that carry information about the day/night environmental cycle. Moreover, it has been suggested that social rhythms can function as zeitgebers for the internal system [12]. However, many critics raise questions over whether these social factors can really affect circadian rhythms independently of those controlled by environmental light.

## 3.3 PERIPHERAL CLOCK OF ADIPOSE TISSUE

Many studies have shown the existence of a peripheral circadian clock in adipose tissue [13,14]. Although research in this area is recent, the peripheral circadian clock of the adipose tissue seems to play a fundamental role in adipose tissue physiology and consequently in glucose and lipid homeostasis. The importance of new discoveries regarding the peripheral clock of the adipose tissue has been recognized. Some authors have recently developed an in vitro model for studies on circadian biology of human adipose tissue, using differentiated adipocytes derived from stem cells [15].

The adipocyte governs essential metabolic functions of the organism, not only working as an energy store but also as an endocrine organ that secrets hormones and cytokines that regulate many metabolic activities. Although circadian variations of adipose tissue metabolism have been shown to be influenced by external neuro-humoral factors [13,16], they can also be influenced internally by a peripheral circadian clock that acts on tissue metabolism and can alter adipocyte responsiveness in response to different stimuli during the day (for example, levels of glucose, insulin, fatty acids, melatonin) or can alter the capacity of lipolysis and lipogenesis [17,18].

Many adipocytokines produced in adipose tissue present circadian rhythmicity. Leptin and adiponectin show opposite patterns of circadian secretion: the peak for leptin occurs during the sleep phase of the sleep/wake cycle while adiponectin falls during the night and peaks in secretion during the morning [19-21]. In addition, it has been demonstrated that plasmatic concentrations of leptin and adiponectin also present secretion patterns of ultradian pulsatility [20,22]. Ultradian rhythms (fast repetitive oscillations within 20-hour periods) are also a significant part of the organism's temporal organization, allowing more precise adjustment of cellular and tissue responses at optimal time points for best improvement in cellular functions [23].

Adipogenesis, adipocyte differentiation and lipogenesis also appear to be directly regulated by the circadian clock. Shimba et al. (2005) demonstrated that adipocyte differentiation is directly regulated by BMAL1 [24], since embryo fibroblasts from *Bmal1* knockout mice showed deficiency in the ability to become mature adipocytes, whose deficiency was restored by the transfection of an adenovirus containing the original Bmal1. Additionally, in the same study, when *Bmal1* was knocked-down in cultured pre-adipocytes, the cells were unable to accumulate intracellular lipids and demonstrated decreased expression of genes related to differentiation, including the *C/ebp* family of transcriptional factors such as *Srebp1a* and *Pparγ2*, proving the importance of the circadian clock in adipocyte physiology. It was also demonstrated that *Reverbα* is a target gene for *Pparγ* [25], and that *C/ebpβ* and *Reverbα* genes are critical factors for adipocyte differentiation, showing a circadian rhythmic expression in epididymis and subcutaneous adipose tissue in mice [26].

Besides evidence showing the influence of the circadian clock on cellular proliferation and differentiation processes of adipose tissue, it has been demonstrated that hormonal and metabolic functions in adipose tissue are synchronized in circadian rhythms by the presence of melatonin in circulation [18]. Melatonin induces alterations in gene expression of the adipocyte clock genes that are translated into different cellular responses. This means that the role of the circadian clock in adipose tissue is relevant for the functioning of the tissue, modulating adipocyte intracellular responses related to external factors while also influencing overall metabolism.

## 3.4 ROLE OF CIRCADIAN CLOCKS IN METABOLISM

It is well known that circadian clocks are involved in glucose and lipid homeostasis since many metabolic factors present circadian variations including enzymes, substrate transporters and hormones.

Evidence has demonstrated that biological rhythms and metabolism closely resemble each other. Kennaway et al. (2007) showed this connection [27] in a recent study on transgenic mice that presented non-rhythmical expression of clock genes in liver and skeletal muscle. The mice however, had preserved rhythmicity in the SCN and pineal gland. Although these animals did not develop obesity or fatty acid augmentation, they had an increased plasmatic adiponectin, decreased glucose transporter *Glut4* mRNA in skeletal muscle, low glucose tolerance, low insulin levels, and a decrease in gene expression with loss of rhythmicity in enzymes related to hepatic glycolysis and gluconeogenesis.

In humans, the relationship between clock genes and metabolism has been previously demonstrated. Studies involving obese humans for instance, have found that circadian clock gene expression in adipose tissue was related to abdominal fat content and with risk factors for cardiovascular disease, since it was associated to plasmatic LDL levels, total cholesterol and with abdominal circumference [28]. The same group studied isolated adipocytes from morbid obese individuals and demonstrated that the circadian clock genes continued oscillating in a 24 hour pattern, independently of the central circadian clock, for at least 48 hours in vitro, and that genes directly related to adipose tissue metabolism such as *PPARγ*, are controlled by clock genes [29]. Moreover, it was shown that clock gene expression depends on metabolic conditions, even in healthy subjects with normal body weight [30]. It is evident that there is a direct association among rhythms at different levels of metabolism and the regulation of glucose and lipid homeostasis. We can conclude that circadian regulation is essential for maintaining metabolism balance in the organism, even though the mechanisms involved in this process are not yet well defined.

Concerning molecular mechanisms, components of the circadian clock are linked with metabolic pathways. The gene expression of Bmal1 is negatively regulated by REVERBα and positively by RORα (retinoic acid receptor-related orphan receptor α), through RORE (ROR-response element) [31]. In skeletal muscle, RORα regulates lipogenesis and lipid storage [32] whereas REVERBα is stimulated during adipogenesis [33]. By contrast, the heterodimer CLOCK/BMAL1 regulates the gene expression of *Reverbα, Rora* and *Ppar* (peroxisome proliferator-activated receptor family, principally α and γ) [34]. PPARα, which is involved in the regulation of lipid and glucose metabolism, participates in the regulation of *Bmal1* transcription, since it is linked to the gene promoter. In addition, many other nuclear receptors directly involved in glucose and lipid metabolisms show circadian rhythmicity [35], proving the participation of different molecular mechanisms in the relationship between circadian clocks and metabolism (Figure 2).

Different biological rhythms synchronize physiological processes with daily environmental changes, allowing the organism to anticipate and adapt, generating responses in a rapid and appropriate manner. A failure in this mechanism of synchronization between rhythms and metabolism can have serious consequences, allowing or inducing metabolic pathologies such as obesity and diabetes.

Turek et al. (2005) have demonstrated that clock knockout mice developed obesity and showed alterations in feeding behavior such as hyperphagia, as well as hormonal abnormalities associated to metabolic syndrome, including hyperlipidemia, hyperleptinemia, hepatic steatosis, hyperglycemia and hypoinsulinemia [36]. *Bmal1* knockout mice showed weight loss from 10 weeks of age due to a decrease in adipose and muscle tissue mass [24]. These animals also showed loss of circadian rhythm and altered metabolic phenotypes, including modified glycemic homeostasis and reduced lifetime [24,37]. Akin to *Bmal1* knockout animals, *Per1* knockout (*Per1$^{Brd}$*) mice had reduced body mass compared to wild type animals, despite the same food intake [38]. The *Per1$^{Brd}$* mice also had increased diurnal concentrations of glucocorticoids and higher fasting glucose clearance, suggesting that PER1 directly alters metabolic behavior. These results demonstrate that a disturbance in the circadian clock mechanism leads to significant alterations in glucose and lipid homeostasis and body weight maintenance.

## 3.5 CIRCADIAN CLOCKS AND FEEDING BEHAVIOR

Feeding behavior directly influences changes in body weight and is also under the circadian clocks control. Inversely, food ingestion, meals times, types of nutrient intake and metabolism can also synchronize the circadian clocks and stimulate specific responses.

Food restriction (FR) is an experimental model in which time and duration of food availability is restricted without reducing calories. Animals submitted to this regimen, being fed ad libitum at the same time of day for just a few hours, adjust their feeding behavior for that specific time of day within only a few days [39,40]. Thus, FR promotes physiological and behavioral modifications that show anticipatory responses from 2 to 4 hours before the feeding period. These changes are evidenced by multiple systems influenced by circadian clocks that show an increase in locomotor activity, cardiac frequency, body temperature, gastrointestinal motility and activity of digestive enzymes.

However, FR affects the peripheral circadian clocks without altering the central circadian clock, since animals without SCN submitted to FR maintain circadian rhythms independently of the light/dark cycle [41,42]. This means that FR desynchronizes peripheral and central circadian clocks yet when the feeding behavior reverts to normal, the peripheral circadian clocks are resynchronized by the central circadian clock. The hypothalamic dorsomedial nucleus, involved in central hunger and satiety regulation, is considered the food-entrainable oscillator (FEO) that acts in conjunction with the SCN to coordinate circadian feeding behavior [43].

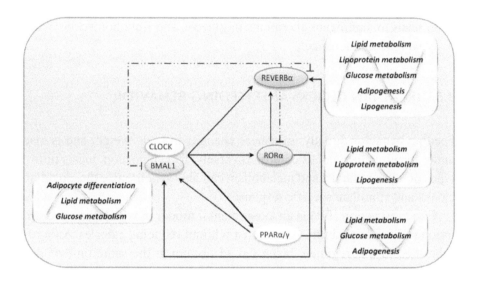

**FIGURE 2:** Molecular mechanisms underlying the association between circadian clock and metabolic pathways. CLOCK/BMAL1 heterodimer activates transcription of genes directly related to metabolism, especially nuclear receptors *Reverbα* and *Rorα* (members of clock machinery) and *Ppar* family of transcriptional factors (clock-controlled genes; do not participate of clock machinery itself). RORα and PPARα activate *Bmal1* and *Reverbα* expressions. REVERBα represses *Bmal1, Rorα* and its own transcription. PPAR family and BMAL1 are involved in glucose and lipid metabolism and adipogenesis. REVERBα and RORα are implicated in the regulation of glucose, lipid and lipoprotein metabolism, adipogenesis and lipogenesis. They can also cross-talk with other important genes of metabolism such as PGC-1α (PPARγ- coactivator- 1α). Straight lines: stimulation. Dashed lines: inhibition.

It is known that food nutritional value also affects anticipatory responses. When rats are fed daily with two meals containing two or three macronutrients (protein + fat or protein + carb), they show anticipatory feeding behavior, a state which does not occur with free access to food containing all macronutrients [44].

Calorie restriction (CR) consists of reducing the amount of calories from lipids, carbohydrates and protein diet by 25 to 60% without causing malnutrition. In contrast, CR affects the central circadian clock, suggesting that a low calorie diet can alter physiological and behavioral rhythms. It also alters clock gene expression since it modifies the SCN function and its responsiveness to the light/dark cycle, thereby impairing circadian responses [45,46]. CR has been shown to prolong lifetime and can postpone the onset of many diseases such as obesity and diabetes [47,48].

Moreover, it was also observed that high calorie diets can influence many systems controlled by the circadian clock [49]. Animals submitted to high calorie diets develop symptoms similar to metabolic syndrome, including insulin resistance and increased body weight gain, because several hormonal and behavioral rhythms are altered by this intake [49,50]. A high fat diet also directly affects clock synchronization to environmental light carried out by the SCN [51].

The kind of food and regular feeding schedules are important synchronizers of circadian clocks since they are capable of inducing anticipatory responses and rhythms of food ingestion. The understanding of all mechanisms by which these synchronizations occur is relevant for better comprehension of the physiological processes involved in body weight and hunger/satiety regulation.

## 3.6 CIRCADIAN RHYTHMS, BODY WEIGHT AND OBESITY

Generally, knowledge on body weight control is centered on the understanding of the mechanisms by which animals sense and respond to nutritional signs. In this context, circadian clocks act directly on energy balance and food intake control and consequently regulate body weight.

The season of the year influences body weight, food intake, energy consumption, body temperature among other parameters that are common in mammals as a result of evolutionary adaptations. This advantage allows animals to adapt to environment variations, optimizing their endogenous responses.

Several studies in animals have demonstrated the presence of seasonal rhythms, suggesting the importance of circadian clocks in body weight rhythmicity. Hamsters from Siberia show well-defined seasonal rhythms for body weight, food intake and reproduction. Through photoperiod modifications, i.e. length of the daylight period, seasonal alterations can be induced by melatonin secretion [52]. In the winter phenotype for instance (shorter days and longer nights) there is a decrease in food intake, lethargy, body weight loss of up to 35% (especially intra-abdominal fat loss), change to a clearer pelage and differentiated body temperature control, avoiding excessive energy expenditure [53]. There is also a decrease in leptin gene expression in adipose tissue and its concentration in circulation [54]. Studies on bird circannual rhythms have demonstrated that those exposed to shorter photoperiods exhibited lower daily energy expenditure [55]. It was also observed that, during the winter period, reindeers (arctic ruminants) exhibit lower plasmatic concentrations of leptin and insulin, together with reductions in body weight, total serum proteins and urea [56]. These, and other studies, have indicated that the photoperiod duration is associated to body weight alterations and that circadian clocks play a key role in its regulation.

It is known that light exposition at night and sleeplessness lead to an increase in adiposity and to other factors conducive to metabolic syndrome prevalence, including obesity, diabetes and cardiovascular disease.

Studies in children and young adults have shown a direct association between fewer hours of sleep and weight gain, and individuals that sleepless have an increased chance of developing obesity in adult life [57,58]. This association also holds for elderly people, and has been proven recently in a study with men and women over 65 years old [59]: individuals who slept less than 5 hours per day exhibited higher body mass index (BMI), being an average of 2.5 kg/m$^2$ higher in men, and 1.8 kg/m$^2$ greater in women.

These data were also confirmed in lab studies. One such study compared subjects submitted to 4 or 10 hours of sleep for 2 consecutive nights, and found that sleep restriction was associated with an average reduction of 18% in leptin concentration, an elevation of 28% in the orexigenic factor ghrelin, and increases in hunger (24%) and appetite (23%), especially for calorie-dense foods with high carbohydrate content [60]. Given that hunger increases during sleep restriction lead to increased food intake, individuals who sleep less are expected to experience greater weight gain over time.

Laposky et al. [61,62] performed studies with leptin-deficient obese *ob/ob* mice, and obese and diabetic *db/db* mice (they do not express a particular isoform of leptin receptor) and demonstrated that these animals had disturbed wake/sleep cycles, slept less and had reduced locomotor activity. Therefore, fewer sleep hours can contribute to increased prevalence of overweight and obesity through changes in regulation of appetite, increased availability of feeding and/or stimulating a decrease in energy expenditure. All these factors are influenced by the control of circadian clocks.

Night shift workers have different patterns of sleep due to changes in synchronization of their endogenous rhythms with the light/dark cycle. These sleep alterations are associated with metabolic disturbances, cardiovascular disease, diabetes and obesity. In a study involving approximately 27,500 individuals, it was observed that obesity, increased triglycerides and decreased HDL cholesterol were more prevalent in night shift workers compared to day shift workers [63]. Another study demonstrated that night workers also exhibited increased fasting glucose, free fatty acids, arterial blood pressure, abdominal circumference and BMI [64,65]. Regarding the nutritional status of night workers, different eating patterns were found: 1. total intake of calories and the presence of three major groups of nutrients in one meal did not differ from day laborers, except for a 10% higher consumption of saturated fat for night workers, 2. food intake was more fragmented during the day, being lower at breakfast and lunch, and higher at dinner and in snacks between meals, especially evening and night [65].

It is important to highlight that obese individuals report less total sleep time per night, with a difference of one hour of sleep per week corresponding to an increase of 5.4 kg/m$^2$ in BMI [1]. Sleep disorders such as insomnia and obstructive sleep apnea are very common in individuals with metabolic and endocrine pathologies, but often remain undiagnosed. This can lead to the onset of obesity and diabetes [66]. Treatment of sleep disorders has a potential to improve glucose metabolism and energy balance.

Another point to consider is that even in altered metabolic states, circadian rhythms of hormones, receptors, transporters, etc are maintained. For example, in obese subjects, circadian rhythms of leptin and adiponectin are still present, albeit changed. In a 24-hour period, obese individuals showed increased plasmatic leptin concentrations with higher peaks of secretion. On the other hand, adiponectin concentrations were lower where this was associated with smaller and shorter peaks of secretion [67]. Ghrelin (hormone involved in body weight regulation) concentrations are decreased in the obese while no increase is seen in the evening in contrast to lean subjects [67].

Recently, Kaneko et al. (2009) [68] demonstrated that obesity modifies clock gene circadian expression in the central nervous system. Moreover, it alters the expression of target genes of circadian clocks that can participate in mechanisms involved in the rhythmic alterations and neuronal dysfunctions observed in obese individuals such as PPARα.

Expression of peripheral clock gene components in adipose tissue are also altered in obese subjects, as demonstrated by Loboda et al. in 2009 [14]. The authors studied subcutaneous adipose tissue (obtained from biopsies collected in the morning, afternoon or evening) from obese patients submitted to fasting and/or treated with sibutramine. Results showed that 25% of the expressed genes in adipose tissue presented circadian rhythm, including those essentially involved in energy metabolism and tissue physiology. Thus, they hypothesized that circadian rhythms showed by the genes involved in energy metabolism may be reflecting in the adipocyte, a transition from a state of energy expenditure in the morning to a state of energy storage during the night. This mechanism was indeed demonstrated by the delay of this transition observed after fasting and treatment with sibutramine.

Therefore, obesity is closely related to circadian clock disturbances, both central and peripheral. This highlights the importance of circadian rhythms in adipose tissue physiology and energy metabolism regulation of the body. Circadian clocks play a key role in body weight control and in mechanisms implicated in this control, such as hunger/satiety cycle, feeding behavior, wake/sleep cycle, energy expenditure/storage and hormonal secretion.

## 3.7 GENETICS AND THE LINK BETWEEN OBESITY, BODY WEIGHT AND CIRCADIAN CLOCKS

Genetic factors are important contributors to obesity development, as demonstrated by several studies in humans and animals. Some authors have suggested four levels of genetic determination of obesity: genetic obesity, strong genetic predisposition, slight genetic predisposition, and genetically resistant [69].

The heritability of common obesity is usually due to an interaction of multiple candidate genes found at different locations on the gene map and is therefore polygenic in nature [70]. Candidate genes either predispose to obesity or promote body weight loss. Genes either interact with each other (gene- gene interactions) or with various environmental factors (gene- environment interactions). Interactions between biological (genes, hormones, neurotransmitters, etc.), psychobehavioral and environmental factors influence body fat accumulation and fat distribution and can also increase other elements related to body weight gain.

Most of the genes discovered to date chiefly impact hunger, satiety and food intake [71]. Mutations in the leptin gene (LEP), leptin receptor (LEPR), pro-opiomelanocortin (POMC), proconvertase 1 (PC1), melanocortin receptor 4 (MC4R), melanocortin receptor 3 (MC3R), neurotrophic tyrosine kinase receptor type 2 (NTRK2) and many others have been recognized as promoters of morbid obesity and rare forms of human obesity [72].

Studies evaluating twins and adopted children compared to their biological relatives showed heritability of BMI [73]. A recent study involving 5,092 British twins aged from 8 to 11 years revealed that genetic influences were extremely significant in BMI (77%) and abdominal circumference, whereby 60% of abdominal adiposity heritability was from the same genes in BMI, and the remaining 40% were attributed to different genetic factors [74].

Several human genetic polymorphisms have been described in circadian clock genes as have their associations with metabolic disturbances. For example, studies in different populations demonstrated some associations between polymorphisms in the clock gene and metabolic syndrome, hepatic steatosis, obesity predisposition, eating disorder, sleep disorders, schizophrenia and bipolar disease [75-78]. Other studies have revealed associations between: polymorphisms in BMAL1 with hypertension and type 2 diabetes [79], hypertension and NPAS2 (CLOCK gene analogous) [80], and glucose and PER2 [81].

Recent research has shown differences in the distribution of circadian clock gene polymorphism frequencies among populations in different parts of the world including Chinese, African-American, Caucasian-African individuals [82]. Population genetic analyses suggest these differences stem more from genetic factors than natural selection. These results point to the fact that each population presents variations in circadian clock genes that allow metabolic and behavioral adaptations according to their ambient, cultural and social environment.

## 3.8 CONCLUSIONS

A large body of evidence suggests that obesity can cause alterations in circadian rhythms and vice-versa, since desynchronized rhythms can induce the onset of obesity and other metabolic diseases. It is clear that perfect synchronization between central and peripheral clocks and correct functioning of the adipose tissue clock are essential in regulating hunger, adiposity, energy balance and body weight. Further studies are needed to investigate the molecular and physiological mechanisms involved in this control. This knowledge can contribute to the development of new therapies for the treatment of obesity and other metabolic disorders.

## REFERENCES

1.  Vorona RD, Winn MP, Babineau TW, Eng BP, Feldman HR, Ware JC: Overweight and obese patients in a primary care population report less sleep than patients with a normal body mass index. Arch Intern Med 2005, 165(1):25-30.
2.  Rao MN, Blackwell T, Redline S, Stefanick ML, Ancoli-Israel S, Stone KL: Osteoporotic Fractures in Men (MrOS) Study Group. Association between sleep architecture and measures of body composition. Sleep 2009, 32(4):483-90.
3.  Albrecht U, Eichele G: The mammalian circadian clock. Curr Opin Genet Dev 2003, 13(3):271-7.

4.  Reppert SM, Weaver DR: Molecular analysis of mammalian circadian rhythms. Annu Rev Physiol 2001, 63:647-76.
5.  Van Esseveldt KE, Lehman MN, Boer GJ: The suprachiasmatic nucleus and the circadian time-keeping system revisited. Brain Res Brain Res Rev 2000, 33(1):34-77.
6.  Gekakis N, Staknis D, Nguyen HB, Davis FC, Wilsbacher LD, King DP, et al.: Role of the CLOCK protein in the mammalian circadian mechanism. Science 1998, 280(5369):1564-9.
7.  Yoshitane H, Takao T, Satomi Y, Du NH, Okano T, Fukada Y: Roles of CLOCK phosphorylation in suppression of E-box-dependent transcription. Mol Cell Biol 2009, 29(13):3675-86.
8.  Froy O: Metabolism and circadian rhythms- Implications for obesity. Endocrine Reviews 2010, 31(1):1-24.
9.  Cipolla-Neto J, Afeche SC: Glândula pineal: fisiologia celular e função. In Fisiologia. Edited by Guanabara Koogan. Rio de Janeiro: Aires; 2007::83-93.
10. Damiola F, Le Minh N, Preitner N, Kornmann B, Fleury-Olela F, Schibler U: Restricted feeding uncouples circadian oscillators in peripheral tissues from the central pacemaker in the suprachiasmatic nucleus. Genes Dev 2000, 14(23):2950-61.
11. Balsalobre A, Brown SA, Marcacci L, Tronche F, Kellendonk C, Reichardt HM, et al.: Resetting of circadian time in peripheral tissues by glucocorticoid signaling. Science 2000, 289(5488):2344-7.
12. Mistlberger RE, Skene DS: Social influences on mammalian circadian rhythms: animal and human studies. Biol Rev 2004, 79:533-56.
13. Zvonic S, Ptitsyn AA, Conrad SA, Scott LK, Floyd ZE, Kilroy G, et al.: Characterization of peripheral circadian clocks in adipose tissues. Diabetes 2006, 55:962-70.
14. Loboda A, Kraft WK, Fine B, Joseph J, Nebozhyn M, Zhang C, et al.: Diurnal variation of the human adipose transcriptome and the link to metabolic disease. BMC Medical Genomics 2009, 9:2-7.
15. Wu X, Zvonic S, Floyd ZE, Kilroy G, Goh BC, Hernandez TL, et al.: Induction of circadian gene expression in human subcutaneous adipose-derived stem cells. Obesity (Silver Spring) 15(11):2560-70. 200
16. Suzuki M, Shimomura Y, Satoh Y: Diurnal changes in lipolytic activity of isolated fat cells and their increased responsiveness to epinephrine and theophylline with meal feeding in rats. J Nutr Sci Vitaminol 1983, 29:399-411.
17. Chawla A, Lazar MA: Induction of Rev-ErbA alpha, an orphan receptor encoded on the opposite strand of the alpha-thyroid hormone receptor gene, during adipocyte differentiation. J Biol Chem 1993, 268:16265-9.
18. Alonso-Vale MI, Andreotti S, Mukai PY, Borges-Silva CN, Peres SB, Cipolla-Neto J, et al.: Melatonin and the circadian entrainment of metabolic and hormonal activities in primary isolated adipocytes. J Pineal Res 2008, 45(4):422-9.
19. Ando H, Yanagihara H, Hayashi Y, Obi Y, Tsuruoka S, Takamura T, et al.: Rhythmic messenger ribonucleic acid expression of clock genes and adipocytokines in mouse visceral adipose tissue. Endocrinology 2005, 146(12):5631-6.
20. Saad MF, Riad-Gabriel MG, Khan A, Sharma A, Michael R, Jinagouda SD, et al.: Diurnal and ultradian rhythmicity of plasma leptin: effects of gender and adiposity. J Clin Endocrinol Metab 1998, 83:453-9.

21.  Kalra SP, Bagnasco M, Otukonyong EE, Dube MG, Kalra OS: Rhythmic, reciprocal ghrelin and leptin signaling: new insight in the development of obesity. Regul Pept 2003, 111:1-11.
22.  Gavrila A, Peng CK, Chan JL, Mietus JE, Goldberger AL, Mantzoros CS: Diurnal and ultradian dynamics of serum adiponectin in healthy men: comparison with leptin, circulating soluble leptin receptor, and cortisol patterns. J Clin Endocrinol Metab 2003, 88(6):2838-43.
23.  Brodsky VY: Direct cell-cell communication: a new approach derived from recent data on the nature and self-organisation of ultradian (circahoralian) intracellular rhythms. Biol Rev Camb Philos Soc 2006, 81(1):143-62.
24.  Shimba S, Ishii N, Ohta Y, Ohno T, Watabe Y, Hayashi M, et al.: Brain and muscle Arnt-like protein-1 (BMAL1), a component of the molecular clock, regulates adipogenesis. Proc Natl Acad Sci USA 2005, 102:12071-6.
25.  Fontaine C, Dubois G, Duguay Y, Helledie T, Vu-Dac N, Gervois P, et al.: The orphan nuclear receptor Rev-Erbalpha is a peroxisome proliferator-activated receptor (PPAR) gamma target gene and promotes PPARgamma-induced adipocyte differentiation. J Biol Chem 2003, 278(39):37672-80.
26.  Bray MS, Young ME: Circadian rhythms in the development of obesity: Potential role for the circadian clock within the adipocyte. Obes Rev 2006, 8:169-81.
27.  Kennaway DJ, Owens JA, Voultsios A, Boden MJ, Varcoe TJ: Metabolic homeostasis in mice with disrupted Clock gene expression in peripheral tissues. Am J Physiol Regul Integr Comp Physiol 2007, 293:R1528-37.
28.  Gómez-Abellán P, Hernández-Morante JJ, Luján JA, Madrid JA, Garaulet M: Clock genes are implicated in the human metabolic syndrome. Int J Obes 2008, 32(1):121-8.
29.  Gómez-Santos C, Gómez-Abellán P, Madrid JA, Hernández-Morante JJ, Lujan JA, Ordovas JM, Garaulet M: Circadian Rhythm of Clock Genes in Human Adipose Explants. Obesity (Silver Spring) 2009, 17(8):1481-5.
30.  Ando H, Ushijima K, Kumazaki M, Eto T, Takamura T, Irie S, Kaneko S, Fujimura A: Associations of metabolic parameters and ethanol consumption with messenger RNA expression of clock genes in healthy men. Chronobiol Int 2010, 27:194-203.
31.  Sato TK, Panda S, Miraglia LJ, Reyes TM, Rudic RD, McNamara P, et al.: A functional genomics strategy reveals Rora as a component of the mammalian circadian clock. Neuron 2004, 43:527-37.
32.  Lau P, Nixon SJ, Parton RG, Muscat GE: RORalpha regulates the expression of genes involved in lipid homeostasis in skeletal muscle cells: caveolin-3 and CPT-1 are direct targets of ROR. J Biol Chem 2004, 279:36828-40.
33.  Canaple L, Rambaud J, Dkhissi-Benyahya O, Rayet B, Tan NS, Michalik L, et al.: Reciprocal regulation of brain and muscle Arnt-like protein 1 and peroxisome proliferator-activated receptor alpha defines a novel positive feedback loop in the rodent liver circadian clock. Mol Endocrinol 2006, 20:1715-27.
34.  Duez H, Staels B: The nuclear receptors Rev-erbs and RORs integrate circadian rhythms and metabolism. Diab Vasc Dis Res 2008, 5:82-8.
35.  Teboul M, Guillaumond F, Gréchez-Cassiau A, Delaunay F: The nuclear hormone receptor family round the clock. Mol Endocrinol 2008, 22(12):2573-82.

36. Turek FW, Joshu C, Kohsaka A, Lin E, Ivanova G, McDearmon E, et al.: Obesity and metabolic syndrome in circadian Clock mutant mice. Science 2005, 308:1043-5.
37. Kondratov RV, Antoch MP: The clock proteins, aging, and tumorigenesis. Cold Spring Harb Symp Quant Biol 2007, 72:477-82.
38. Dallmann R, Touma C, Palme R, Albrecht U, Steinlechner S: Impaired daily glucocorticoid rhythm in Per1 (Brd) mice. J Comp Physiol A Neuroethol Sens Neural Behav Physiol 2006, 192:769-75.
39. Schibler U, Ripperger J, Brown SA: Peripheral circadian oscillators in mammals: time and food. J Biol Rhythms 2003, 18(3):250-260.
40. Angeles-Castellanos M, Salgado-Delgado R, Rodríguez K, Buijs RM, Escobar C: Expectancy for food or expectancy for chocolate reveals timing systems for metabolism and reward. Neuroscience 2008, 155(1):297-307.
41. Stephan FK: Circadian rhythm dissociation induced by periodic feeding in rats with suprachiasmatic lesions. Behav Brain Res 1983, 7(1):81-98.
42. Mistlberger RE: Circadian rhythms: perturbing a food-entrained clock. Curr Biol 2006, 16(22):R968-9.
43. Mieda M, Williams SC, Richardson JA, Tanaka K, Yanagisawa M: The dorsomedial hypothalamic nucleus as a putative food-entrainable circadian pacemaker. Proc Natl Acad Sci USA 2006, 103(32):12150-5.
44. Mistlberger RE, Houpt TA, Moore-Ede MC: Food-anticipatory rhythms under 24-hour schedules of limited access to single macronutrients. J Biol Rhythms 1990, 5(1):35-46.
45. Challet E, Pévet P, Vivien-Roels B, Malan A: Phase-advanced daily rhythms of melatonin, body temperature, and locomotor activity in food-restricted rats fed during daytime. J Biol Rhythms 1997, 12(1):65-79.
46. Mendoza J, Pévet P, Challet E: Circadian and photic regulation of clock and clock-controlled proteins in the suprachiasmatic nuclei of calorie-restricted mice. Eur J Neurosci 2007, 25(12):3691-701.
47. Zanquetta MM, Seraphim PM, Sumida DH, Cipolla-Neto J, Machado UF: Calorie restriction reduces pinealectomy-induced insulin resistance by improving GLUT4 gene expression and its translocation to the plasma membrane. J Pineal Res 2003, 35(3):141-8.
48. Ravussin E, Redman LM: Adiposity and comorbidities: favorable impact of caloric restriction. Nestle Nutr Workshop Ser Pediatr Program 2009, 63:135-46. discussion 147-50, 259-68
49. Bartol-Munier I, Gourmelen S, Pevet P, Challet E: Combined effects of high-fat feeding and circadian desynchronization. Int J Obes 2006, 30(1):60-7.
50. Kohsaka A, Laposky AD, Ramsey KM, Estrada C, Joshu C, Kobayashi Y, et al.: High-fat diet disrupts behavioral and molecular circadian rhythms in mice. Cell Metab 2007, 6:414-21.
51. Mendoza J, Pévet P, Challet E: High-fat feeding alters the clock synchronization to light. J Physiol 2008, 586(Pt24):5901-10.
52. Morgan PJ, Ross AW, Mercer JG, Barrett P: Photoperiodic programming of body weight through the neuroendocrine hypothalamus. J Endocrinol 2003, 177:27-34.
53. Bartness TJ, Hamilton JM, Wade GN, Goldman BD: Regional differences in fat pad responses to short days in Siberian hamsters. Am J Physiol 1989, 257:R1533-40.

54. Klingenspor M, Dickopp A, Heldmaier G, Klaus S: Short photoperiod reduces leptin gene expression in white and brown adipose tissue of Djungarian hamsters. FEBS Letters 1996, 399:290-4.

55. Wikelski M, Martin LB, Scheuerlein A, Robinson MT, Robinson ND, Helm B, et al.: Avian circannual clocks: adaptive significance and possible involvement of energy turnover in their proximate control. Philos Trans R Soc Lond B Biol Sci 2008, 363(1490):411-23.

56. Soppela P, Saarela S, Heiskari U, Nieminen M: The effects of wintertime undernutrition on plasma leptin and insulin levels in an arctic ruminant, the reindeer. Comp Biochem Physiol B Biochem Mol Biol 2008, 149(4):613-21.

57. Cappuccio FP, Taggart FM, Kandala NB, Currie A, Peile E, Stranges S, et al.: Meta-analysis of short sleep duration and obesity in children and adults. Sleep 2008, 31:619-26.

58. Van Cauter E, Knutson KL: Sleep and the epidemic of obesity in children and adults. Eur J Endocrinol 2008, 159(Suppl 1):S59-66.

59. Patel SR, Blackwell T, Redline S, Ancoli-Israel S, Cauley JA, Hillier TA, et al.: The association between sleep duration and obesity in older adults. Int J Obes 2008, 32(12):1825-34.

60. Spiegel K, Tasali E, Penev P, Van Cauter E: Brief communication: sleep curtailment in healthy young men is associated with decreased leptin levels, elevated ghrelin levels, and increased hunger and appetite. Ann Intern Med 2004, 141(11):846-50.

61. Laposky AD, Shelton J, Bass J, Dugovic C, Perrino N, Turek FW: Altered sleep regulation in leptin-deficient mice. Am J Physiol Regul Integr Comp Physiol 2006, 290(4):R892-3.

62. Laposky AD, Bradley MA, Williams DL, Bass J, Turek FW: Sleep-wake regulation is altered in leptin-resistant (db/db) genetically obese and diabetic mice. Am J Physiol Regul Integr Comp Physiol 2008, 295(6):R2059-66.

63. Karlsson B, Knutsson A, Lindahl B: Is there an association between shift work and having a metabolic syndrome? Results from a population based study of 27,485 people. Occup Environ Med 2001, 58(11):747-52.

64. Biggi N, Consonni D, Galluzzo V, Sogliani M, Costa G: Metabolic syndrome in permanent night workers. Chronobiol Int 2008, 25(2):443-54.

65. Esquirol Y, Bongard V, Mabile L, Jonnier B, Soulat JM, Perret B: Shift work and metabolic syndrome: respective impacts of job strain, physical activity, and dietary rhythms. Chronobiol Int 2009, 26(3):544-59.

66. Spiegel K, Tasali E, Leproult R, Van Cauter E: Effects of poor and short sleep on glucose metabolism and obesity risk. Nat Rev Endocrinol 2009, 5(5):253-61.

67. Yildiz BO, Suchard MA, Wong ML, McCann SM, Licinio J: Alterations in the dynamics of circulating ghrelin, adiponectin, and leptin in human obesity. Proc Natl Acad Sci USA 2004, 101(28):10434-9.

68. Kaneko K, Yamada T, Tsukita S, Takahashi K, Ishigaki Y, Oka Y, et al.: Obesity alters circadian expressions of molecular clock genes in the brainstem. Brain Res 2009, 1263:58-68.

69. Loos RJ, Bouchard C: Obesity- is it a genetic disorder? J Intern Med 2003, 254(5):401-25.

70. Hainer V, Zamrazilová H, Spálová J, Hainerová I, Kunesová M, Aldhoon B, et al.: Role of Hereditary Factors in Weight Loss and Its Maintenance. Physiol Res 2008, 57(Suppl 1):S1-15.
71. O'Rahilly S, Farooqi IS: Human obesity as a heritable disorder of the central control of energy balance. Int J Obes 2008, 32(Suppl 7):S55-61.
72. Rankinen T, Zuberi A, Chagnon YC, Weisnagel SJ, Argyropoulos G, Walts B, et al.: The human obesity gene map: the 2005 update. Obesity (Silver Spring) 2006, 14(4):529-644.
73. Schousboe K, Visscher PM, Erbas B, Kyvik KO, Hopper JL, Henriksen JE, et al.: Twin study of genetic and environmental influences on adult body size, shape, and composition. Int J Obes Relat Metab Disord 2004, 28:39-48.
74. Wardle J, Carnell S, Haworth CM, Plomin R: Evidence for a strong genetic influence on childhood adiposity despite the force of the obesogenic environment. Am J Clin Nutr 2008, 87:398-404.
75. Sookoian S, Castaño G, Gemma C, Gianotti TF, Pirola CJ: Common genetic variations in CLOCK transcription factor are associated with nonalcoholic fatty liver disease. World J Gastroenterol 2007, 13(31):4242-8.
76. Tortorella A, Monteleone P, Martiadis V, Perris F, Maj M: The 3111T/C polymorphism of the CLOCK gene confers a predisposition to a lifetime lower body weight in patients with anorexia nervosa and bulimia nervosa: a preliminary study. Am J Med Genet B Neuropsychiatr Genet 2007, 144B(8):992-5.
77. Benedetti F, Dallaspezia S, Fulgosi MC, Lorenzi C, Serretti A, Barbini B, Benedetti F, et al.: Actimetric evidence that CLOCK 3111 T/C SNP influences sleep and activity patterns in patients affected by bipolar depression. Am J Med Genet B Neuropsychiatr Genet 2007, 144B(5):631-5.
78. Monteleone P, Tortorella A, Docimo L, Maldonato MN, Canestrelli B, De Luca L, et al.: Investigation of 3111T/C polymorphism of the CLOCK gene in obese individuals with or without binge eating disorder: association with higher body mass index. Neurosci Lett 2008, 435(1):30-3.
79. Woon PY, Kaisaki PJ, Bragança J, Bihoreau MT, Levy JC, Farrall M, et al.: Aryl hydrocarbon receptor nuclear translocator-like (BMAL1) is associated with susceptibility to hypertension and type 2 diabetes. Proc Natl Acad Sci USA 2007, 104(36):14412-7.
80. DeBruyne JP, Weaver DR, Reppert SM: CLOCK and NPAS2 have overlapping roles in the suprachiasmatic circadian clock. Nat Neurosci 2007, 10(5):543-5.
81. Englund A, Kovanen L, Saarikoski ST, Haukka J, Reunanen A, Aromaa A, et al.: NPAS2 and PER2 are linked to risk factors of the metabolic syndrome. J Circadian Rhythms 2009, 7:5.
82. Ciarleglio CM, Ryckman KK, Servick SV, Hida A, Robbins S, Wells N, et al.: Genetic differences in human circadian clock genes among worldwide populations. J Biol Rhythms 2008, 23(4):330-40.

# PART II

# METABOLISM AT NIGHT VERSUS THE MORNING

# CHAPTER 4

# CIRCADIAN DESYNCHRONY PROMOTES METABOLIC DISRUPTION IN A MOUSE MODEL OF SHIFTWORK

JOHANNA L. BARCLAY, JANA HUSSE, BRID BODE, NADINE NAUJOKAT, JUDIT MEYER-KOVAC, SEBASTIAN M. SCHMID, HENDRIK LEHNERT, AND HENRIK OSTER

## 4.1 INTRODUCTION

Shiftwork refers to a job schedule in which employees work hours other than the standard hours, e.g. in the early morning or during the night. Chronic shiftwork is correlated to increased body mass index (BMI) and risk of developing metabolic syndrome [1]–[5]. It further affects the secretion of endocrine factors such as melatonin, growth hormone, prolactin, leptin and glucocorticoids, all of which impinge on metabolic homeostasis [6]–[10]. It has been proposed that chronic sleep disruption may be causal in the incidence of metabolic dysregulation and obesity in shift workers [3], [7], [11]. In rodents, four weeks of enforced daytime activity causes altered diurnal rhythms of food uptake, blood glucose and neuronal activation [12], [13], suggesting an effect of sleep timing on circadian clock

This chapter was originally published under the Creative Commons Attribution License. Barclay JL, Husse J, Bode B, Naujokat N, Meyer-Kovac J, Schmid SM, Lehnert H, and Oster H. Circadian Desynchrony Promotes Metabolic Disruption in a Mouse Model of Shiftwork. PLoS ONE 7,5 (2012). doi:10.1371/journal.pone.0037150.

function. However, the molecular mechanisms underlying these observations remain unclear.

Circadian clocks provide a mechanism by which external time is interpreted and translated into time-of-day appropriate physiology, with the overall aim of promoting fitness and energy efficiency of an organism [14]. In mammals, circadian physiological rhythms are regulated by a hierarchical system of tissue clocks, with a master pacemaker situated in the suprachiasmatic nuclei (SCN) of the hypothalamus. The SCN receive external time information predominately in the form of light via the retinohypothalamic tract. They then transmit this information via neurohumoral signals to subsidiary oscillators in other regions of the brain and in the periphery. Peripheral clocks can also be directly entrained by food, independent of the SCN [15].

At the cellular level circadian clocks are organized into a system of interlocking transcriptional translational feedback loops (TTLs) [16]. The positive arm of the core TTL in mammals is formed by the transcriptional activators circadian locomotor output cycles kaput (CLOCK) and brain and muscle ARNT-like protein 1 (BMAL1 or ARNTL), which dimerize and bind to E-Box cis-elements on target gene promoters. Transcription of three period (*Per1-3*) and two cryptochrome genes (*Cry1* and *2*) is initiated by the CLOCK:BMAL1 complex. The resulting CRY and PER proteins inhibit CLOCK:BMAL1 activity, thus forming a negative feedback loop impinging on their own transcription. The clock machinery translates time information into physiologically meaningful signals by the regulation of hundreds of clock-controlled output genes (CCGs). While the nature of core clock genes is preserved among different tissues, CCGs are highly tissue-specific. It is estimated that up to 10% of the transcriptome of each cell is regulated in a circadian fashion [17]. In this way, physiological processes can be sequestered to the appropriate time of the day.

The rhythmic mammalian transcriptome of various tissues is enriched for genes involved in metabolic processes, indicating a major role for the clock in metabolic regulation [17]. In humans, circadian disruption correlates with metabolic dysfunction [5], [14], [16]. Genetic clock disruption in rodents has similar effects. *Bmal*$^{-/-}$ mice show impaired glucose tolerance, gluconeogenesis, altered triglyceride rhythms and increased body fat [18], [19]. *Clock*$^{\Delta 19}$ mice display impaired gluconeogenesis in addition to hyperphagy and obesity [20], [21], and *Per2* mutant mice are also obese [22].

Given that sleep and clock dysfunction share the same metabolic end-point, it was hypothesized that shiftwork-induced metabolic deregulation may be a direct result of circadian clock disturbance. This study demonstrates that two weeks of timed sleep restriction (TSR) leads to clock disruption and global diurnal desynchrony at the transcriptional level in the liver, while metabolic functions are still only moderately affected. Molecular and metabolic effects of TSR can be alleviated by timed food access, a strong synchronizer of peripheral clocks, emphasizing the therapeutic potential of behavioral chronotherapy to combat the metabolic consequences of shiftwork.

## 4.2 RESULTS

### 4.2.1 TSR IN MICE RESULTS IN PERTURBATIONS OF DIURNAL BEHAVIORAL RHYTHMS

Young adult male C57Bl6/J mice were subjected to a two-week regime of TSR designed to mimic common human night shiftwork schedules. Mice were housed under 12 h light: 12 h dark (LD) conditions with food and water given ad libitum at all times. During TSR animals were kept awake during the first 6 hours of the light phase (Zeitgeber time (ZT) 0–6) on Days 1 through 5 and Days 8 through 12 using a 'gentle handling' approach designed to minimize stress effects and intervention by the experimenter [23], [24] (boxes in Figure 1A and 1B). At all other times mice were left undisturbed. To assess stress levels in TSR mice plasma corticosterone was measured at 8 different times during the day. No overall increase in diurnal corticosterone release was observed, but corticosterone peak phase was found to be advanced by 6 h in TSR mice (Figure 1C). As expected, during TSR mice displayed increased activity from ZT0 to ZT6 relative to control animals (Figure 1A and 1B). In addition, activity during the dark phase gradually declined during the course of TSR (Figure 1D).

In parallel, TSR animals developed altered feeding rhythms, with light phase food intake increasing relative to controls (Figure 1E). Of note, no overall changes in activity or food intake, and no significant effects on body weight were recorded during 2 weeks of TSR (Figure 1D, 1E and S1). On Day 12 central clock function was assessed by quantifying clock gene expression profiles in the SCN using $^{35}$S-UTP labeled ISH on sections. An upregulation of mRNA levels was observed in TSR animals in the early light phase (ZT1) for *Bmal1, Per1* and *Dbp*, and mid light phase (ZT7) for *Rev-erbα* (Figure 1F). However, overall diurnal rhythmicity and peak phasing of clock gene transcripts in the SCN was maintained. In line with this, when TSR mice were released into constant darkness (DD), thus avoiding photic masking effects on activity rhythms [25], activity profiles were virtually indistinguishable from control mice that had been allowed to sleep ad libitum prior to release into DD (Figure 1G).

### 4.2.2 TSR RESETS LIVER CLOCKS

The marked effect of TSR on food intake and corticosterone rhythms prompted us to assess circadian clock function in the liver, a key peripheral tissue involved in energy metabolism. Diurnal clock gene expression profiles in the liver were analyzed using qPCR. A marked dampening of diurnal transcriptional rhythms was observed for *Bmal1, Per1* and *Npas2* with changes in expression peak times for *Bmal1* and *Per1*, while little effect was seen for *Rev-erbα* (Figure 2A). To examine the significance of these changes for hepatic clock function in the absence of external entrainment signals, liver slice cultures from TSR and control *PER2::LUC* circadian clock reporter mice were compared for phase and period. Slices from TSR animals showed delayed phasing and decreased period lengths of luciferase activity rhythms relative to control animals (Figure 2B–D).

### 4.2.3 TSR DISRUPTS TRANSCRIPTOME RHYTHMICITY IN THE LIVER

Because of the strong effect of TSR on liver clock regulation we speculated that TSR would have a broad impact on transcriptome regulation in this

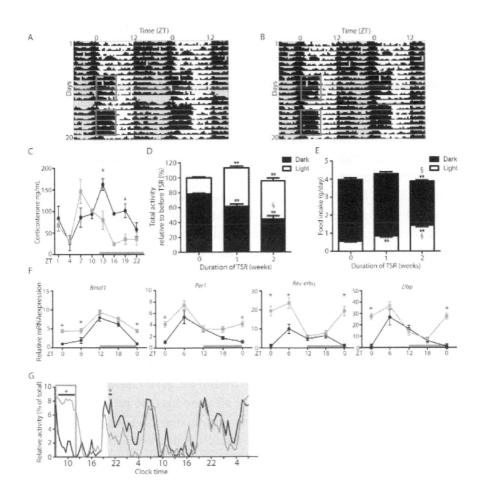

**FIGURE 1:** TSR results in perturbations of diurnal behavioral rhythms. (A and B) Representative activity recordings of TSR mice. Actograms are double-plotted. Grey shadings indicate dark phases, red boxes indicate period of TSR. (C) Plasma corticosterone in control and TSR mice on Day12 of TSR (n = 3–5). (D) Distribution of light and dark activity during TSR expressed as % of total activity of the same set of animals during control conditions (n = 5 cages of 4 mice each), * indicates p<0.05 and **p<0.01 relative to 0 weeks of TSR, § indicates p<0.05 relative to 1 week of TSR. (E) Food intake during light and dark phase during TSR, * indicates p<0.05 and **p<0.01 relative to 0 weeks of TSR (n = 10–23), § indicates p<0.05 relative to 1 week of TSR determined by 2-way ANOVA. (F) Quantitation of clock gene mRNA by ISH in the SCN of control and TSR mice expressed relative to controls at ZT0 (n = 3 at each time point). (G) Activity of control and TSR mice upon release into DD (n = 3 cages). Grey bars indicate dark phase, box indicates last period of gentle handling. Control mice represented by black lines, TSR mice by grey lines; * indicates p<0.05 determined by 2-way ANOVA.

tissue. To test this, cRNA preparations from liver samples harvested at 4 different time points from TSR and control mice were hybridized to whole genome expression microarrays (Affymetrix Mouse Gene 1.0 ST Arrays). Under control conditions, and in accordance with previous reports, we found a large number of genes with diurnal changes in expression levels (Figure 3A). After TSR the vast majority of previously rhythmic genes no longer showed diurnal variation and the normal phase relationship between different transcripts was lost (Figure 3A). When rhythmic genes from both treatment groups were sorted for expression peak time, profound changes in the overall distribution of transcriptional activity were observed. While expression peaks were evenly distributed along the day in the liver of control animals, a bimodal distribution pattern was observed in TSR animals, with most genes peaking in the early light phase or the early dark phase (ZT1 and ZT13, respectively; Figure 3B). Interestingly, although a general desynchrony of a formerly rhythmic transcriptome organization was observed during TSR, at the same time an additional array of changes in expression profiles for specific transcripts including phase shifts, alterations to baseline expression of non-rhythmic genes, and the induction of rhythmic gene expression in previously non-rhythmic genes was observed. TSR-induced changes in diurnal gene regulation are summarized and compared in Figure 3C. Full gene lists are provided in Table S1. In order to confirm that the array expression data was reliable, we directly compared our array results to the qPCR data on clock gene expression (Figure 2). A good correlation between both data sets was observed (Figure S2).

## 4.2.4 METABOLIC GENE RHYTHMICITY IS AFFECTED BY TSR

Previous studies in humans and rodents show that chronic shiftwork has profound effects on metabolism. Supporting this, gene ontology (GO) analysis of our array data revealed that the genes that lost rhythmicity following TSR were enriched for transcripts involved in metabolic processes (Table S2). To further investigate this phenomenon, expression profiles of all genes rhythmically expressed under control conditions and associated with metabolism (i.e. listed under the GO categories 'Carbohydrate Me-

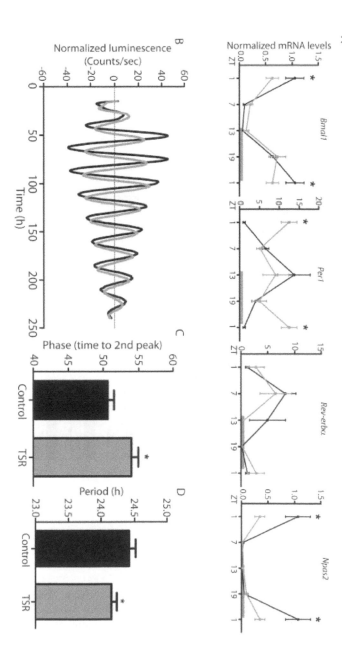

**FIGURE 2:** TSR resets the hepatic circadian clock. (A) qPCR analysis of diurnal clock gene mRNA profiles in the liver of control and TSR mice (n = 3 at each time point). (B) Luciferase activity in liver slice cultures from control and TSR PER2::LUC mice (n = 8) and (C) quantitation of phase and (D) period. Control mice are represented by black lines, TSR mice by grey lines; * indicates p<0.05 determined by 2-way ANOVA.

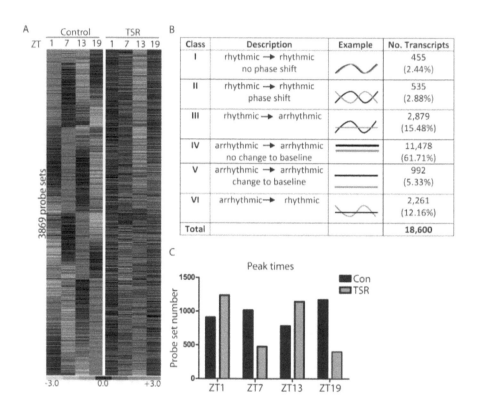

**FIGURE 3:** TSR causes global disruption of transcriptome rhythmicity in the liver. (A) Heat map illustrating diurnal expression of rhythmically expressed genes sorted for phase in control animals, and their corresponding expression profiles in TSR animals in liver (n = 3 at each time point). (B) Summary of transcriptional effects seen in liver following TSR. (C) Peak times of rhythmically expressed genes under control and TSR conditions. Black bars and lines indicate controls, grey bars and lines indicate TSR.

tabolism' - GO:0005975, 'Lipid Metabolism' - GO:0006629 or 'Amino Acid Metabolism' - GO:0006520) were compared. A profound loss of metabolic gene rhythmicity was seen for genes peaking at all time points (Figure 4A–D). Of note, no directional shift in expression peaks was observed for metabolic genes that were rhythmic both under control and TSR conditions (Figure S3), indicating that TSR had a disruptive, but not a phase resetting effect on liver metabolism.

Among the affected genes were a number of important regulators of carbohydrate metabolism (Figure 4E), such as the glucose transporter 2 (*Slc2a2*), glucose-responsive forkhead box O1 (*Foxo1*) and insulin receptor substrate 2 (*Irs2*). There appeared to be a particular emphasis on regulators of the glycolysis/gluconeogenesis pathway, such as liver pyruvate kinase (*Pklr*), pyruvate dehydrogenase kinase 4 (*Pdk4*), the pyruvate transporter Slc16a7, the glycerol transporter aquaporin 9 (*Aqp9*), fructose-2,6-biphosphatase 1 (*Pfkfb1*) and pyruvate carboxylase (*Pcx*). Glycerol phosphate dehydrogenase 2 (*Gpd2*) and glycerol kinase (*Gyk*), regulators of glycerol biosynthesis, and glutamic-pyruvate transaminase (*Gpt*), a regulator of pyruvate production from alanine, were also affected. Together, these findings suggested a marked effect of TSR on glucose metabolism, particularly gluconeogenesis. Supporting this, TSR animals showed profoundly impaired gluconeogenic capacity, determined by a pyruvate tolerance test (Figure 5A). Hepatic glycogen storage rhythms were also altered with increased levels at the beginning of the dark phase (ZT13) in TSR mice, and circulating glycerol was increased at ZT13, while diurnal triglyceride rhythms were dampened with lower levels at ZT1, indicating that TSR had further effects on lipid metabolism (Figure 5B–D). Finally, decreased leptin levels were observed in the light phase in TSR animals, correlating to increased food intake observed during this period (Figure 1E).

## 4.2.5 DARK PHASE RESTRICTED FEEDING PREVENTS TSR-INDUCED PERIPHERAL CLOCK AND METABOLIC DISRUPTION

Although 2 weeks of TSR did not result in significant changes in overall food intake, insulin sensitivity or weight gain as has been reported for

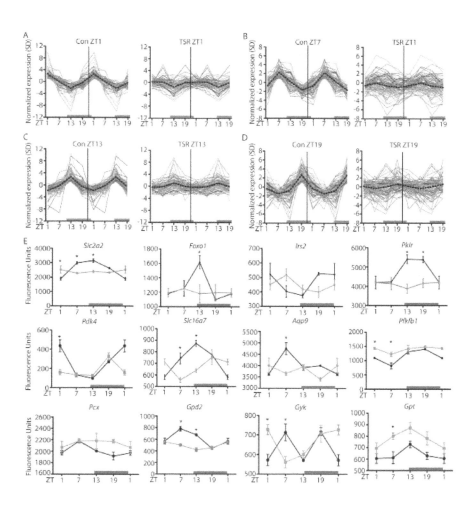

**FIGURE 4:** Metabolic gene rhythmicity in the liver is affected by shiftwork. Double plotted expression profiles of rhythmic genes associated with the GO terms 'Carbohydrate Metabolism', 'Lipid Metabolism' and 'Amino Acid Metabolism' sorted for peak time ((A) ZT1, (B) ZT7, (C) ZT13 and (D) ZT19) for both control and TSR groups. (E) Array expression profiles of selected metabolically relevant genes with altered expression profiles in the livers of TSR mice. Control mice are represented by black lines, TSR mice by grey lines; * indicates p<0.05 determined by 2-way ANOVA.

human shift workers or for longer shiftwork-like protocols in rodents, the perturbations to glucose and lipid handling observed in this study could be considered as early signs of future metabolic dysfunction. Given the hepatic transcriptional desynchrony observed in TSR animals we speculated that stabilizing liver clock regulation during TSR would potentially prevent, or at least alleviate, the emergence of metabolic effects. Indeed, when food access was restricted to the dark phase during TSR (NF-TSR) marked effects on both the molecular and metabolic level were observed. In NF-TSR animal diurnal expression peak times for *Bmal1, Npas2* and *Rev-erbα* in the liver were undistinguishable from control animals, however, some dampening effect of TSR on *Rev-erbα* and *Per1* expression was preserved (Figure 6A, compare Figure 2A). Moreover, TSR perturbations to plasma glycerol and triglyceride profiles were rescued in NF-TSR mice (Figure 6B and 6C, compare Figure 5B and 5C) together with improved gluconeogenic potential (Figure 6D). Finally, the phase of plasma corticosterone rhythms was restored in NF-TSR mice (Figure 6E, compare Figure 1C). In summary, restricting food intake during TSR to the normal active phase rescued peripheral clock gene rhythmicity and subsequently improved glucose and lipid handling. This marked effect of feeding time on TSR effects prompted us to test if altered food intake rhythms may play a causative role in the metabolic pathophysiology of shiftwork [26]. To test this, mice were subjected to two weeks of timed feeding schedules mimicking the light/dark food intake pattern observed in the second week of TSR (Figure 1E), followed by a pyruvate tolerance test on the last day. These animals showed no changes to gluconeogenic potential (Figure 6F), indicating that alterations in food uptake rhythms are necessary, but not sufficient for the induction of metabolic effects of TSR.

## 4.3 DISCUSSION

The current study employs a 2 week schedule of TSR in mice to examine the early molecular and physiological responses to altered activity timing preceding the metabolic consequences of chronic shiftwork. Profound disruption in the diurnal regulation of core clock genes and CCGs was observed in liver, with a strong emphasis on metabolic transcripts, while only moderate effects were seen at the level of the circadian pacemaker of the SCN. The physiological significance of these changes was demonstrated by early alterations in lipid and glucose handling, while bodyweight regulation was not yet affected. Both peripheral clock gene rhythmicity and metabolic physiology were rescued by concurrent dark phase restricted food access, suggesting meal timing as a possible therapeutic intervention for the treatment of shiftwork-associated metabolic disorders.

### 4.3.1 TSR EFFECTS ON SCN CLOCK RHYTHMS

Changes to core clock gene expression were evident following TSR. In the SCN, moderate effects on *Bmal1, Per1, Rev-erbα* and *Dbp* were observed, while overall rhythmicity was preserved. At the behavioral level, however, decreased activity was observed in the dark phase, accompanied by a shift of food intake to the light phase. These activity phase shifts appear to be acute effects of the TSR procedure, perhaps in response to increased light input, and alterations in activity rhythms ceased when animals were released into DD conditions after the end of TSR (Figure 1). Collectively this suggests that TSR has only a moderate effect on the central clock, despite an overall disruption of diurnal activity, although it is not possible to conclusively rule out changes to CCGs in the SCN. These findings correlate with a recent study of 4 weeks of enforced daytime activity in rats which showed no changes of PER1 protein expression in the SCN, but marked disruption of PER1 rhythms in other hypothalamic nuclei [13]. It would therefore be interesting to extend our analysis to CCGs in the SCN, and other clocks in the brain, or to analyze clock gene effects after longer periods of TSR. Given the late onset of metabolic disturbances in human shift workers it is tempting to speculate that SCN clock disruption may become more apparent at a later time point. In a combined review of six studies of permanent night shift workers describing melatonin rhythms—generally considered a reliable readout of the circadian pacemaker in humans—it was concluded that very few people ever show an adaptation of their internal clock to the altered activity schedule [27].

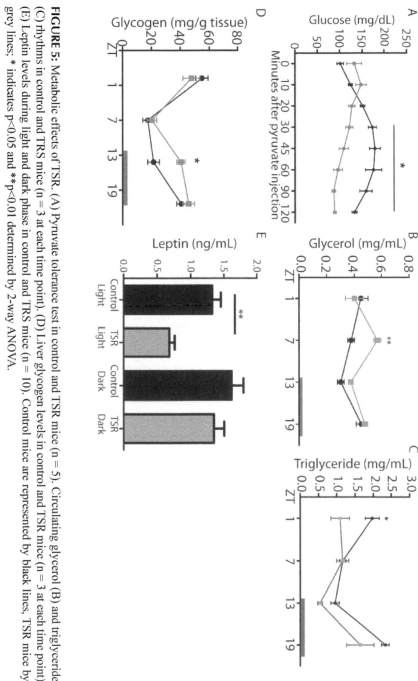

**FIGURE 5:** Metabolic effects of TSR. (A) Pyruvate tolerance test in control and TSR mice (n = 5). Circulating glycerol (B) and triglyceride (C) rhythms in control and TRS mice (n = 3 at each time point). (D) Liver glycogen levels in control and TSR mice (n = 3 at each time point) (E) Leptin levels during light and dark phase in control and TRS mice (n = 10). Control mice are represented by black lines, TSR mice by grey lines; * indicates p<0.05 and **p<0.01 determined by 2-way ANOVA.

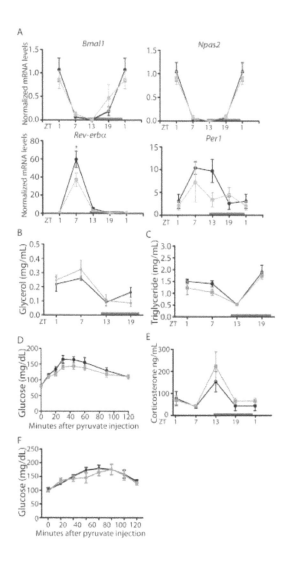

**FIGURE 6:** Dark phase feeding rescues TSR-induced disruption of peripheral clock gene expression and gluconeogenesis. (A) qPCR analysis of clock gene expression in the liver of control/dark phase fed (DF) and TSR/dark phase fed (DF-TSR) mice. (B) Plasma glycerol and (C) triglyceride rhythms in control/DF and DF-TSR mice. (D) Pyruvate tolerance test in control/DF and DF-TSR mice (n = 5). (E) Plasma corticosterone control/DF fed and DF-TSR mice. (F) Pyruvate tolerance test in non-TRS mice under a TSR-like feeding regimen (n = 5). (A-E) Control mice are represented by black lines, TSR mice by grey lines. (F) Ad libitum fed mice are represented by black lines, TSR-like fed mice are represented by grey lines; * indicates p<0.05 determined by 2-way ANOVA, n = 3 at each time point, unless stated otherwise.

## 4.3.2 TSR CAUSES GLOBAL DISRUPTION OF THE LIVER CLOCK AND CCGS

The effect of TSR on clock gene expression in the liver was much more pronounced than in the SCN (Figure 2), with a consequent global disruption of normal transcriptome rhythmicity (Figure 3). Genes from Class III ("rhythmic to arrhythmic") showed ontology enrichment for metabolic processes, correlating with a marked dampening of rhythms in metabolism-associated (Figure 4). TSR also impinges on the regulation of several non-rhythmic genes in which rhythmic expression was induced following TSR (Class VI). These genes may be directly affected by changes in food uptake [28] or activity [29]. If one assumes that rest and activity roughly corresponds to fasting and feeding, the strong increase in early light phase activity during TSR would indicate a profound increase in food intake during this time which would then drive gene expression rhythms. In this particular case this assumption would be misleading, as the increased activity can be largely attributed to exploration of the novel objects placed in the cage as part of the gentle handling protocol. This is supported by the observation that the effects of TSR on feeding rhythmicity are far less pronounced than those on locomotor activity (Figure 1D and 1E). Alternately these genes may be directly sleep-responsive and may therefore be classified as "acutely sleep (-loss) regulated". In a study by Maret et al. which employed the same gentle handling method used in the current study, a number of genes specifically responsive to sleep-loss were identified for the brain as well as the liver [30], some of which encoded heat shock proteins which the authors hypothesized to be part of a tissue-independent stress response. A number of heat shock protein gene were also identified in the current study (Table S1). However, it should be noted that sleep was not directly measured in either the Maret study or ours—with the notable exception of during the TSR protocol when the animals were continually observed for wakefulness—and therefore any possible "sleep-related" changes are inferred from activity and must be very cautiously considered.

### 4.3.3 TSR EFFECTS ON CARBOHYDRATE METABOLISM IN LIVER

Genes involved in carbohydrate metabolism were deregulated in the liver. Under normal conditions hepatic glucose uptake and glycolysis are enhanced during the active phase, corresponding with high *Slc2a2* and *Pklr* expression at ZT13/19 in our control animals. There was an emphasis on gluconeogenesis in the late part of the rest period at ZT7 and ZT13, indicated by high *Slc16a7* and *Aqp9* (substrate uptake), high *Pcx* (conversion of pyruvate to oxaloacetate), high *Gpd2* and *Gyk* (glycerol de novo biosynthesis), and low *PDK4* mRNA levels (inhibition of glycolysis). TSR resulted in most of these genes being reduced, in some cases remaining at basal expression levels throughout the day, indicating profound changes to diurnal carbohydrate utilization (Figure 4). Downregulation of hepatic *Scl2a2* has been previously reported in mice with genetic liver-specific clock disruption (*L-Bmal1$^{-/-}$*) [18], which supports our hypothesis that alterations in liver clock regulation may underlie the molecular perturbations brought about by TSR. Molecular disruption could also be correlated with physiology, with TSR mice displaying severely retarded gluconeogenic potential as measured using a pyruvate tolerance test (PTT). This phenotype was observed previously in *Clock$^{Δ19}$* and *Bmal1$^{-/-}$* mice, suggesting a direct effect of the circadian clock on this process [21]. Liver-specific *L-Foxo1$^{-/-}$* mice similarly display reduced hepatic glucose production [31], [32].

Circulating glycerol, a product of lipolysis and a substrate for gluconeogenesis, was high directly after the sleep restriction period (ZT7) following TSR (Figure 1), suggesting increased energy demands at this time, further emphasized by the impaired utilization of glycerol by the liver. Hepatic glycogen storage was increased at the beginning of the nocturnal active period (ZT13) following TSR. In the absence of gluconeogenic potential, despite adequate substrate availability, more emphasis is placed on glycogen. Once glycogen stores are depleted under resting, i.e. fasting, conditions (light phase), in the absence of efficient gluconeogenesis, increased food intake would be necessary to meet glucose demands. In TSR mice leptin is decreased at this time, relieving normal appetite suppression and coinciding with increased food consumption (Figure 1). Under sustained shiftwork conditions this would presumably promote hyperphagy [12]. In human shift workers – who, unlike rodents, have access to a range of food options – abnormal eating behavior with an increased tendency to consume high caloric carbohydrate-rich foods is reported [33]–[37]. In summary, the observed metabolic effects in TSR mice suggest a desynchronization of hepatic energy utilization, which under control conditions should employ glycogen breakdown at the beginning of the resting phase and move to gluconeogenesis when glycogen stores are depleted towards the end of the resting phase. In TSR glucose utilization from liver stores is altered and may promote carbohydrate craving and increased food intake during normal rest hours.

### 4.3.4 PERIPHERAL CLOCK DISRUPTION PRECEDES METABOLIC DISORDERS

Collectively, the observed molecular disruption seen in the liver can be directly correlated to changes in physiology. However, given the short duration of the model used, the full-blown metabolic phenotype characterized by obesity, insulin and leptin resistance seen in more chronic models of sleep restriction and in human shiftwork were not observed. Similarly for rodents, in which 4 weeks of night work results in hyperphagy and obesity, after only 2 weeks the effects on food intake are still relatively mild [12]. Therefore it may be concluded that TSR-induced clock disruption precedes metabolic pathophysiology. This is reminiscent of findings in leptin-deficient ob/ob mice, showing that circadian disruption precedes the development of obesity in these animals [38]. Additionally, clock disruption in humans can confound the effects of shiftwork. In a recent study by Gamble et al., it was shown that clock gene polymorphisms in nurses were correlated with adverse adaptation to shiftwork, culminating in increased alcohol and caffeine consumption and the likelihood to doze [39]. This scenario could be extended to rotating shiftwork conditions, which would presumably lead to chronic circadian desynchrony, and result in the most severe pathophysiology [40], [41]. These findings strongly support a causal role of clock desynchrony on metabolism following sleep disruption.

## 4.3.5 PERIPHERAL CLOCK RESTORATION PREVENTS METABOLIC TSR EFFECTS

In order to strengthen the link between the circadian clock and shiftwork-induced metabolic effects, a regime of normocaloric dark phase restricted feeding was employed concurrent to TSR to stabilize the peripheral clock machinery. Dark phase restricted feeding has been shown previously to reset clock gene rhythms in subsidiary oscillators, but not the SCN master clock [15], [28]. Further, Dark phase feeding stabilizes body temperature and glucose rhythms in a model of night work in rats [12]. Indeed, Dark phase feeding ameliorated the effects of TSR on clock gene rhythms in the liver (Figure 6). Concurrently, disrupted triglyceride, glycerol and corticosterone rhythms were rescued, as was gluconeogenic potential. Together, these findings suggest that TSR-induced metabolic resetting is a result of clock perturbation, and altered feeding patterns might, at least in part, underlie this phenomenon. Adverse effects of dark phase eating have been reported in studies of shift workers, resulting in decreased glucose and lipid tolerance [42]–[44]. However, merely enforcing an altered food consumption schedule to mimic that seen during TSR did not result in compromised gluconeogenic potential (Figure 6). Collectively these data suggest that alterations in feeding rhythmicity observed during TSR may promote, but are not sufficient to explain the metabolic pathophysiology of shiftwork. Nevertheless, imposing a strict dark phase feeding rhythm can be employed to reset peripheral clocks and alleviate metabolic perturbations.

## 4.3.6 CONCLUSION

This study examines the early effects of extended timed sleep restriction as an experimental model of shiftwork on behavior, physiology and transcriptional regulation, with an emphasis on the circadian aspects of metabolism. While it is clear that causal interpretations from studies on complex interacting processes such as diurnal activities, feeding, sleep, metabolism, and circadian mechanisms are always limited, our liver transcriptome analyses indicate a direct effect of sleep timing on the molecular circadian machinery and on clock controlled genes involved in carbohydrate and lipid utilization. Importantly, disruption to circadian gene rhythmicity appears early compared to the adverse metabolic disturbances seen with chronic shiftwork in both rodents and humans, suggesting a causal role of clock disruption in the progression of shiftwork-induced metabolic syndrome. Resetting peripheral circadian clocks by nighttime feeding rescues physiological parameters altered during timed sleep restriction, implying that peripheral clocks may be attractive therapeutic targets for combating the metabolic effects of shiftwork.

## 4.4 MATERIALS AND METHODS

### 4.4.1 ANIMALS

Male C67Bl6/J mice, 10–14 weeks old, were entrained to a 12 h (50 lux) light: 12 h dark (LD) schedule with lights on (ZT0) at 7:00am. Activity measurements were recorded using custom-made infra-red detectors fitted to the roof of the cages and analyzed using ClockLab software (Actimetrics, Evanston, IL). Mice were housed in groups of 3–6 animals per cage, and kept under constant temperature (20.0+/−0.5°C) and humidity (50–60%) conditions with ad libitum access to standard chow (Ssniff V1126, Soest, Germany) and water. All animal experiments were approved by the Office for Consumer Protection and Food Safety (LAVES) of the State of Lower Saxony and executed in accordance with the German Law on Animal Welfare.

### 4.4.2 TIMED SLEEP RESTRICTION (TSR) AND FEEDING SCHEDULES

During TSR mice were kept awake using a gentle handling method between ZT0 and ZT6 from Days 1 to 5, and Days 8 to 12 [23]. Briefly, animals were constantly watched and novel objects were introduced into the cages to induce alertness only when mice assumed a position suggestive of intended sleep. At all other times mice were able to sleep ad libitum. Control mice were kept under the same conditions in separate compartments, without intervention. Starting in the evening of Day 11, control and TSR mice were sacrificed by cervical dislocation at 6 hour intervals. In the dark phase, a 5 W safety red light was used to avoid light effects. Plasma, liver, epididymal adipose (WAT) and brains were collected and frozen. In the case of TSR with high light intensity, 500 lux light was used in the same LD schedule. In the case of TSR with dark phase restricted feeding (DF-TSR), food was removed from the cages at ZT0 (7:00am) on each day and replaced at ZT12 (7:00pm) on each day. In the case of altered food rhythmicity in control mice, mice were provided with 1.6 g of food at the start of the light/inactive phase and 2.2 g of food at the start of the dark/active phase. Each time food was given, any remaining uneaten food was removed to prevent hoarding.

### 4.4.3 PYRUVATE TOLERANCE TESTING

Pyruvate tolerance tests were performed in the week prior to TSR, and on Day 12 of TSR. Mice were starved for 13 h overnight, and injected with 2 g/kg pyruvate i.p. at ZT1. Glucose measurements were taken from tail vein blood at indicated time points.

### 4.4.4 PLASMA ANALYSIS

Leptin was determined using the Mouse Leptin ELISA Kit (Crystal Chem, Downers Grove, IL), and insulin was determined using the Ultrasensitive Mouse Insulin ELISA (Mercodia, Uppsala, Sweden). Circulating glycerol and triglycerides were determined using the Serum Triglyceride Determination Kit (Sigma, St. Louis, MO), and glycogen was determined using anthrone reagent as described previously [45]. Corticosterone was measured from plasma samples using the ImmuChem Double Antibody 125I-Radioimmunoassay Kit (MP Biomedicals, Solon, OH).

## 4.4.5 IN SITU HYBRIDIZATION

In situ hybridization using digoxigenin or [35]S-labeled probes on frozen sections was performed as described [46]. Probe details are available on request.

## 4.4.6 QUANTITATIVE REAL-TIME PCR (QPCR)

Relative quantification of mRNA levels by qPCR was done as previously described [47]. Total RNA was extracted using Trizol reagent (Invitrogen, Carlsbad, CA), and cleaned of genomic DNA contamination using TURBO DNase (Ambion, Austin, TX) as per manufacturer's instructions. cDNA synthesis was performed using Superscript III (Invitrogen) and random hexamer primers, and qPCR was performed using iQ SYBR Green Supermix (Bio-Rad, Hercules, CA) on an Bio-Rad C1000 Thermal Cycler and a CFX96 Real-Time system (95°C for 3 min, 40 cycles at 94°C for 15 sec, 60°C for 15 sec and 72°C for 20 sec, 95°C 10 sec, then 95°C for 10 sec followed by a melt curve from 65°C to 95°C at 0.5°C increments for 5 sec) Primer sequences are available on request. Eef1a was used as a reference gene, and data was expressed as relative quantitation ($\Delta\Delta$-CT method).

## 4.4.7 LIVER SLICE CULTURE AND LUCIFERASE MEASUREMENTS

Control and TSR heterozygous PER2::LUC (n = 6) [48] animals were scarified at ZT6 and 300 µm vibratome slices were prepared from agarose embedded liver lobes and cultured on Millicell culture membranes (PIC-MORG50, Millipore, Billerica, MA) in DMEM medium (high glucose, w/o L-glutamine), supplemented with 10 mM Hepes (pH 7.2), 2% B27, 25 units/ml penicillin, 25 µg/ml streptomycin, 352.5 mg/ml sodium carbonate, 2 mM L-glutamine and 0.1 mM luciferin (all from Invitrogen) in a Lumicycle luminometer (Actimetrics). For each animal 3 liver sections were analyzed.

## 4.4.8 MICROARRAY ANALYSIS

Microarray experiments using liver and adipose tissue total RNA preparations were performed at the Transcriptome Analysis Lab (TAL) of the University of Göttingen, Germany. cRNA samples were hybridized to Mo-Gene ST1.0 gene expression arrays (Affimetrix, Santa Clara, CA). Three chips per time point, condition and tissue were used. Gene expression was normalized using d-Chip Software [49] and rhythmic gene expression and expression phases were determined using CircWave Software (University of Groningen, The Netherlands) as described [50]. Rhythmic genes were grouped and heat maps were generated using d-Chip Software [49]. These sequence data have been submitted to the GEO databases under accession number GSE33381. Gene ontology analysis was performed using DAVID (NIAID, NIH) [51], [52].

## 4.4.9 STATISTICAL ANALYSIS

Unless otherwise noted in the figure legend, all data are shown as mean +/− SEM. Statistical comparisons were performed using GraphPad Prism software (GraphPad, La Jolla, CA) for single gene expression profiles and physiological parameters or using the Bioconductor/R software package [53] for comparing multiple data sets from the microarray experiments. T-tests, one-way or two-way ANOVA with Bonferroni post-hoc test were used to compare single transcript profiles or physiological parameters. For large scale multiple comparisons two-tailed t-tests with Benjamini-Hochberg corrections were used [54]. P-values below 0.05 were considered significant.

## REFERENCES

1. Baron KG, Reid KJ, Kern AS, Zee PC (2011) Role of Sleep Timing in Caloric Intake and BMI. Obesity 19: 1374–1381.
2. Karlsson B, Knutsson A, Lindahl B (2001) Is there an association between shift work and having a metabolic syndrome? Results from a population based study of 27,485 people. Occup Environ Med 58: 747–752.

3.  Fonken LK, Workman JL, Walton JC, Weil ZM, Morris JS, et al. (2010) Light at night increases body mass by shifting the time of food intake. Proceedings of the National Academy of Sciences 107: 18664–18669.
4.  Li Y, Sato Y, Yamaguchi N (2011) Shift work and the risk of metabolic syndrome: a nested case-control study. Int J Occup Environ Health 17: 154–160.
5.  Garaulet M, Ortega FB, Ruiz JR, Rey-Lopez JP, Beghin L, et al. (2011) Short sleep duration is associated with increased obesity markers in European adolescents: effect of physical activity and dietary habits. The HELENA study. Int J Obes.
6.  Rehman J-u, Brismar K, Holmbäck U, Åkerstedt T, Axelsson J (2010) Sleeping during the day: effects on the 24-h patterns of IGF-binding protein 1, insulin, glucose, cortisol, and growth hormone. European Journal of Endocrinology 163: 383–390.
7.  Arendt J (2010) Shift work: coping with the biological clock. Occupational Medicine 60: 10–20.
8.  Wu H, Zhao Z, Stone WS, Huang L, Zhuang J, et al. (2008) Effects of sleep restriction periods on serum cortisol levels in healthy men. Brain Research Bulletin 77: 241–245.
9.  Crispim CA, Waterhouse J, Damaso AR, Zimberg IZ, Padilha HG, et al. (2011) Hormonal appetite control is altered by shift work: a preliminary study. Metabolism 60: 1726–1735.
10. Van Cauter E, Knutson KL (2008) Sleep and the epidemic of obesity in children and adults. Eur J Endocrinol 159: S59–66.
11. Korkmaz A, Topal T, Tan D-X, Reiter R (2009) Role of melatonin in metabolic regulation. Reviews in Endocrine & Metabolic Disorders 10: 261–270.
12. Salgado-Delgado R, Angeles-Castellanos M, Saderi N, Buijs RM, Escobar C (2010) Food Intake during the Normal Activity Phase Prevents Obesity and Circadian Desynchrony in a Rat Model of Night Work. Endocrinology 151: 1019–1029.
13. Salgado-Delgado R, Nadia S, Angeles-Castellanos M, Buijs RM, Escobar C (2010) In a Rat Model of Night Work, Activity during the Normal Resting Phase Produces Desynchrony in the Hypothalamus. Journal of Biological Rhythms 25: 421–431.
14. Bass J, Takahashi JS (2010) Circadian Integration of Metabolism and Energetics. Science 330: 1349–1354.
15. Damiola F, Le Minh N, Preitner N, Kornmann B, Fleury-Olela F, et al. (2000) Restricted feeding uncouples circadian oscillators in peripheral tissues from the central pacemaker in the suprachiasmatic nucleus. Genes Dev 14: 2950–2961.
16. Takahashi JS, Hong H-K, Ko CH, McDearmon EL (2008) The genetics of mammalian circadian order and disorder: implications for physiology and disease. Nat Rev Genet 9: 764–775.
17. Panda S, Antoch MP, Miller BH, Su AI, Schook AB, et al. (2002) Coordinated Transcription of Key Pathways in the Mouse by the Circadian Clock. Cell 109: 307–320.
18. Lamia KA, Storch KF, Weitz CJ (2008) Physiological significance of a peripheral tissue circadian clock. Proc Natl Acad Sci U S A 105: 15172–15177.
19. Rudic R, McNamara P, Curtis A, Boston R, Panda S, et al. (2004) BMAL1 and CLOCK, two essential components of the circadian clock, are involved in glucose homeostasis. PLoS Biol 2: e377.
20. Turek FW, Joshu C, Kohsaka A, Lin E, Ivanova G, et al. (2005) Obesity and Metabolic Syndrome in Circadian Clock Mutant Mice. Science 308: 1043–1045.

21. Rudic RD, McNamara P, Curtis A-M, Boston RC, Panda S, et al. (2004) BMAL1 and CLOCK, Two Essential Components of the Circadian Clock, Are Involved in Glucose Homeostasis. PLoS Biol 2: e377.

22. Yang S, Liu A, Weidenhammer A, Cooksey RC, McClain D, et al. (2009) The Role of mPer2 Clock Gene in Glucocorticoid and Feeding Rhythms. Endocrinology 150: 2153–2160.

23. Tobler I, Borbely A, Groos G (1983) The effect of sleep deprivation on sleep in rats with suprachiasmatic lesions. Neurosci Lett 42: 49–54.

24. Hasan S, Dauvilliers Y, Mongrain V, Franken P, Tafti M (2012) Age-related changes in sleep in inbred mice are genotype dependent. Neurobiol Aging 33: 195 e113–126:

25. Mrosovsky N (1999) Masking: History, Definitions, and Measurement. Chronobiology International 16: 415–429.

26. Arble DM, Bass J, Laposky AD, Vitaterna MH, Turek FW (2009) Circadian timing of food intake contributes to weight gain. Obesity (Silver Spring) 17: 2100–2102.

27. Folkard S (2008) Do Permanent Night Workers Show Circadian Adjustment? A Review Based on the Endogenous Melatonin Rhythm. Chronobiology International 25: 215–224.

28. Vollmers C, Gill S, DiTacchio L, Pulivarthy SR, Le HD, et al. (2009) Time of feeding and the intrinsic circadian clock drive rhythms in hepatic gene expression. Proc Natl Acad Sci U S A 106: 21453–21458.

29. Yamanaka Y, Honma S, Honma K-I (2008) Scheduled exposures to a novel environment with a running-wheel differentially accelerate re-entrainment of mice peripheral clocks to new light–dark cycles. Genes to Cells 13: 497–507.

30. Maret S, Dorsaz S, Gurcel L, Pradervand S, Petit B, et al. (2007) Homer1a is a core brain molecular correlate of sleep loss. Proceedings of the National Academy of Sciences 104: 20090–20095.

31. Puigserver P, Rhee J, Donovan J, Walkey CJ, Yoon JC, et al. (2003) Insulin-regulated hepatic gluconeogenesis through FOXO1-PGC-1[alpha] interaction. Nature 423: 550–555.

32. Haeusler RA, Kaestner KH, Accili D (2010) FoxOs Function Synergistically to Promote Glucose Production. Journal of Biological Chemistry 285: 35245–35248.

33. Persson M, MÅRtensson J (2006) Situations influencing habits in diet and exercise among nurses working night shift. Journal of Nursing Management 14: 414–423.

34. Wong H, Wong MCS, Wong SYS, Lee A (2010) The association between shift duty and abnormal eating behavior among nurses working in a major hospital: A cross-sectional study. International Journal of Nursing Studies 47: 1021–1027.

35. Morikawa Y, Miura K, Sasaki S, Yoshita K, Yoneyama S, et al. (2008) Evaluation of the Effects of Shift Work on Nutrient Intake: A Cross-sectional Study. Journal of Occupational Health 50: 270–278.

36. Di Lorenzo L, De Pergola G, Zocchetti C, L'Abbate N, Basso A, et al. (2003) Effect of shift work on body mass index: results of a study performed in 319 glucose-tolerant men working in a Southern Italian industry. Int J Obes Relat Metab Disord 27: 1353–1358.

37. Spiegel K, Tasali E, Penev P, Van Cauter E (2004) Brief communication: Sleep curtailment in healthy young men is associated with decreased leptin levels, elevated

ghrelin levels, and increased hunger and appetite. Annals of Internal Medicine 141: 846–850.

38. Ando H, Kumazaki M, Motosugi Y, Ushijima K, Maekawa T, et al. (2011) Impairment of Peripheral Circadian Clocks Precedes Metabolic Abnormalities in ob/ob Mice. Endocrinology 152: 1347–1354.

39. Gamble KL, Motsinger-Reif AA, Hida A, Borsetti HM, Servick SV, et al. (2011) Shift Work in Nurses: Contribution of Phenotypes and Genotypes to Adaptation. PLoS ONE 6: e18395.

40. Sookoian S, Gemma C, Fernández Gianotti T, Burgueño A, Alvarez A, et al. (2007) Effects of rotating shift work on biomarkers of metabolic syndrome and inflammation. Journal of Internal Medicine 261: 285–292.

41. Gibbs M, Hampton S, Morgan L, Arendt J (2007) Predicting Circadian Response to Abrupt Phase Shift: 6-Sulphatoxymelatonin Rhythms in Rotating Shift Workers Offshore. Journal of Biological Rhythms 22: 368–370.

42. Al-Naimi S, Hampton SM, Richard P, Tzung C, Morgan LM (2004) Postprandial Metabolic Profiles Following Meals and Snacks Eaten during Simulated Night and Day Shift Work. Chronobiology International 21: 937–947.

43. Lund J, Arendt J, Hampton S, English J, Morgan L (2001) Postprandial hormone and metabolic responses amongst shift workers in Antarctica. Journal of Endocrinology 171: 557–564.

44. Ribeiro D, Hampton S, Morgan L, Deacon S, Arendt J (1998) Altered postprandial hormone and metabolic responses in a simulated shift work environment. Journal of Endocrinology 158: 305–310.

45. Roe JH, Dailey RE (1966) Determination of glycogen with the anthrone reagent. Analytical Biochemistry 15: 245–250.

46. Oster H, Baeriswyl S, van der Horst GTJ, Albrecht U (2003) Loss of circadian rhythmicity in aging mPer1−/− mCry2−/− mutant mice. Genes & Development 17: 1366–1379.

47. Oster H, Damerow S, Kiessling S, Jakubcakova V, Abraham D, et al. (2006) The circadian rhythm of glucocorticoids is regulated by a gating mechanism residing in the adrenal cortical clock. Cell Metabolism 4: 163–173.

48. Yoo S, Yamazaki S, Lowrey P, Shimomura K, Ko C, et al. (2004) PERIOD2::LUCIFERASE real-time reporting of circadian dynamics reveals persistent circadian oscillations in mouse peripheral tissues. Proc Natl Acad Sci USA 101: 5339–5346.

49. Li C, Wong WH (2001) Model-based analysis of oligonucleotide arrays: Expression index computation and outlier detection. Proceedings of the National Academy of Sciences 98: 31–36.

50. Oster H, Damerow S, Hut RA, Eichele G (2006) Transcriptional Profiling in the Adrenal Gland Reveals Circadian Regulation of Hormone Biosynthesis Genes and Nucleosome Assembly Genes. Journal of Biological Rhythms 21: 350–361.

51. Huang DW, Sherman BT, Lempicki RA (2009) Bioinformatics enrichment tools: paths toward the comprehensive functional analysis of large gene lists. Nucleic Acids Research 37: 1–13.

52. Huang DW, Sherman BT, Lempicki RA (2008) Systematic and integrative analysis of large gene lists using DAVID bioinformatics resources. Nat Protocols 4: 44–57.

53. Gentleman R, Carey V, Bates D, Bolstad B, Dettling M, et al. (2004) Bioconductor: open software development for computational biology and bioinformatics. Genome Biology 5: R80.
54. Hochberg Y, Benjamini Y (1990) More powerful procedures for multiple significance testing. Statistics in Medicine 9: 811–818.

*There are several supplemental files that are not available in this version of the article. To view this additional information, please use the citation information cited on the first page of this chapter.*

# CHAPTER 5

# CIRCADIAN RHYTHMS AND OBESITY IN MAMMALS

OREN FROY

## 5.1 INTRODUCTION

Obesity has become a serious and growing public health problem [1]. Attempts to develop new therapeutic strategies have mostly focused on energy expenditure and caloric intake. Recent studies link energy homeostasis to the circadian clock at the behavioral, physiological, and molecular levels [2–5], emphasizing that certain nutrients and the timing of food intake may play a significant role in weight gain [6]. Therefore, it is plausible that resetting of the circadian clock can be used as a new approach to attenuate obesity.

## 5.2 CIRCADIAN RHYTHMS

Our planet revolves around its axis causing light and dark cycles of 24 hours. Organisms on our planet evolved to predict these cycles by developing an endogenous circadian (circa: about and dies: day) clock, which is synchronized to external time cues. This way, organisms ensure that physi-

*This chapter was originally published under the Creative Commons Attribution License. Froy O. Circadian Rhythms and Obesity in Mammals. ISRN Obesity 2012, (2012). http://dx.doi. org/10.5402/2012/437198.*

ological processes are carried out at the right time of the circadian cycle [7]. All aspects of physiology, including sleep-wake cycles, cardiovascular activity, endocrine system, body temperature, renal activity, gastrointestinal tract motility, and metabolism, are influenced by the circadian clock [7, 8]. Indeed, 10–20% of all cellular transcripts are cyclically expressed, most of which are tissue-specific [2, 9–13].

## 5.3 THE CIRCADIAN CLOCK

The central circadian clock is located in the suprachiasmatic nuclei (SCN) of the brain anterior hypothalamus. The SCN clock is composed of multiple, single-cell oscillators synchronized to generate circadian rhythms [8, 14–16]. The endogenous period of the SCN oscillation is approximately, but not exactly, 24 h. Therefore, it requires resetting each day to the external light-dark cycle to prevent drifting out of phase. Light is a strong synchronizer for the brain clock, perceived by the retina and transmitted via the retinohypothalamic tract (RHT) to the SCN [17–19]. Similar clocks are found in peripheral tissues, such as the liver, intestine, and retina [20–22] (Figure 1). Complete destruction of the SCN abolishes circadian rhythmicity in the periphery leading to arrhythmicity [23, 24]. The SCN transmits the information to peripheral oscillators to prevent the dampening of circadian rhythms via neuronal connections or circulating factors. In turn, SCN rhythms can be altered by neuronal and endocrine inputs [25].

## 5.4 PHYSIOLOGICAL EFFECTS OF RESET VERSUS DISRUPTED CIRCADIAN RHYTHMS

Disruption of circadian rhythms has negative effects on physiology. Certain pathologies, such as myocardial infarction, pulmonary edema, hypertensive crises, and asthma and allergic attacks, peak at certain times during the circadian cycle [26–28]. These findings emphasize the prominent influence of the circadian clock on human physiology and pathophysiology [8]. Living in a Western society requires us to extend wakefulness or repeatedly invert the normal sleep-wake cycle, for example, during shift work or transmeridian flights. These usually cause fatigue, disorientation, insomnia, altered nighttime melatonin levels, and hormone-related diseases [29]. Sleep disorders are also associated with impaired functioning of the central circadian clock exacerbating the disruption [8]. Disruption of circadian coordination has also been found to accelerate cancer proneness, malignant growth, and tumor progression [29–31]. Recently, the circadian clock has been linked to energy homeostasis and its disruption leads to metabolic disorders (see below). Thus, disruption of circadian coordination leads to hormone imbalance, sleep disorders, cancer proneness, and reduced life span [8, 29–33], whereas reset circadian rhythms leads to improved health and increased longevity [34–36]. Indeed, longevity in hamsters is decreased with rhythmicity disruption and is increased in old animals given fetal brain implants that restore robust rhythms [34]. Circadian rhythms also change dramatically with the age, including a shift in the phase and decrease in amplitude [20, 37–39].

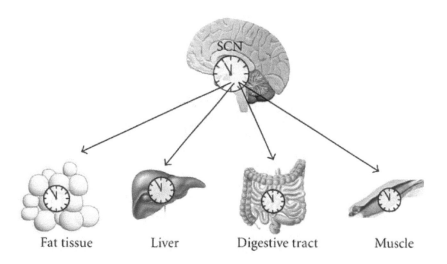

Fat tissue    Liver    Digestive tract    Muscle

**FIGURE 1:** Effect of the SCN clock on peripheral clocks. The suprachiasmatic (SCN) clock resets signals in peripheral tissues, such as muscle, fat tissue, digestive tract, and liver.

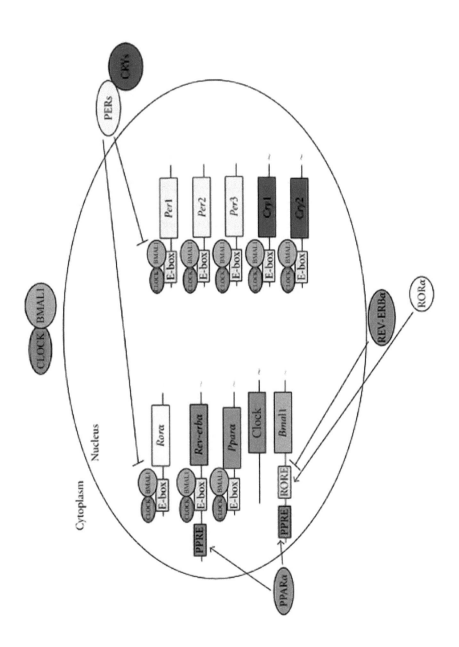

**FIGURE 2:** The core mechanism of the mammalian circadian clock and its link to energy metabolism. The cellular oscillator is composed of a positive limb (CLOCK and BMAL1) and a negative limb (CRYs and PERs). CLOCK and BMAL1 dimerize in the cytoplasm and translocate to the nucleus. The CLOCK:BMAL1 heterodimer then binds to enhancer (E-box) sequences located in the promoter region of Per and Cry genes, activating their transcription. After translation, PERs and CRYs undergo nuclear translocation and inhibit CLOCK:BMAL1, resulting in decreased transcription of their own genes. CLOCK:BMAL1 heterodimer also induces the transcription of *Rev-erbα* and *Rora*. RORα and REV-ERBα regulate lipid metabolism and adipogenesis, and also participate in the regulation of *Bmal1* expression. RORα stimulates and REV-ERBα inhibits *Bmal1* transcription, acting through RORE. CLOCK:BMAL1 heterodimer also mediates the transcription of *Ppara*, a nuclear receptor involved in glucose and lipid metabolism. PPARα activates transcription of *Rev-erbα* by binding to a peroxisome proliferator-response element (PPRE). PPARα also induces *Bmal1* expression, acting through PPRE located in its promoter.

## 5.5 THE MOLECULAR CLOCK

The circadian clock is a cellular mechanism of gene transcription, translation, and posttranslational modifications [40]. The mechanism itself exists in both the central clock and peripheral tissues. In all tissues, generation of circadian rhythms requires the coexpression of specific clock genes. The mechanism includes several key players. The transcription factor CLOCK dimerizes with BMAL1 to activate transcription upon binding to E-box (5'-CACGTG-3') promoter elements [11]. CLOCK:BMAL1 heterodimer mediates transcription of a large number of genes including Pers and Crys. The PERIOD proteins (PER1, PER2, and PER3) and the two CRYPTOCHROMEs (CRY1 and CRY2) operate as negative regulators [41–43]. When PERs and CRYs are produced, they oligomerize, translocate to the nucleus, and inhibit CLOCK:BMAL1-mediated transcription (Figure 2). In addition, casein kinase I epsilon(CKIε) phosphorylates the PER proteins and, thereby, enhances their instability and degradation [44–46]. CKIε also phosphorylates and partially activates BMAL1 [47].

## 5.6 THE CIRCADIAN CLOCK AND METABOLIC HOMEOSTASIS

The circadian clock regulates metabolism and energy homeostasis in peripheral tissues [2, 48]. The expression and/or activity of certain enzymes and transport systems [49, 50] involved in the various metabolic pathways, such as cholesterol metabolism, amino acid regulation, drug and toxin metabolism, the citric acid cycle, and glycogen and glucose metabolism, exhibit circadian expression [2, 48, 51–54]. Similarly, glucose uptake and adenosine triphosphate (ATP) concentrations exhibit circadian fluctuations in brain and peripheral tissues [52, 55, 56]. Indeed, lesions of rat SCN clock abolishes daily changes in glucose homeostasis [57], altering rhythms in glucose utilization rates and hepatic glucose production. This is because the SCN projects to the preautonomic paraventricular nucleus (PVN) neurons that control hepatic glucose production [55].

One of the key tissues that regulate metabolism is the adipose tissue. Circadian clocks have been shown to be present in white and brown adipose tissues [58, 59]. Adipose tissue secretes metabolic mediators, such as adiponectin, resistin, visfatin, and leptin that are clock controlled [60]. In addition, key metabolic factors in adipocytes exhibit diurnal variations in expression [61]. In addition, many hormones that regulate metabolism, such as insulin [53], glucagon [62], adiponectin [60], corticosterone [63], leptin, and ghrelin [64, 65], exhibit circadian oscillation. Leptin, secreted from adipose tissue, plays an important role in appetite suppression in the brain. Plasma leptin levels are circadian with leptin peaking early in the nonactive phase, that is during the early dark phase in diurnal animals, such as monkeys and humans [66, 67], and during the early to mid-light phase in nocturnal animals, such as rats and mice [68, 69]. Neither feeding time nor adrenalectomy affects the rhythmicity of leptin release. However, ablation of the SCN eliminates leptin circadian rhythmicity in rodents, suggesting that the central circadian clock regulates leptin expression [68]. Leptin receptors are present on SCN neurons [70–72], suggesting that leptin binds directly to SCN neurons. It seems that leptin may affect the central circadian clock directly via its receptors on SCN neurons and/ or through its effect on the arcuate nucleus (ARC), a region nearby the

SCN involved in appetite regulation. These findings place leptin as a major bridge linking energy homeostasis and circadian control.

## 5.7 CIRCADIAN RHYTHMS OF HORMONE AND METABOLIC DISORDERS

### 5.7.1 INSULIN

Daily oscillation of insulin secretion and glucose tolerance are lost in patients with type 2 diabetes [73, 74], as are daily variations in plasma corticosterone levels and locomotor activity in streptozotocin-induced diabetic rats [75, 76]. These results suggest that loss of circadian rhythmicity of glucose metabolism may contribute to the development of metabolic disorders, such as type 2 diabetes [74–78].

### 5.7.2 LEPTIN

In obese subjects, leptin retains diurnal variation in release, but with lower amplitude [79, 80]. Circadian patterns of leptin concentration were distinctly different between adult women with upper-body or lower-body obesity, with a delay in peak values of leptin of approximately 3 h in women with upper-body obesity [81].

### 5.7.3 ADIPONECTIN

The rhythmic expression of resistin and adiponectin, two cytokines secreted from adipose tissue, was greatly blunted in obese (KK) and obese, diabetic (KK-Ay) mice [60]. In humans, circulating adiponectin levels exhibit both ultradian pulsatility and a diurnal variation. The expression of many adipokines is blunted in obese patients [68, 82, 83]. In obese subjects, adiponectin levels were significantly lower than lean controls, although the obese group had significantly higher average peak of secretion [84].

## 5.8 MUTUAL REGULATION OF KEY METABOLIC FACTORS AND CLOCK MECHANISM

### 5.8.1 BMAL1

Recent molecular studies established the involvement of the activity of the positive circadian transcription factor BMAL1 in the control of adipogenesis and lipid metabolism in mature adipocytes via Wnt signaling pathway [85, 86]. Embryonic fibroblasts from *Bmal1*$^{-/-}$ knockout mice failed to differentiate into adipocytes. Loss of BMAL1 expression led to a significant decrease in adipogenesis and gene expression of several key adipogenic/lipogenic factors. *Bmal1*$^{-/-}$ mice exhibited a metabolic syndrome-like onset, that is, elevation of the level of circulating fatty acids, including triglycerides, free fatty acids, and low-density lipoprotein (LDL)-cholesterol. In addition, ectopic fat formation was observed in the liver and skeletal muscle. This could be due to loss of the functions of adipose tissue, since ectopic fat formation was not observed in tissue-specific *Bmal1*$^{-/-}$ mice even under high fat diet [87]. Furthermore, overexpression of BMAL1 in adipocytes increased lipid synthesis activity. Thus, BMAL1, a master regulator of circadian rhythms, plays important roles in the regulation of adipose differentiation and lipogenesis in mature adipocytes [86]. These findings may explain in part why clock disruption leads to obesity. However, recently it was reported that disruption of *Bmal1*, in mice led to increased adipogenesis, adipocyte hypertrophy, and obesity, compared to wild-type mice. Attenuation of *Bmal1* function resulted in downregulation of genes in the canonical Wnt pathway, known to suppress adipogenesis and its overexpression to augmentation [85]. Clearly, BMAL1 plays a role in adipogenesis, however, more studies are merited.

## 5.8.2 REV-ERBS AND RORS

Two other important families of factors that link the circadian clock with lipid metabolism are the REV-ERB and ROR families. REV-ERBs and RORs, which are crucial for adipocyte differentiation [88], lipogenesis and lipid storage exhibit striking circadian rhythm [61, 89]. In addition to their role in lipid metabolism and adipocyte differentiation, REV-ERBs are a negative regulator of *Bmal1* expression [90, 91]. In contrast, retinoic acid-related orphan receptor α (RORα) is a positive regulator of *Bmal1* expression [92, 93]. In addition, the CLOCK:BMAL1 heterodimer regulates the expression of both *Rev-erbα* and *Rorα* [91, 92, 94] (Figure 2). Treatment of diet-induced obese mice with aREV-ERBagonist decreased obesity by reducing fat mass and markedly improving dyslipidaemia and hyperglycaemia [95], suggesting that inhibition of BMAL1 expression is beneficial for obesity (see above).

## 5.8.3 PPARα

Peroxisome proliferator-activated receptor α (PPARα) is a member of the nuclear receptor family. PPARα serves also as a link between metabolism and the circadian clock. PPARα plays a key role in the transcription of genes involved in lipid and glucose metabolism upon binding of endogenous free fatty acids [96, 97]. Its expression is mediated by the CLOCK:BMAL heterodimer. In turn, PPARα binds to the peroxisome-proliferator response element (PPRE) to activate *Bmal1* expression [4, 98, 99]. We recently showed that a PPARα agonist advanced locomotor activity and feeding daily rhythms in mice [100].

## 5.8.4 PPARγ COACTIVATOR (PGC-1α)

PGC-1α, a transcriptional coactivator that regulates energy metabolism, exhibits circadian expression. In turn, PGC-1α stimulates the expression of *Bmal1* and *Rev-erbα*, through coactivation of the ROR family of orphan nuclear receptors [101, 102]. The role of PGC-1α in the circadian system is emphasized by null mice that show abnormal diurnal rhythms of activity, body temperature, and metabolic rate, due to aberrant expression of clock genes and those involved in energy metabolism. Indeed, analyses of PGC-1α-deficient fibroblasts and mice with liver-specific knockdown of PGC-1α indicate that it is required for cell-autonomous clock function [102].

## 5.8.5 AMP-ACTIVATED PROTEIN KINASE (AMPK)

AMPK is a sensor of the energy status within cells, whose activation leads to increased catabolism [103, 104]. AMPK has been found to directly phosphorylate Ser-389 of CKIε, resulting in increased CKIε activity leading to PERs degradation [105]. AMPK also phosphorylates and, as a result, destabilizes CRY1 in mouse fibroblasts [106]. PERs and CRYs degradation causes the relief of CLOCK:BMAL1-mediated expression leading to a phase advance in the circadian expression in some tissues [107]. Recently, it was shown that metformin, an indirect AMPK activator, leads to phase changes in a tissue-specific manner, mainly phase advances in the liver but phase delays in muscle tissue [108]. The major role of AMPK in the core clock mechanism merits further study.

## 5.8.6 SIRT1

Another protein found to link metabolism with the circadian clock is SIRT1, an $NAD^+$-dependent histone deacetylase involved in transcriptional silencing [109, 110]. It was recently found that AMPK modulates $NAD^+$ levels and SIRT1 activity [109]. Nonhistone substrates of SIRT1 include regulatory molecules that modulate energy metabolism, such as PPARγ and PGC-1α [111], key regulators of the core molecular clock (see above). It turns out that SIRT1 interacts directly with CLOCK and deacetylates BMAL1 and PER2 [112, 113] affecting their stability. Deacetylated PER2 is further phosphorylated and degraded relieving the inhibition of

CLOCK:BMAL1 heterodimer. CLOCK:BMAL1 heterodimer also regulates the circadian expression of NAMPT (nicotinamide phosphoribosyltransferase), a rate-limiting enzyme in the $NAD^+$ salvage pathway. SIRT1 is recruited to the *Nampt* promoter and contributes to the circadian synthesis of its own coenzyme [114]. In addition, CLOCK and its homolog NPAS2 can bind efficiently to BMAL1 and consequently to E-box sequences in the presence of NADH and NADPH. On the other hand, $NAD^+$ and $NADP^+$ inhibit DNA binding of CLOCK:BMAL1 or NPAS2:BMAL1 [115, 116]. Thus, the levels of $NAD^+$ together with the cycling of SIRT1 can determine the activity and robustness of clock gene transcription.

## 5.9 CLOCK MUTANTS AND METABOLIC DISORDERS

Although disruption of circadian expression leads to metabolic disorders, the most compelling linkage between metabolic disorders and the circadian clock is demonstrated by the phenotypes of clock gene mutants and knockouts.

### 5.9.1 CLOCK

Mice with a truncated exon 18 and deleted exon 19 of the *Clock* gene (*Clock*$^{Δ19}$ mice) have a greatly attenuated diurnal feeding rhythm, are hyperphagic and obese, and develop a metabolic syndrome of hyperleptinemia, hyperlipidemia, hepatic steatosis, and hyperglycemia [5]. However, some studies found that *Clock* mutant mice have lower serum triglyceride and free fatty acids than wild-type mice [117]. Combination of the *Clock*$^{Δ19}$ mutation with the leptin knockout (*ob/ob*) resulted in significantly heavier mice than the *ob/ob* phenotype [118], reiterating the contribution of clock disruption to the obese phenotype [2, 11, 48].

### 5.9.2 BMAL1

*Bmal1*$^{-/-}$ knockout mice, similarly to *Clock* mutant mice, exhibited suppressed diurnal variations in glucose and triglycerides as well as abolished gluconeogenesis. Although recovery from insulin-induced hypoglycemia was impaired in Clock mutant and Bmal1−/− knockout mice, the counter-regulatory response of corticosterone and glucagon was retained [119].

### 5.9.3 PER2

The diurnal feeding rhythm in *Per2*−/− mice is absent and these mice exhibit no glucocorticoid rhythm even though the corticosterone response to hypoglycemia is intact. Interestingly, although food consumption was similar during the light and dark periods, *Per2*−/− mice fed a high-fat diet developed significant obesity [120].

## 5.10 EFFECT OF RESTRICTED FEEDING (RF) ON CIRCADIAN RHYTHMS

RF limits the time and duration of food availability without calorie reduction, that is, food is provided ad libitum for about 3–5 h at the same time every day, usually at daytime [40, 49, 121, 122]. Rodents on RF, although nocturnal, adjust to the diurnal feeding period within a few days and learn to eat their daily food intake during that limited time [123–125]. Restricting food to a particular time of day has profound effects on the behavior and physiology of animals. Many physiological activities normally dictated by the SCN, such as body temperature, locomotor activity, and heart rate, are altered by RF [126–129]. 2–4 h before the meal, the animals display food anticipatory behavior, which is demonstrated by an increase in locomotor activity, body temperature, corticosterone secretion, gastrointestinal motility, and activity of digestive enzymes [122, 125, 130, 131], all are known output systems of the biological clock. RF is dominant over the SCN and is effective in all lighting conditions including in SCN-lesioned animals [122, 127, 129, 132–134]. RF affects circadian oscillators in peripheral tissues, such as liver, kidney, heart, and pancreas, with no effect on the central pacemaker in the SCN [40, 49, 121, 127, 133, 135, 136]. Thus, RF uncouples the SCN from the periphery, suggesting that nutritional regulation of clock oscillators in peripheral tissues may

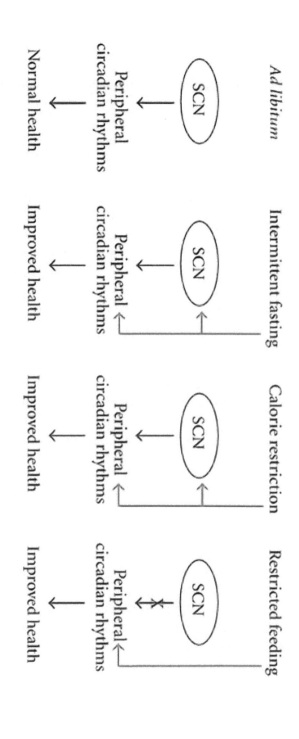

**FIGURE 3:** Effect of feeding regimens on circadian rhythms and health. SCN: suprachiasmatic nuclei.

play a direct role in coordinating metabolic oscillations [137]. As soon as food availability returns to be ad libitum, the SCN clock, whose phase remains unaffected, resets the peripheral oscillators [135]. It has recently been shown that long-term day-time RF can increase the amplitude of clock gene expression, increase expression of catabolic factors, and reduce the levels of disease markers leading to better health [138] (Figure 3). Moreover, timed high-fat diet led to reduced body weight and improved metabolism compared to animals that consumed the same caloric intake spread out throughout the day [139] (see below).

Because timed feeding is dominant in resetting circadian rhythms even in animals with lesioned SCN, it has been suggested that there is a food-entrainable oscillator (FEO). However, the location of this FEO has been elusive. Lesions in brain regions involved in feeding, such as the dorsomedial hypothalamic nucleus (DMH) [140–143], the brain stem parabrachial nuclei (PBN) [140, 144], and the core and shell regions of nucleus accumbens [145, 146], revealed that these nuclei may be involved in FEO output, but they cannot fully account for the oscillation [147]. Neither vagal signals nor leptin are critical for the entrainment [130, 148]. CLOCK [149] or BMAL1 [150] and other clock genes [151] have been shown not to be necessary for food anticipatory activity. However, it has recently been demonstrated that *Per2* mutant mice did not exhibit wheel-running food anticipation [152, 153]. Thus, how RF entrains circadian rhythms remains an extremely important topic for research.

## 5.11 EFFECT OF CALORIE RESTRICTION (CR) ON CIRCADIAN RHYTHMS

CR refers to a dietary regimen low in calories without malnutrition. CR restricts the amount of calories derived from carbohydrates, fats, or proteins to 60–75% of ad libitum-fed animals [154]. It has been documented that calorie restriction significantly extends the life span of rodents by up to 50% [155, 156]. In addition to the increase in life span, CR also delays the occurrence of age-associated pathophysiological changes, such as cancer, diabetes, kidney disease, and cataracts [156–159]. Theories on how

CR modulates aging and longevity abound, but the exact mechanism is still unknown [156]. As opposed to RF, CR entrains the clock in the SCN [160–163], indicating that calorie reduction could affect the central oscillator. CR during the daytime affects the temporal organization of the SCN clockwork and circadian outputs in mice under light/dark cycle. In addition, CR affects responses of the circadian system to light, indicating that energy metabolism modulates gating of photic inputs in mammals [164]. These findings suggest that synchronization of peripheral oscillators during CR could be achieved directly due to the temporal eating, as has been reported for RF [127, 135, 136], or by synchronizing the SCN [160–162], which, in turn, sends humoral or neuronal signals to synchronize the peripheral tissues [107, 165] (Figure 3).

## 5.12 EFFECT OF INTERMITTENT FASTING (IF) ON CIRCADIAN RHYTHMS

During IF, food is available ad libitum every other day. IF-treated mice eat on the days they have access to food approximately twice as much as those having continuous access to food [166, 167]. Similarly to calorically restricted animals, IF-fed animals exhibit increased life span in comparison with the ad libitum-fed control [168] as well as improved glucose metabolism, cardioprotection, neuroprotection [166, 169–173], and increased resistance to cancer [167]. The IF-induced beneficial effects are thought to occur independently of the overall caloric intake, but the underlying mechanisms are still unknown. One suggested mechanism is stimulation of cellular stress pathways induced by the IF regimen [166, 174, 175]. Recently it has been shown that when food was introduced during the light period, mice exhibited almost arrhythmicity in clock gene expression in the liver. Unlike daytime feeding, nighttime feeding yielded rhythms similar to those generated during ad libitum feeding [176]. The fact that IF can affect circadian rhythms differently depending on the timing of food availability suggests that this regimen affects the SCN clock, similarly to CR. SCN resetting by IF and CR could be involved in the health benefits conferred by these regimens [107] (Figure 3).

## 5.13 EFFECT OF HIGH-FAT DIET ON CIRCADIAN RHYTHMS

Few studies show that a high-fat diet leads to minimal effects on the rhythmic expression of clock genes in visceral adipose tissue and liver [177]. However, recent studies have shown that introduction of a high-fat diet to animals leads to rapid changes in both the period of locomotor activity in constant darkness and to increased food intake during the normal rest period under light-dark conditions [178]. These changes in behavioral rhythmicity correlated with disrupted clock gene expression within hypothalamus, liver, and adipose tissue, and as well as with altered cycling of hormones and nuclear hormone receptors involved in fuel utilization, such as leptin, thyroid stimulating hormone (TSH), and testosterone in mice, rats, and humans [178–183]. Furthermore, a high-fat diet modulates carbohydrate metabolism by amplifying circadian variation in glucose tolerance and insulin sensitivity [119].

In addition to the disruption of clock gene expression, high-fat diet induced a phase delay in clock and clock-controlled genes [179, 180]. As mentioned above, AMPK activation leads to CKIε activity, degradation of PERs, and to a phase advance. As the levels of AMPK decline under HF diet [179, 180], it is plausible that the changes seen in the expression phase of genes under HF diet are mediated by changes in AMPK levels. In addition to its effect on gene expression, high-fat feeding led to impaired adjustment to local time by light resetting, including slower rate of reentrainment of behavioral and body temperature rhythms after "jet-lag" tests (6 h advanced light-dark cycle) and reduced phase-advance responses to light. These results correlated with reduction in c-FOS and phosphor-ERK expression in the SCN in response to light-induced phase shifts [184].

Recently, it was shown that timed high-fat diet can prevent obesity [139, 185]. Timed HF diet led to decreased body weight, cholesterol and TNFα levels and improved insulin sensitivity compared with mice fed HF diet ad libitum. Timed HF-fed mice exhibited a better satiated and less stressed phenotype of low ghrelin and corticosterone compared with mice fed timed low-fat diet [139]. In addition, timed HF diet improved metabolic pathway function and oscillations of the circadianclockand their target gene expression. These changes in catabolic and anabolic pathways altered liver metabolome and improved nutrient utilization and energy expenditure [185]. Altogether, these findings suggest that timing can prevent obesity and rectify the harmful effects of HF diet.

## 5.14 CONCLUSION

1. Western lifestyle leads to high food consumption, inactivity during the active period, enhanced activity in the rest period, and shortened sleep period.
2. Disrupted biological rhythms might lead to attenuated circadian feeding rhythms, disrupted metabolism, cancer proneness, and reduced life expectancy.
3. Resetting the biological clock by food or feeding time may lead to better functionality of physiological systems, preventing metabolic disorders, promoting well being, and extending life span.
4. Feeding time has the ability to reset bodily rhythms.

## REFERENCES

1. S. B. Wyatt, K. P. Winters, and P. M. Dubbert, "Overweight and obesity: prevalence, consequences, and causes of a growing public health problem," American Journal of the Medical Sciences, vol. 331, no. 4, pp. 166–174, 2006.
2. O. Froy, "Metabolism and circadian rhythms—implications for obesity," Endocrine Reviews, vol. 31, no. 1, pp. 1–24, 2010.
3. B. Marcheva, K. M. Ramsey, E. D. Buhr et al., "Disruption of the clock components CLOCK and BMAL1 leads to hypoinsulinaemia and diabetes," Nature, vol. 466, no. 7306, pp. 627–631, 2010.
4. K. Oishi, H. Shirai, and N. Ishida, "CLOCK is involved in the circadian transactivation of peroxisome- proliferator-activated receptor α (PPARα) in mice," Biochemical Journal, vol. 386, no. 3, pp. 575–581, 2005.
5. F. W. Turek, C. Joshu, A. Kohsaka et al., "Obesity and metabolic syndrome in circadian clock mutant nice," Science, vol. 308, no. 5724, pp. 1043–1045, 2005.
6. D. M. Arble, J. Bass, A. D. Laposky, M. H. Vitaterna, and F. W. Turek, "Circadian timing of food intake contributes to weight gain," Obesity, vol. 17, no. 11, pp. 2100–2102, 2009.
7. S. Panda, J. B. Hogenesch, and S. A. Kay, "Circadian rhythms from flies to human," Nature, vol. 417, no. 6886, pp. 329–335, 2002.

8.  S. M. Reppert and D. R. Weaver, "Coordination of circadian timing in mammals," Nature, vol. 418, no. 6901, pp. 935–941, 2002.

9.  R. A. Akhtar, A. B. Reddy, E. S. Maywood et al., "Circadian cycling of the mouse liver transcriptome, as revealed by cDNA microarray, is driven by the suprachiasmatic nucleus," Current Biology, vol. 12, no. 7, pp. 540–550, 2002.

10. G. E. Duffield, J. D. Best, B. H. Meurers, A. Bittner, J. J. Loros, and J. C. Dunlap, "Circadian programs of transcriptional activation, signaling, and protein turnover revealed by microarray analysis of mammalian cells," Current Biology, vol. 12, no. 7, pp. 551–557, 2002.

11. C. B. Green, J. S. Takahashi, and J. Bass, "The meter of metabolism," Cell, vol. 134, no. 5, pp. 728–742, 2008.

12. B. Kornmann, N. Preitner, D. Rifat, F. Fleury-Olela, and U. Schibler, "Analysis of circadian liver gene expression by ADDER, a highly sensitive method for the display of differentially expressed mRNAs," Nucleic Acids Research, vol. 29, no. 11, article E51, 2001.

13. K. F. Storch, O. Lipan, I. Leykin et al., "Extensive and divergent circadian gene expression in liver and heart," Nature, vol. 417, pp. 78–83, 2002.

14. E. D. Herzog, J. S. Takahashi, and G. D. Block, "Clock controls circadian period in isolated suprachiasmatic nucleus neurons," Nature Neuroscience, vol. 1, no. 8, pp. 708–713, 1998.

15. C. Liu, D. R. Weaver, S. H. Strogatz, and S. M. Reppert, "Cellular construction of a circadian clock: period determination in the suprachiasmatic nuclei," Cell, vol. 91, no. 6, pp. 855–860, 1997.

16. D. K. Welsh, D. E. Logothetis, M. Meister, and S. M. Reppert, "Individual neurons dissociated from rat suprachiasmatic nucleus express independently phased circadian firing rhythms," Neuron, vol. 14, no. 4, pp. 697–706, 1995.

17. J. J. Gooley, J. Lu, T. C. Chou, T. E. Scammell, and C. B. Saper, "Melanopsin in cells of origin of the retinohypothalamic tract," Nature Neuroscience, vol. 4, no. 12, p. 1165, 2001.

18. R. J. Lucas, M. S. Freedman, D. Lupi, M. Munoz, Z. K. David-Gray, and R. G. Foster, "Identifying the photoreceptive inputs to the mammalian circadian system using transgenic and retinally degenerate mice," Behavioural Brain Research, vol. 125, no. 1-2, pp. 97–102, 2001.

19. J. E. Quintero, S. J. Kuhlman, and D. G. McMahon, "The biological clock nucleus: a multiphasic oscillator network regulated by light," Journal of Neuroscience, vol. 23, no. 22, pp. 8070–8076, 2003.

20. O. Froy, "Circadian rhythms, aging, and life span in mammals," Physiology (Bethesda), vol. 26, pp. 225–235, 2011.

21. O. Froy and N. Chapnik, "Circadian oscillation of innate immunity components in mouse small intestine," Molecular Immunology, vol. 44, no. 8, pp. 1954–1960, 2007.

22. C. Lee, J. P. Etchegaray, F. R. A. Cagampang, A. S. I. Loudon, and S. M. Reppert, "Posttranslational mechanisms regulate the mammalian circadian clock," Cell, vol. 107, no. 7, pp. 855–867, 2001.

23. D. K. Welsh, S. H. Yoo, A. C. Liu, J. S. Takahashi, and S. A. Kay, "Bioluminescence imaging of individual fibroblasts reveals persistent, independently phased circadian

rhythms of clock gene expression," Current Biology, vol. 14, no. 24, pp. 2289–2295, 2004.

24. S. H. Yoo, S. Yamazaki, P. L. Lowrey et al., "PERIOD2::LUCIFERASE real-time reporting of circadian dynamics reveals persistent circadian oscillations in mouse peripheral tissues," Proceedings of the National Academy of Sciences of the United States of America, vol. 101, no. 15, pp. 5339–5346, 2004.

25. K. Saeb-Parsy, S. Lombardelli, F. Z. Khan, K. McDowall, I. T. H. Au-Yong, and R. E. J. Dyball, "Neural connections of hypothalamic neuroendocrine nuclei in the rat," Journal of Neuroendocrinology, vol. 12, no. 7, pp. 635–648, 2000.

26. N. Burioka, Y. Fukuoka, M. Takata et al., "Circadian rhythms in the CNS and peripheral clock disorders: function of clock genes: influence of medication for bronchial asthma on circadian gene," Journal of Pharmacological Sciences, vol. 103, no. 2, pp. 144–149, 2007.

27. B. J. Maron, J. Kogan, M. A. Proschan, G. M. Hecht, and W. C. Roberts, "Circadian variability in the occurrence of sudden cardiac death in patients with hypertrophic cardiomyopathy," Journal of the American College of Cardiology, vol. 23, no. 6, pp. 1405–1409, 1994.

28. B. Staels, "When the Clock stops ticking, metabolic syndrome explodes," Nature Medicine, vol. 12, no. 1, pp. 54–55, 2006.

29. S. Davis and D. K. Mirick, "Circadian disruption, shift work and the risk of cancer: a summary of the evidence and studies in Seattle," Cancer Causes and Control, vol. 17, no. 4, pp. 539–545, 2006.

30. E. Filipski, V. M. King, X. M. Li et al., "Disruption of circadian coordination accelerates malignant growth in mice," Pathologie Biologie, vol. 51, no. 4, pp. 216–219, 2003.

31. L. Fu, H. Pelicano, J. Liu, P. Huang, and C. C. Lee, "The circadian gene period2 plays an important role in tumor suppression and DNA-damage response in vivo," Cell, vol. 111, pp. 41–50, 2002.

32. R. V. Kondratov, A. A. Kondratova, V. Y. Gorbacheva, O. V. Vykhovanets, and M. P. Antoch, "Early aging and age-related pathologies in mice deficient in BMAL1, the core component of the circadian clock," Genes and Development, vol. 20, no. 14, pp. 1868–1873, 2006.

33. P. D. Penev, D. E. Kolker, P. C. Zee, and F. W. Turek, "Chronic circadian desynchronization decreases the survival of animals with cardiomyopathic heart disease," American Journal of Physiology, vol. 275, no. 6, pp. H2334–H2337, 1998.

34. M. W. Hurd and M. R. Ralph, "The significance of circadian organization for longevity in the golden hamster," Journal of Biological Rhythms, vol. 13, no. 5, pp. 430–436, 1998.

35. M. Karasek, "Melatonin, human aging, and age-related diseases," Experimental Gerontology, vol. 39, no. 11-12, pp. 1723–1729, 2004.

36. A. Klarsfeld and F. Rouyer, "Effects of circadian mutations and LD periodicity on the life span of drosophila melanogaster," Journal of Biological Rhythms, vol. 13, no. 6, pp. 471–478, 1998.

37. M. A. Hofman and D. F. Swaab, "Living by the clock: the circadian pacemaker in older people," Ageing Research Reviews, vol. 5, no. 1, pp. 33–51, 2006.

38. K. Scarbrough, S. Losee-Olson, E. P. Wallen, and F. W. Turek, "Aging and photoperiod affect entrainment and quantitative aspects of locomotor behavior in Syrian hamsters," American Journal of Physiology, vol. 272, no. 4, pp. R1219–R1225, 1997.

39. S. Yamazaki, M. Straume, H. Tei, Y. Sakaki, M. Menaker, and G. D. Block, "Effects of aging on central and peripheral mammalian clocks," Proceedings of the National Academy of Sciences of the United States of America, vol. 99, no. 16, pp. 10801–10806, 2002.

40. U. Schibler, J. Ripperger, and S. A. Brown, "Peripheral circadian oscillators in mammals: time and food," Journal of Biological Rhythms, vol. 18, no. 3, pp. 250–260, 2003.

41. O. Froy, D. C. Chang, and S. M. Reppert, "Redox potential: differential roles in dCRY and mCRY1 functions," Current Biology, vol. 12, no. 2, pp. 147–152, 2002.

42. S. M. Reppert and D. R. Weaver, "Molecular analysis of mammalian circadian rhythms," Annual Review of Physiology, vol. 63, pp. 647–676, 2001.

43. M. J. Zylka, L. P. Shearman, D. R. Weaver, and S. M. Reppert, "Three period homologs in mammals: differential light responses in the suprachiasmatic circadian clock and oscillating transcripts outside of brain," Neuron, vol. 20, no. 6, pp. 1103–1110, 1998.

44. E. J. Eide and D. M. Virshup, "Casein kinase I: another cog in the circadian clockworks," Chronobiology International, vol. 18, no. 3, pp. 389–398, 2001.

45. E. J. Eide, M. F. Woolf, H. Kang et al., "Control of mammalian circadian rhythm by CKIε-regulated proteasome-mediated PER2 degradation," Molecular and Cellular Biology, vol. 25, no. 7, pp. 2795–2807, 2005.

46. D. Whitmore, N. Cermakian, C. Crosio et al., "A clockwork organ," Biological Chemistry, vol. 381, no. 9-10, pp. 793–800, 2000.

47. E. J. Eide, H. Kang, S. Crapo, M. Gallego, and D. M. Virshup, "Casein kinase I in the mammalian circadian clock," Methods in Enzymology, vol. 393, article no. 19, pp. 408–418, 2005.

48. M. Garaulet and J. A. Madrid, "Chronobiological aspects of nutrition, metabolic syndrome and obesity," Advanced Drug Delivery Reviews, vol. 62, no. 9-10, pp. 967–978, 2010.

49. T. Hirota and Y. Fukada, "Resetting mechanism of central and peripheral circadian clocks in mammals," Zoological Science, vol. 21, no. 4, pp. 359–368, 2004.

50. A. Kohsaka and J. Bass, "A sense of time: how molecular clocks organize metabolism," Trends in Endocrinology and Metabolism, vol. 18, no. 1, pp. 4–11, 2007.

51. A. J. Davidson, O. Castañón-Cervantes, and F. K. Stephan, "Daily oscillations in liver function: diurnal vs circadian rhythmicity," Liver International, vol. 24, no. 3, pp. 179–186, 2004.

52. S. E. la Fleur, "Daily rhythms in glucose metabolism: suprachiasmatic nucleus output to peripheral tissue," Journal of Neuroendocrinology, vol. 15, no. 3, pp. 315–322, 2003.

53. S. E. La Fleur, A. Kalsbeek, J. Wortel, and R. M. Buijs, "A suprachiasmatic nucleus generated rhythm in basal glucose concentrations," Journal of Neuroendocrinology, vol. 11, no. 8, pp. 643–652, 1999.

54. K. M. Ramsey, B. Marcheva, A. Kohsaka, and J. Bass, "The clockwork of metabolism," Annual Review of Nutrition, vol. 27, pp. 219–240, 2007.
55. A. Kalsbeek, M. Ruiter, S. E. La Fleur, C. Cailotto, F. Kreier, and R. M. Buijs, "Chapter 17: the hypothalamic clock and its control of glucose homeostasis," Progress in Brain Research, vol. 153, pp. 283–307, 2006.
56. S. Yamazaki, Y. Ishida, and S. I. Inouye, "Circadian rhythms of adenosine triphosphate contents in the suprachiasmatic nucleus, anterior hypothalamic area and caudate putamen of the rat—negative correlation with electrical activity," Brain Research, vol. 664, no. 1-2, pp. 237–240, 1994.
57. C. Cailotto, S. E. La Fleur, C. Van Heijningen et al., "The suprachiasmatic nucleus controls the daily variation of plasma glucose via the autonomic output to the liver: are the clock genes involved?" European Journal of Neuroscience, vol. 22, no. 10, pp. 2531–2540, 2005.
58. S. Zvonic, Z. E. Floyd, R. L. Mynatt, and J. M. Gimble, "Circadian rhythms and the regulation of metabolic tissue function and energy homeostasis," Obesity, vol. 15, no. 3, pp. 539–543, 2007.
59. S. Zvonic, A. A. Ptitsyn, S. A. Conrad et al., "Characterization of peripheral circadian clocks in adipose tissues," Diabetes, vol. 55, no. 4, pp. 962–970, 2006.
60. H. Ando, H. Yanagihara, Y. Hayashi et al., "Rhythmic messenger ribonucleic acid expression of clock genes and adipocytokines in mouse visceral adipose tissue," Endocrinology, vol. 146, no. 12, pp. 5631–5636, 2005.
61. M. S. Bray and M. E. Young, "Circadian rhythms in the development of obesity: potential role for the circadian clock within the adipocyte," Obesity Reviews, vol. 8, no. 2, pp. 169–181, 2007.
62. M. Ruiter, S. E. La Fleur, C. Van Heijningen, J. Van der Vliet, A. Kalsbeek, and R. M. Buijs, "The daily rhythm in plasma glucagon concentrations in the rat is modulated by the biological clock and by feeding behavior," Diabetes, vol. 52, no. 7, pp. 1709–1715, 2003.
63. S. F. De Boer and J. Van Der Gugten, "Daily variations in plasma noradrenaline, adrenaline and corticosterone concentrations in rats," Physiology and Behavior, vol. 40, no. 3, pp. 323–328, 1987.
64. R. S. Ahima, D. Prabakaran, and J. S. Flier, "Postnatal leptin surge and regulation of circadian rhythm of leptin by feeding: implications for energy homeostasis and neuroendocrine function," Journal of Clinical Investigation, vol. 101, no. 5, pp. 1020–1027, 1998.
65. B. Bodosi, J. Gardi, I. Hajdu, E. Szentirmai, F. Obal Jr., and J. M. Krueger, "Rhythms of ghrelin, leptin, and sleep in rats: effects of the normal diurnal cycle, restricted feeding, and sleep deprivation," American Journal of Physiology, vol. 287, no. 5, pp. R1071–R1079, 2004.
66. J. L. Downs and H. F. Urbanski, "Aging-related sex-dependent loss of the circulating leptin 24-h rhythm in the rhesus monkey," Journal of Endocrinology, vol. 190, no. 1, pp. 117–127, 2006.
67. S. P. Kalra, M. Bagnasco, E. E. Otukonyong, M. G. Dube, and P. S. Kalra, "Rhythmic, reciprocal ghrelin and leptin signaling: new insight in the development of obesity," Regulatory Peptides, vol. 111, no. 1–3, pp. 1–11, 2003.

68. A. Kalsbeek, E. Fliers, J. A. Romijn et al., "The suprachiasmatic nucleus generates the diurnal changes in plasma leptin levels," Endocrinology, vol. 142, no. 6, pp. 2677–2685, 2001.

69. S. Sukumaran, R. R. Almon, D. C. DuBois, and W. J. Jusko, "Circadian rhythms in gene expression: relationship to physiology, disease, drug disposition and drug action," Advanced Drug Delivery Reviews, vol. 62, no. 9-10, pp. 904–917, 2010.

70. X. M. Guan, J. F. Hess, H. Yu, P. J. Hey, and L. H. T. Van Der Ploeg, "Differential expression of mRNA for leptin receptor isoforms in the rat brain," Molecular and Cellular Endocrinology, vol. 133, no. 1, pp. 1–7, 1997.

71. C. X. Yi, J. Van Der Vliet, J. Dai, G. Yin, L. Ru, and R. M. Buijs, "Ventromedial arcuate nucleus communicates peripheral metabolic information to the suprachiasmatic nucleus," Endocrinology, vol. 147, no. 1, pp. 283–294, 2006.

72. J. M. Zigman, J. E. Jones, C. E. Lee, C. B. Saper, and J. K. Elmquist, "Expression of ghrelin receptor mRNA in the rat and the mouse brain," Journal of Comparative Neurology, vol. 494, no. 3, pp. 528–548, 2006.

73. G. Boden, X. Chen, and M. Polansky, "Disruption of circadian insulin secretion is associated with reduced glucose uptake in first-degree relatives of patients with type 2 diabetes," Diabetes, vol. 48, no. 11, pp. 2182–2188, 1999.

74. E. Van Cauter, K. S. Polonsky, and A. J. Scheen, "Roles of circadian rhythmicity and sleep in human glucose regulation," Endocrine Reviews, vol. 18, no. 5, pp. 716–738, 1997.

75. M. H. Oster, T. W. Castonguay, C. L. Keen, and J. S. Stern, "Circadian rhythm of corticosterone in diabetic rats," Life Sciences, vol. 43, no. 20, pp. 1643–1645, 1988.

76. A. Velasco, I. Huerta, and B. Marin, "Plasma corticosterone, motor activity and metabolic circadian patterns in streptozotocin-induced diabetic rats," Chronobiology International, vol. 5, no. 2, pp. 127–135, 1988.

77. Y. Shimomura, M. Takahashi, H. Shimizu et al., "Abnormal feeding behavior and insulin replacement in STZ-induced diabetic rats," Physiology and Behavior, vol. 47, no. 4, pp. 731–734, 1990.

78. V. Spallone, L. Bernardi, L. Ricordi et al., "Relationship between the circadian rhythms of blood pressure and sympathovagal balance in diabetic autonomic neuropathy," Diabetes, vol. 42, no. 12, pp. 1745–1752, 1993.

79. R. Heptulla, A. Smitten, B. Teague, W. V. Tamborlane, Y. Z. Ma, and S. Caprio, "Temporal patterns of circulating leptin levels in lean and obese adolescents: relationships to insulin, growth hormone, and free fatty acids rhythmicity," Journal of Clinical Endocrinology and Metabolism, vol. 86, no. 1, pp. 90–96, 2001.

80. J. Licinio, "Longitudinally sampled human plasma leptin and cortisol concentrations are inversely correlated," Journal of Clinical Endocrinology and Metabolism, vol. 83, no. 3, p. 1042, 1998.

81. F. Perfetto, R. Tarquini, G. Cornélissen et al., "Circadian phase difference of leptin in android versus gynoid obesity," Peptides, vol. 25, no. 8, pp. 1297–1306, 2004.

82. M. F. Saad, M. G. Riad-Gabriel, A. Khan, et al., "Diurnal and ultradian rhythmicity of plasma leptin: effects of gender and adiposity," The Journal of Clinical Endocrinology & Metabolism, vol. 83, no. 2, pp. 453–459, 1998.

83. A. Gavrila, C. K. Peng, J. L. Chan, J. E. Mietus, A. L. Goldberger, and C. S. Mantzoros, "Diurnal and ultradian dynamics of serum adiponectin in healthy men: compari-

son with leptin, circulating soluble leptin receptor, and cortisol patterns," The Journal of Clinical Endocrinology & Metabolism, vol. 88, no. 6, pp. 2838–2843, 2003.

84. B. O. Yildiz, M. A. Suchard, M. L. Wong, S. M. McCann, and J. Licinio, "Alterations in the dynamics of circulating ghrelin, adiponectin, and leptin in human obesity," Proceedings of the National Academy of Sciences of the United States of America, vol. 101, no. 28, pp. 10434–10439, 2004.

85. B. Guo, S. Chatterjee, L. Li et al., "The clock gene, brain and muscle Arnt-like 1, regulates adipogenesis via Wnt signaling pathway," FASEB Journal, vol. 26, pp. 3453–3463, 2012.

86. S. Shimba, N. Ishii, Y. Ohta et al., "Brain and muscle Arnt-like protein-1 (BMAL1), a component of the molecular clock, regulates adipogenesis," Proceedings of the National Academy of Sciences of the United States of America, vol. 102, no. 34, pp. 12071–12076, 2005.

87. S. Shimba, T. Ogawa, S. Hitosugi, et al., "Deficient of a clock gene, brain and muscle Arnt-like protein-1 (BMAL1), induces dyslipidemia and ectopic fat formation," PLoS One, vol. 6, article e25231, 2011.

88. A. Chawla and M. A. Lazar, "Induction of Rev-ErbAα, an orphan receptor encoded on the opposite strand of the α-thyroid hormone receptor gene, during adipocyte differentiation," Journal of Biological Chemistry, vol. 268, no. 22, pp. 16265–16269, 1993.

89. I. P. Torra, V. Tsibulsky, F. Delaunay et al., "Circadian and glucocorticoid regulation of Rev-erbα expression in liver," Endocrinology, vol. 141, no. 10, pp. 3799–3806, 2000.

90. H. Cho, X. Zhao, M. Hatori et al., "Regulation of circadian behaviour and metabolism by REV-ERB-alpha and REV-ERB-beta," Nature, vol. 485, pp. 123–127, 2012.

91. N. Preitner, F. Damiola, Luis-Lopez-Molina et al., "The orphan nuclear receptor REV-ERBα controls circadian transcription within the positive limb of the mammalian circadian oscillator," Cell, vol. 110, no. 2, pp. 251–260, 2002.

92. T. K. Sato, S. Panda, L. J. Miraglia, et al., "A functional genomics strategy reveals Rora as a component of the mammalian circadian clock," Neuron, vol. 43, no. 4, pp. 527–537, 2004.

93. P. Lau, S. J. Nixon, R. G. Parton, and G. E. Muscat, "RORalpha regulates the expression of genes involved in lipid homeostasis in skeletal muscle cells: caveolin-3 and CPT-1 are direct targets of ROR," The Journal of Biological Chemistry, vol. 279, no. 35, pp. 36828–36840, 2004.

94. H. R. Ueda, W. Chen, A. Adachi, et al., "A transcription factor response element for gene expression during circadian night," Nature, vol. 418, no. 6897, pp. 534–539, 2002.

95. L. A. Solt, Y. Wang, S. Banerjee, et al., "Regulation of circadian behaviour and metabolism by synthetic REV-ERB agonists," Nature, vol. 485, pp. 62–68, 2012.

96. S. Kersten, B. Desvergne, and W. Wahli, "Roles of PPARS in health and disease," Nature, vol. 405, no. 6785, pp. 421–424, 2000.

97. P. Lefebvre, G. Chinetti, J. C. Fruchart, and B. Staels, "Sorting out the roles of PPARα in energy metabolism and vascular homeostasis," Journal of Clinical Investigation, vol. 116, no. 3, pp. 571–580, 2006.

98. L. Canaple, J. Rambaud, O. Dkhissi-Benyahya et al., "Reciprocal regulation of brain and muscle Arnt-like protein 1 and peroxisome proliferator-activated receptor α de-

fines a novel positive feedback loop in the rodent liver circadian clock," Molecular Endocrinology, vol. 20, no. 8, pp. 1715–1727, 2006.

99. I. Inoue, Y. Shinoda, M. Ikeda et al., "CLOCK/BMAL1 is involved in lipid metabolism via transactivation of the peroxisome proliferator-activated receptor (PPAR) response element," Journal of Atherosclerosis and Thrombosis, vol. 12, no. 3, pp. 169–174, 2005.

100. R. Gutman, M. Barnea, L. Haviv, N. Chapnik, and O. Froy, "Peroxisome proliferator-activated receptor alpha (PPARalpha) activation advances locomotor activity and feeding daily rhythms in mice," International Journal of Obesity, vol. 36, pp. 1131–1134, 2012.

101. B. Grimaldi and P. Sassone-Corsi, "Circadian rhythms: metabolic clockwork," Nature, vol. 447, no. 7143, pp. 386–387, 2007.

102. C. Liu, S. Li, T. Liu, J. Borjigin, and J. D. Lin, "Transcriptional coactivator PGC-1α integrates the mammalian clock and energy metabolism," Nature, vol. 447, no. 7143, pp. 477–481, 2007.

103. D. Carling, "AMP-activated protein kinase: balancing the scales," Biochimie, vol. 87, no. 1, pp. 87–91, 2005.

104. D. G. Hardie, S. A. Hawley, and J. W. Scott, "AMP-activated protein kinase—development of the energy sensor concept," Journal of Physiology, vol. 574, no. 1, pp. 7–15, 2006.

105. H. U. Jee, S. Yang, S. Yamazaki et al., "Activation of 5′-AMP-activated kinase with diabetes drug metformin induces casein kinase Iε (CKIε)-dependent degradation of clock protein mPer2," Journal of Biological Chemistry, vol. 282, no. 29, pp. 20794–20798, 2007.

106. K. A. Lamia, U. M. Sachdeva, L. Di Tacchio et al., "AMPK regulates the circadian clock by cryptochrome phosphorylation and degradation," Science, vol. 326, no. 5951, pp. 437–440, 2009.

107. O. Froy and R. Miskin, "Effect of feeding regimens on circadian rhythms: implications for aging and longevity," Aging, vol. 2, no. 1, pp. 7–27, 2010.

108. M. Barnea, L. Haviv, R. Gutman, N. Chapnik, Z. Madar, and O. Froy, "Metformin affects the circadian clock and metabolic rhythms in a tissue-specific manner," Biochim Biophys Acta, vol. 1822, pp. 1796–1180, 2012.

109. C. Canto and J. Auwerx, "Caloric restriction, SIRT1 and longevity," Trends in Endocrinology and Metabolism, vol. 20, no. 7, pp. 325–331, 2009.

110. M. C. Haigis and L. P. Guarente, "Mammalian sirtuins—emerging roles in physiology, aging, and calorie restriction," Genes and Development, vol. 20, no. 21, pp. 2913–2921, 2006.

111. C. Cantó, Z. Gerhart-Hines, J. N. Feige et al., "AMPK regulates energy expenditure by modulating NAD+ metabolism and SIRT1 activity," Nature, vol. 458, no. 7241, pp. 1056–1060, 2009.

112. G. Asher, D. Gatfield, M. Stratmann et al., "SIRT1 regulates circadian clock gene expression through PER2 deacetylation," Cell, vol. 134, no. 2, pp. 317–328, 2008.

113. Y. Nakahata, M. Kaluzova, B. Grimaldi et al., "The NAD+-dependent deacetylase SIRT1 modulates CLOCK-mediated chromatin remodeling and circadian control," Cell, vol. 134, no. 2, pp. 329–340, 2008.

114. Y. Nakahata, S. Sahar, G. Astarita, M. Kaluzova, and P. Sassone-Corsi, "Circadian control of the NAD+ salvage pathway by CLOCK-SIRT1," Science, vol. 324, no. 5927, pp. 654–657, 2009.

115. J. Rutter, M. Reick, L. C. Wu, and S. L. McKnight, "Regulation of clock and NPAS2 DNA binding by the redox state of NAD cofactors," Science, vol. 293, no. 5529, pp. 510–514, 2001.

116. J. Rutter, M. Reick, and S. L. McKnight, "Metabolism and the control of circadian rhythms," Annual Review of Biochemistry, vol. 71, pp. 307–331, 2002.

117. K. Oishi, G. I. Atsumi, S. Sugiyama et al., "Disrupted fat absorption attenuates obesity induced by a high-fat diet in Clock mutant mice," FEBS Letters, vol. 580, no. 1, pp. 127–130, 2006.

118. K. Oishi, N. Ohkura, M. Wakabayashi et al., "CLOCK is involved in obesity-induced disordered fibrinolysis in ob/ob mice by regulating PAI-1 gene expression," Journal of Thrombosis and Haemostasis, vol. 4, no. 8, pp. 1774–1780, 2006.

119. R. D. Rudic, P. McNamara, A. M. Curtis et al., "BMAL1 and CLOCK, two essential components of the circadian clock, are involved in glucose homeostasis," PLoS Biology, vol. 2, no. 11, article e377, 2004.

120. S. Yang, A. Liu, A. Weidenhammer et al., "The role of mPer2 clock gene in glucocorticoid and feeding rhythms," Endocrinology, vol. 150, no. 5, pp. 2153–2160, 2009.

121. V. M. Cassone and F. K. Stephan, "Central and peripheral regulation of feeding and nutrition by the mammalian circadian clock: implications for nutrition during manned space flight," Nutrition, vol. 18, no. 10, pp. 814–819, 2002.

122. F. K. Stephan, "The "other" circadian system: food as a Zeitgeber," Journal of Biological Rhythms, vol. 17, no. 4, pp. 284–292, 2002.

123. O. Froy, N. Chapnik, and R. Miskin, "Long-lived αMUPA transgenic mice exhibit pronounced circadian rhythms," American Journal of Physiology, vol. 291, no. 5, pp. E1017–E1024, 2006.

124. B. Grasl-Kraupp, W. Bursch, B. Ruttkay-Nedecky, A. Wagner, B. Lauer, and R. Schulte-Hermann, "Food restriction eliminates preneoplastic cells through apoptosis and antagonizes carcinogenesis in rat liver," Proceedings of the National Academy of Sciences of the United States of America, vol. 91, no. 21, pp. 9995–9999, 1994.

125. K. I. Honma, S. Honma, and T. Hiroshige, "Critical role of food amount for prefeeding corticosterone peak in rats," The American Journal of Physiology, vol. 245, no. 3, pp. R339–R344, 1983.

126. A. Boulamery-Velly, N. Simon, J. Vidal, J. Mouchet, and B. Bruguerolle, "Effects of three-hour restricted food access during the light period on circadian rhythms of temperature, locomotor activity, and heart rate in rats," Chronobiology International, vol. 22, no. 3, pp. 489–498, 2005.

127. R. Hara, K. Wan, H. Wakamatsu et al., "Restricted feeding entrains liver clock without participation of the suprachiasmatic nucleus," Genes to Cells, vol. 6, no. 3, pp. 269–278, 2001.

128. J. Hirao, S. Arakawa, K. Watanabe, K. Ito, and T. Furukawa, "Effects of restricted feeding on daily fluctuations of hepatic functions including P450 monooxygenase activities in rats," Journal of Biological Chemistry, vol. 281, no. 6, pp. 3165–3171, 2006.

129. R. E. Mistlberger, "Circadian food-anticipatory activity: formal models and physiological mechanisms," Neuroscience and Biobehavioral Reviews, vol. 18, no. 2, pp. 171–195, 1994.

130. C. A. Comperatore and F. K. Stephan, "Entrainment of duodenal activity to periodic feeding," Journal of Biological Rhythms, vol. 2, no. 3, pp. 227–242, 1987.

131. M. Saito, E. Murakami, and M. Suda, "Circadian rhythms in disaccharidases of rat small intestine and its relation to food intake," Biochimica et Biophysica Acta, vol. 421, no. 1, pp. 177–179, 1976.

132. K. Horikawa, Y. Minami, M. Iijima, M. Akiyama, and S. Shibata, "Rapid damping of food-entrained circadian rhythm of clock gene expression in clock-defective peripheral tissues under fasting conditions," Neuroscience, vol. 134, no. 1, pp. 335–343, 2005.

133. K. Oishi, K. Miyazaki, and N. Ishida, "Functional CLOCK is not involved in the entrainment of peripheral clocks to the restricted feeding: entrainable expression of mPer2 and BMAL1 mRNAs in the heart of Clock mutant mice on Jcl:ICR background," Biochemical and Biophysical Research Communications, vol. 298, no. 2, pp. 198–202, 2002.

134. F. K. Stephan, J. M. Swann, and C. L. Sisk, "Anticipation of 24-hr feeding schedules in rats with lesions of the suprachiasmatic nucleus," Behavioral and Neural Biology, vol. 25, no. 3, pp. 346–363, 1979.

135. F. Damiola, N. Le Minli, N. Preitner, B. Kornmann, F. Fleury-Olela, and U. Schibler, "Restricted feeding uncouples circadian oscillators in peripheral tissues from the central pacemaker in the suprachiasmatic nucleus," Genes and Development, vol. 14, no. 23, pp. 2950–2961, 2000.

136. K. A. Stokkan, S. Yamazaki, H. Tei, Y. Sakaki, and M. Menaker, "Entrainment of the circadian clock in the liver by feeding," Science, vol. 291, no. 5503, pp. 490–493, 2001.

137. J. D. Lin, C. Liu, and S. Li, "Integration of energy metabolism and the mammalian clock," Cell Cycle, vol. 7, no. 4, pp. 453–457, 2008.

138. H. Sherman, I. Frumin, R. Gutman et al., "Long-term restricted feeding alters circadian expression and reduces the level of inflammatory and disease markers," Journal of Cellular and Molecular Medicine, vol. 15, pp. 2745–2759, 2011.

139. H. Sherman, Y. Genzer, R. Cohen, N. Chapnik, Z. Madar, and O. Froy, "Timed high-fat diet resets circadian metabolism and prevents obesity," FASEB Journal, vol. 26, pp. 3493–3502, 2012.

140. J. J. Gooley, A. Schomer, and C. B. Saper, "The dorsomedial hypothalamic nucleus is critical for the expression of food-entrainable circadian rhythms," Nature Neuroscience, vol. 9, no. 3, pp. 398–407, 2006.

141. G. J. Landry, M. M. Simon, I. C. Webb, and R. E. Mistlberger, "Persistence of a behavioral food-anticipatory circadian rhythm following dorsomedial hypothalamic ablation in rats," American Journal of Physiology, vol. 290, no. 6, pp. R1527–R1534, 2006.

142. G. J. Landry, G. R. Yamakawa, I. C. Webb, R. J. Mear, and R. E. Mistlberger, "The dorsomedial hypothalamic nucleus is not necessary for the expression of circadian food-anticipatory activity in rats," Journal of Biological Rhythms, vol. 22, no. 6, pp. 467–478, 2007.

143. M. Mieda, S. C. Williams, J. A. Richardson, K. Tanaka, and M. Yanagisawa, "The dorsomedial hypothalamic nucleus as a putative food-entrainable circadian pacemaker," Proceedings of the National Academy of Sciences of the United States of America, vol. 103, no. 32, pp. 12150–12155, 2006.

144. A. J. Davidson, S. L. T. Cappendijk, and F. K. Stephan, "Feeding-entrained circadian rhythms are attenuated by lesions of the parabrachial region in rats," American Journal of Physiology, vol. 278, no. 5, pp. R1296–R1304, 2000.

145. J. Mendoza, M. Angeles-Castellanos, and C. Escobar, "Differential role of the accumbens Shell and Core subterritories in food-entrained rhythms of rats," Behavioural Brain Research, vol. 158, no. 1, pp. 133–142, 2005.

146. R. E. Mistlberger and D. G. Mumby, "The limbic system and food-anticipatory circadian rhythms in the rat: ablation and dopamine blocking studies," Behavioural Brain Research, vol. 47, no. 2, pp. 159–168, 1992.

147. A. J. Davidson, "Search for the feeding-entrainable circadian oscillator: a complex proposition," American Journal of Physiology, vol. 290, no. 6, pp. R1524–R1526, 2006.

148. R. E. Mistlberger and E. G. Marchant, "Enhanced food-anticipatory circadian rhythms in the genetically obese Zucker rat," Physiology and Behavior, vol. 66, no. 2, pp. 329–335, 1999.

149. S. Pitts, E. Perone, and R. Silver, "Food-entrained circadian rhythms are sustained in arrhythmic Clk/Clk mutant mice," American Journal of Physiology, vol. 285, no. 1, pp. R57–R67, 2003.

150. J. S. Pendergast, W. Nakamura, R. C. Friday, F. Hatanaka, T. Takumi, and S. Yamazaki, "Robust food anticipatory activity in BMAL1-deficient mice," PLoS ONE, vol. 4, no. 3, Article ID e4860, 2009.

151. K. F. Storch and C. J. Weitz, "Daily rhythms of food-anticipatory behavioral activity do not require the known circadian clock," Proceedings of the National Academy of Sciences of the United States of America, vol. 106, no. 16, pp. 6808–6813, 2009.

152. C. A. Feillet, J. A. Ripperger, M. C. Magnone, A. Dulloo, U. Albrecht, and E. Challet, "Lack of food anticipation in Per2 mutant mice," Current Biology, vol. 16, no. 20, pp. 2016–2022, 2006.

153. R. E. Mistlberger, "Circadian rhythms: perturbing a food-entrained clock," Current Biology, vol. 16, no. 22, pp. R968–R969, 2006.

154. E. J. Masoro, I. Shimokawa, Y. Higami, C. A. McMahan, and B. P. Yu, "Temporal pattern of food intake not a factor in the retardation of aging processes by dietary restriction," Journals of Gerontology A, vol. 50, no. 1, pp. B48–B53, 1995.

155. J. Koubova and L. Guarente, "How does calorie restriction work?" Genes and Development, vol. 17, no. 3, pp. 313–321, 2003.

156. E. J. Masoro, "Overview of caloric restriction and ageing," Mechanisms of Ageing and Development, vol. 126, no. 9, pp. 913–922, 2005.

157. G. S. Roth, M. A. Lane, D. K. Ingram et al., "Biomarkers of caloric restriction may predict longevity in humans," Science, vol. 297, no. 5582, p. 811, 2002.

158. G. S. Roth, J. A. Mattison, M. A. Ottinger, M. E. Chachich, M. A. Lane, and D. K. Ingram, "Aging in rhesus monkeys: relevance to human health interventions," Science, vol. 305, no. 5689, pp. 1423–1426, 2004.

159. R. Weindruch and R. S. Sohal, "Caloric intake and aging," The New England Journal of Medicine, vol. 337, no. 14, pp. 986–994, 1997.

160. E. Challet, I. Caldelas, C. Graff, and P. Pévet, "Synchronization of the molecular clockwork by light- and food-related cues in mammals," Biological Chemistry, vol. 384, no. 5, pp. 711–719, 2003.

161. E. Challet, L. C. Solberg, and F. W. Turek, "Entrainment in calorie-restricted mice: conflicting zeitgebers and free- running conditions," American Journal of Physiology, vol. 274, no. 6, pp. R1751–R1761, 1998.

162. J. Mendoza, C. Graff, H. Dardente, P. Pevet, and E. Challet, "Feeding cues alter clock gene oscillations and photic responses in the suprachiasmatic nuclei of mice exposed to a light/dark cycle," Journal of Neuroscience, vol. 25, no. 6, pp. 1514–1522, 2005.

163. D. Resuehr and J. Olcese, "Caloric restriction and melatonin substitution: effects on murine circadian parameters," Brain Research, vol. 1048, no. 1-2, pp. 146–152, 2005.

164. J. Mendoza, K. Drevet, P. Pévet, and E. Challet, "Daily meal timing is not necessary for resetting the main circadian clock by calorie restriction," Journal of Neuroendocrinology, vol. 20, no. 2, pp. 251–260, 2008.

165. O. Froy, N. Chapnik, and R. Miskin, "Relationship between calorie restriction and the biological clock: lessons from long-lived transgenic mice," Rejuvenation Research, vol. 11, no. 2, pp. 467–471, 2008.

166. R. Michael Anson, Z. Guo, R. de Cabo et al., "Intermittent fasting dissociates beneficial effects of dietary restriction on glucose metabolism and neuronal resistance to injury from calorie intake," Proceedings of the National Academy of Sciences of the United States of America, vol. 100, no. 10, pp. 6216–6220, 2003.

167. O. Descamps, J. Riondel, V. Ducros, and A. M. Roussel, "Mitochondrial production of reactive oxygen species and incidence of age-associated lymphoma in OF1 mice: effect of alternate-day fasting," Mechanisms of Ageing and Development, vol. 126, no. 11, pp. 1185–1191, 2005.

168. C. L. Goodrick, D. K. Ingram, M. A. Reynolds, J. R. Freeman, and N. Cider, "Effects of intermittent feeding upon weight and lifespan in inbred mice: interaction of genotype and age," Mechanisms of Ageing and Development, vol. 55, no. 1, pp. 69–87, 1990.

169. I. Ahmet, R. Wan, M. P. Mattson, E. G. Lakatta, and M. Talan, "Cardioprotection by intermittent fasting in rats," Circulation, vol. 112, no. 20, pp. 3115–3121, 2005.

170. A. Contestabile, E. Ciani, and A. Contestabile, "Dietary restriction differentially protects from neurodegeneration in animal models of excitotoxicity," Brain Research, vol. 1002, no. 1-2, pp. 162–166, 2004.

171. D. E. Mager, R. Wan, M. Brown et al., "Caloric restriction and intermittent fasting alter spectral measures of heart rate and blood pressure variability in rats," FASEB Journal, vol. 20, no. 6, pp. 631–637, 2006.

172. M. P. Mattson, "Energy intake, meal frequency, and health: a neurobiological perspective," Annual Review of Nutrition, vol. 25, pp. 237–260, 2005.

173. S. Sharma and G. Kaur, "Neuroprotective potential of dietary restriction against kainate-induced excitotoxicity in adult male Wistar rats," Brain Research Bulletin, vol. 67, no. 6, pp. 482–491, 2005.

174. M. P. Mattson, "Dietary factors, hormesis and health," Ageing Research Reviews, vol. 7, no. 1, pp. 43–48, 2008.

175. M. P. Mattson, W. Duan, R. Wan, and Z. Guo, "Prophylactic activation of neuroprotective stress response pathways by dietary and behavioral manipulations," NeuroRx, vol. 1, no. 1, pp. 111–116, 2004.

176. O. Froy, N. Chapnik, and R. Miskin, "Effect of intermittent fasting on circadian rhythms in mice depends on feeding time," Mechanisms of Ageing and Development, vol. 130, no. 3, pp. 154–160, 2009.

177. H. Yanagihara, H. Ando, Y. Hayashi, Y. Obi, and A. Fujimura, "High-fat feeding exerts minimal effects on rhythmic mRNA expression of clock genes in mouse peripheral tissues," Chronobiology International, vol. 23, no. 5, pp. 905–914, 2006.

178. A. Kohsaka, A. D. Laposky, K. M. Ramsey et al., "High-fat diet disrupts behavioral and molecular circadian rhythms in mice," Cell Metabolism, vol. 6, no. 5, pp. 414–421, 2007.

179. M. Barnea, Z. Madar, and O. Froy, "High-fat diet delays and fasting advances the circadian expression of adiponectin signaling components in mouse liver," Endocrinology, vol. 150, no. 1, pp. 161–168, 2009.

180. M. Barnea, Z. Madar, and O. Froy, "High-fat diet followed by fasting disrupts circadian expression of adiponectin signaling pathway in muscle and adipose tissue," Obesity, vol. 18, no. 2, pp. 230–238, 2010.

181. P. Cano, V. Jimenez-Ortega, A. Larrad, C. F. R. Toso, D. P. Cardinali, and A. I. Esquifino, "Effect of a high-fat diet on 24-h pattern of circulating levels of prolactin, luteinizing hormone, testosterone, corticosterone, thyroid-stimulating hormone and glucose, and pineal melatonin content, in rats," Endocrine, vol. 33, no. 2, pp. 118–125, 2008.

182. M. C. Cha, C. J. Chou, and C. N. Boozer, "High-fat diet feeding reduces the diurnal variation of plasma leptin concentration in rats," Metabolism: Clinical and Experimental, vol. 49, no. 4, pp. 503–507, 2000.

183. P. J. Havel, R. Townsend, L. Chaump, and K. Teff, "High-fat meals reduce 24-h circulating leptin concentrations in women," Diabetes, vol. 48, no. 2, pp. 334–341, 1999.

184. J. Mendoza, P. Pévet, and E. Challet, "High-fat feeding alters the clock synchronization to light," Journal of Physiology, vol. 586, no. 24, pp. 5901–5910, 2008.

185. M. Hatori, C. Vollmers, A. Zarrinpar, et al., "Time-restricted feeding without reducing caloric intake prevents metabolic diseases in mice fed a high-fat diet," Cell Metabolism, vol. 15, pp. 848–860, 2012.

# CHAPTER 6

# FOOD AND THE CIRCADIAN ACTIVITY OF THE HYPOTHALAMIC-PITUITARY-ADRENAL AXIS

A. M. O. LEAL and A. C. MOREIRA

## 6.1 INTRODUCTION

Circadian rhythmicity is present in most organisms living under natural conditions and its most important role is to facilitate adaptation of the organism to periodic fluctuations in the external environment (1). In particular, the food-seeking behavior might have forced the development of specialized functions of the circadian timing system that enable the organism to be prepared for food seeking, digestion and metabolism (2).

Daily variations in plasma corticosteroid levels may be considered a paradigm of circadian rhythms and evidence has been accumulated showing the close relationship between the hypothalamic-pituitary-adrenal (HPA) axis and the nutritional status of mammals, including humans (3).

In this review we focus on the interaction among HPA axis rhythmicity under basal and stress conditions, food ingestion, and different nutritional and endocrine states. In the first part of this paper we introduce the reader to basic concepts of chronobiology (for extensive reviews, see Refs. 1,4-6).

*This chapter was originally published under the Creative Commons Attribution License. Leal AMO and Moreira AC. Food and the Circadian Activity of the Hypothalamic-Pituitary-Adrenal Axis.* Brazilian Journal of Medical and Biological Research *30,12 (1997). http://dx.doi.org/10.1590/S0100-879X1997001200003 .*

## 6.2 CIRCADIAN RHYTHMS

### 6.2.1 GENERAL FEATURES: ANATOMICAL PATHWAYS AND RHYTHM SYNCHRONIZERS

Biological rhythms range extensively in periodicity from a fraction of a second to several years; however, the circadian rhythms (from the Latin circadian meaning "around a day") have a predominant role and can be demonstrated not only in physiological states but also in pathological processes which fluctuate during the course of a day (7).

The daily variations of biological variables are not simply a response to 24-h changes in the environment due to the rotation of the earth on its axis, but rather arise from an internal time-keeping system (4) and persist under constant environmental conditions ("free-running"). The major action of the environment is to synchronize the internal system to a period of exactly 24 h.

In mammals, the suprachiasmatic nucleus (SCN) was initially supposed to be the only master circadian pacemaker (4). The SCN is a complex structure involving two small bilaterally paired nuclei situated in the anterior hypothalamus above the optic chiasm and lateral to the third ventricle (5). The role of the SCN as the circadian clock has been demonstrated by lesion experiments and studies involving transplantation of the SCN (8-10). Although other neural loci have not been identified as sites of the central biological clock, there is evidence demonstrating resynchronization of corticosteroid circadian rhythmicity after SCN destruction. These results may indicate the possibility of the presence of other circadian clocks in brain areas outside the SCN (11). Probably a more complex timing circuitry exists and may support the existence of a multioscillator system where a master oscillator could be responsible for synchronization among other oscillators present in various organs and tissues (12). In addition to the pacemaker hypothesis, the network hypothesis was recently proposed: the interaction between the pacemaker and non-pacemaker cells may be the key factor in the generation of a precise circadian rhythm within the SCN (13).

In mammals the SCN receives entraining information from the light-dark cycle via pathways separated from the visual system. These pathways include the retinohypothalamic tract and the geniculohypothalamic tract which arises from a subdivision of the lateral geniculate nucleus (4). The neurotransmitters and photoreceptors involved in the circadian rhythms of mammals have not been completely established. There are some data suggesting the presence of neurons containing glutamate, gamma-amino-butyric acid, vasoactive intestinal peptide and neuropeptide Y (NPY) in the circadian timing system (13).

The output pathways leaving the SCN project mainly to the medial hypothalamus (14,15) and the localization of the SCN suggests that this nucleus has an important integrative function.

Little is known about the mechanisms whereby nonphotic stimuli influence the circadian clock system and how the SCN exerts its integrative influence. It is generally accepted that the generation of HPA axis periodicity occurs in the central nervous system (CNS) (16). However, specific neuroanatomical pathways and neurotransmitters involved in the expression of pituitary-adrenal circadian rhythmicity have not been clearly demonstrated. Numerous investigators have reported that lesions in various areas of the hypothalamus inhibit daily adrenocorticotropin (ACTH) and corticosterone variation. These procedures include anterior hypothalamic deafferentation and SCN lesions (8,17,18), lesions of ventromedial and dorsomedial nuclei (19), anterior hypothalamic lesions (20) and basal hypothalamic lesions (21). The maintenance of a free-running circadian rhythm for corticosterone in rats with isolation of the medial basal hypothalamus, including the SCN, from the rest of the central nervous system (22) indicates that these neural structures are essential for the manifestation of a light entrainable corticosterone rhythm. In addition, a direct input from the SCN to the paraventricular nucleus (PVN) has been described (14). Catecholaminergic inputs from the brainstem (23,24) and serotonergic projections from the dorsal raphe (25) have also been described as modulators of HPA axis rhythm.

There is evidence that circadian rhythmicity is an inherited characteristic of diverse species, including humans (26). In fact, a period mutation was described in golden hamsters, referred to as the tau mutant, in which the 24-h free-running periods of the activity rhythm are shortened to 20 h and to 22 h, in homozygous and heterozygous animals, respectively (27). However, genetic analysis and identification (cloning) of genes responsible for the determination of circadian rhythm have been restricted to invertebrates (28,29).

Since the endogenous circadian period observed under constant conditions is not exactly 24 h, external physical environmental factors must operate to synchronize (entrain) the internal clock system. The light-dark cycle is the primary agent that synchronizes most circadian rhythms. However, other agents such as food ingestion (30), barometric pressure (31), acoustic stimuli (32) and scents (33) have been cited as synchronizers or "zeitgebers." The effects of these synchronizers on circadian rhythms may differ considerably both in quality and strength between nocturnal and diurnal mammals. In humans, social cues seem to be even stronger stimuli than the light-dark cycle, as clearly observed in experiments with night workers and travelers across time zones (jet lag effect).

Molecular and cellular mechanisms underlying entrainment are poorly defined. However, some studies have shown that light is able to induce the expression of the proto-oncogenes c-fos and jun-B and to influence light entrainment and locomotor activity (34,35).

The role of food presentation as a synchronizer under natural conditions is not yet clear. However, under laboratory conditions, Krieger's first studies (30) showed that periodic meal timing could act as an important rhythm synchronizer in rats. The adaptive feature of food synchronization is of obvious importance for the survival of any species.

## 6.3 DIURNAL RHYTHMS OF THE HYPOTHALAMIC-PITUITARY-ADRENAL AXIS AND THE ROLE OF FOOD

The circadian rhythmicity of the HPA axis is one of the best documented cyclic neuroendocrine activities. Daily variation in plasma corticosteroid has been well characterized in man and in rats, presenting as peak concentrations prior to or at the time of onset of activity, with a decline over the remainder of the 24-h period. After the first description of daily variation in urinary ketosteroid excretion (36), evidence has been accumulated showing daily rhythmicity at every level of the HPA axis.

Even before the corticotropin-releasing hormone (CRH) had been characterized, rhythmicity of hypothalamic CRH activity had been suggested in rats (37-39) by bioassays. After CRH characterization, circadian periodicity in hypothalamic CRH content and plasma CRH was described (40-43). More recently a daily rhythm in CRH mRNA expression was demonstrated by different techniques (44,45). However, these studies showed no consensus about nadirs of the daily CRH pattern and others did not detect daily variation of hypothalamic or plasma CRH (46-48). These controversies may be related to different time sampling and sensitivities of assay methods. In spite of these controversies, the blockade of plasma ACTH rhythm by passive immunization with CRH antiserum and the restoration of the rhythm by pulsatile administration of CRH indicate the participation of CRH in the determination of ACTH rhythm (49,50). The possibility remains that this influence occurs at the pituitary level; however, the data about the daily variation in pituitary responsiveness to CRH are also contradictory (46,47,51-53). In addition, the finding of a persistent daily rhythm of ACTH during continuous administration of CRH (54) suggests that other factors are also involved in the ACTH rhythm. Among these factors, the role of vasopressin was investigated but not well defined (55).

Many studies have confirmed a pattern of plasma ACTH rhythmicity similar to that of corticosteroids (47,56) and have indicated the presence of a daily rhythm in the pituitary secretion of other proopiomelanocortin (POMC)-related peptides, such as ß-lipotropin (57) and ß-endorphin (58,59). In man, the daily rhythm of the corticotropic axis seems to be under the control of amplitude, but not frequency, modulation of ACTH secretion (59,60). In addition, in-phase daily variation of the adrenal responsiveness to ACTH which amplifies the corticosterone rhythm has been well established (21,61). On the other hand, morning cortisol peaks in ACTH-deficient patients treated with exogenous ACTH suggest that extrapituitary factors may act in conjunction with ACTH (62).

The negative feedback mechanism that controls the secretion of ACTH by adrenal steroids also presents daily variation, with higher efficacy at nadir time (46,63). It was demonstrated in rats that the occupation of type I (high affinity) corticosteroid receptors is able to control basal activity in the HPA axis in the morning and that in the evening type I occupation potentiates the inhibition of plasma ACTH by occupation of type II receptors (lower affinity) (64).

Although most evidence indicates that HPA axis rhythmicity is under a hierarchical order, other evidence indicates functional independence at every level of HPA axis organization, including the adrenals. Although the rhythmic secretion of corticosterone in adrenal organ cultures is controversial (47,65,66), the periodicity of corticosterone in hypophysectomized rats implanted with ACTH has been described (67). In addition, it was demonstrated that the rhythm in ACTH, CRH and CRH mRNA persists after adrenalectomy in rats (38,39,68,69). The daily ACTH variation was also maintained in patients with ACTH hypersecretion due to different degrees of cortisol production deficiency as found in Addison's disease (70) or different types of congenital adrenal hyperplasia (71). Thus ACTH rhythmicity is partially independent of negative feedback.

Finally, it should be remembered that variations in the metabolic clearance rate of corticosteroids have been reported and could contribute to its rhythmic pattern (72-74).

Moreover, the circadian variation of the HPA axis changes with the manipulation of rhythm by phase-shifting a synchronizer such as the light-dark, sleep-wake and rest-activity cycles, and food schedule (75). In humans, an adult cortisol circadian pattern (peak of plasma cortisol at early morning) is established and maintained at a mean age of 8 weeks in healthy infants (76). Although it has been suggested that the development of the circadian pattern in adrenocortical activity in humans is parallel to the development of sleeping and feeding patterns and is also related to maternal adrenocortical activity (77), the ontogeny of HPA axis circadian rhythm deserves further investigation both in humans and in rats.

Although neither the mechanism nor the site of feeding-associated daily rhythm is known, studies have indicated feeding as a major organizer of rhythms of HPA axis activity. There are two classes of animals in terms of food behavior. Diurnal mammals, including human beings, are active in the daytime and sleep at night. Nocturnal animals (including many ranging in size from bears to mice) rest in the daytime and are active and take most of their daily food in the dark period. Thus, the feeding synchronizer effect on the HPA axis may differ considerably both in quality and strength between nocturnal and diurnal mammals, especially rats and men.

Rats are nocturnal animals and eat more than 70% of their daily food intake during the night (78). Rats with free access to food manifest a daily peak of plasma corticosterone at 20:00 h, just prior to the time of onset of predominant food intake. Approximately twenty years ago, the pioneering work of Krieger (30) demonstrated that restriction of food access in the morning hours from 9:00 to 11:00 h was able to cause a 12-h shift of plasma corticosterone peak in rats. This observation was initially associated with the changes of locomotor activity and sleep-wake cycle that accompany the eating pattern. Other studies showed that this explanation was not completely correct, since peak corticosterone levels are observed prior to food presentation regardless of its relation to the lighting period (79,80). Furthermore, Honma et al. (22) demonstrated that the rhythm of plasma corticosterone is not a direct consequence of the rhythm of locomotor activity.

Additionally, it was found that food-shifted rhythms of plasma corticosteroid concentrations and of body temperature persisted in animals with SCN lesions and if the animals had become arrhythmic because of SCN lesions, a restricted-feeding schedule could restore circadian rhythmicity. Furthermore, it was observed that daily food cyclicity did not affect SCN neural activity (81,82). These studies indicate the primacy of food as a zeitgeber and suggest the existence of a biological clock other than the SCN. Nevertheless, the abolition of food-shifted daily corticosterone and activity rhythmicity by ventromedial hypothalamic lesions (83,84) indicates the involvement of the hypothalamic area in the generation of food shift rhythms.

Despite much work in the intervening 20 years, our knowledge of the mechanisms and pathways by which food induces synchronization of adrenal axis rhythms is still incomplete. Honma et al. (85) correlated the duration of food restriction and amount of food ingested to the corticosterone rhythm. On the other hand, the prefeeding corticosterone peak does not appear to be related to the availability of certain food constituents (80). Furthermore, the time interval between food presentation and prefeeding corticosterone peak is incompatible with new neurotransmitter synthesis.

We have recently investigated the effect of food restriction on the various functional levels of the HPA axis. Although the 12-h shift of plasma corticosterone peak was clear and plasma ACTH was high in the morning, there was no significant difference between morning and afternoon plasma ACTH levels (47). Furthermore, there was no detectable daily variation of hypothalamic CRH or pituitary ACTH contents and plasma ACTH response to synthetic CRH in free-fed or food-restricted rats. These findings led us to investigate the effect of food restriction on the adrenal responsiveness to ACTH. We demonstrated a 12-h shift in the adrenal response to synthetic ACTH [1-24] induced by the time of feeding as previously suggested by Wilkinson et al. (86). We also originally showed that this shift of corticosterone response to exogenous ACTH may not be influenced by endogenous plasma ACTH levels during the preceding 12 h since it was maintained after dexamethasone pretreatment. This pattern of response, however, was abolished by chlorpromazine-morphine-pentobarbital anesthesia. In addition, in in vitro experiments, incubated adrenal slices obtained from free-fed and food-restricted rats showed no daily variation in adrenal responsiveness to ACTH [1-24]. These results indicate that the daily variation in adrenal responsiveness to ACTH is due to modulation by neural (central or peripheral), vascular or humoral factors other than ACTH.

On the other hand, there is now a considerable body of evidence suggesting the importance of adrenal innervation in the modulation of the HPA axis (87-92), including the adrenal sensitivity to ACTH. Additionally, the pituitary-adrenal axis appears to have a daily pattern of response to stress, with a higher ACTH response in the morning in free-fed rats, that is not dependent on corticosterone (93-96).

As well as the basal activity, the daily variation of the HPA axis stress response appears to be closely related to food intake (96,97). In a previous study we found that food restriction for 2 weeks abolished the a.m.-p.m. difference in plasma ACTH levels attained after immobilization stress in rats by a still uncharacterized mechanism (96). It is suggested that food restriction may also modify the ACTH response to stress along the day.

Although it has been shown that an intact vagus nerve is not necessary for the establishment of the daily rhythmicity of plasma corticosterone in free-fed or food-restricted rats (98), there is extensive evidence indicating the relationship among HPA axis, catecholamines and feeding (99-103). Food intake was shown to be affected by central administration of catecholamines (103) and the permissive role of corticosterone in norepinephrine-elicited feeding which exhibited a circadian pattern has been demonstrated (99,100). Furthermore, the prefeeding increase in paraventricular norepinephrine release and the abolition of the prefeeding corticosterone peak by destruction of catecholaminergic innervation of the PVN in rats under food restriction strongly suggest the participation of catecholamines in the expression of feeding-related corticosterone rhythms (101).

The mechanisms responsible for modulation of the HPA axis by feeding are very complex and probably involve uncharacterized central nervous system pathways, including medial basal hypothalamic nuclei and autonomic pathways. Moreover, feeding patterns result from a balance between anorectic (CRH, cholecystokinin, neurotensin) and orectic (NPY, pancreatic polypeptide, galanine) factors forming a complex circuitry (104-111), many of them being closely related to HPA axis activity.

Neuropeptide Y is a potent orexigenic agent with a dense distribution in hypothalamic nuclei (112,113) and is responsible for stimulating food intake in the rat (104,114). A daily rhythm in NPY content in the parvocellular portion of the PVN with a unimodal peak prior to the onset of dark has been described (115). In rats under food restriction, elevated NPY content and release in the PVN were observed before the introduction of food, with decreasing levels during the course of eating (116). In addition, anatomical and pharmacological studies suggest that NPY can modulate CRH, ACTH and corticosterone secretion (117, 118). On the other hand, glucocorticoids are required for an increase in prepro NPY mRNA levels induced by food deprivation (119,120) and the hypothalamic NPY-feeding system is dependent upon corticosterone. We have investigated the role of vasopressin using the food-restriction model (47). However, we found that the daily patterns of plasma vasopressin and ACTH-corticosterone did not coincide in terms of basal activity and stress response. Vasopressin may not be involved in the pituitary-adrenal adaptations that occur in food restriction (47,96).

We have recently shown a significant correlation between daily variation of plasma atrial natriuretic peptide (ANP) and corticosterone in rats on a free or restricted feeding regimen (121). However, the nature of the relationship between ANP and feeding is far from clear. It is hypothesized that ANP may interact with ACTH and other central neuropeptides (122).

Corticosteroids exert metabolic effects on food intake and intermediary metabolism, which together act to provide an adequate supply of energy (123). The studies of restricted feeding are of considerable importance because they reveal feeding as a synchronizer link between hormonal systems and metabolic machinery. Once the food restriction schedule is set, neurohumoral and metabolic variables are temporarily reorganized to ensure anticipative adaptation of the animal. Thus, rats under food restriction develop high rates of lipogenesis in adipose tissue and in liver (124), resistance to liver glycogen depletion during fasting (125) and increased storage of glycogen in liver, muscle and adipose tissue during the postprandial period (126-128), higher efficiency in food utilization and a higher capacity to recover from hypoglycemia (129,130). In addition, delayed gastric emptying (128) and an increase in intestinal absorbing area due to mucosal hypertrophy have been observed (131). The periodicity of food presentation is an important factor for the establishment of the metabolic changes, since the same amount of food given randomly in time to food-restricted rats promotes a different adaptive metabolic pattern (132). Corticosteroids seem to be required for the metabolic adaptation since adrenalectomized animals do not survive food restriction due to lack of lipogenesis, gluconeogenesis and glucogenolysis (133) to efficiently supply energy in the intermeal period.

Dallman et al. (3) suggest that the interactions among insulin, glucocorticoids and NPY are responsible for the metabolic aspects related to food intake. It was observed that rats under food restriction present higher circulating levels of insulin and greater insulin sensitivity (134). Furthermore, many lines of evidence support the hypothesis that insulin is an afferent central signal which regulates normal energy balance (135). It was recently observed that high-dose dexamethasone administration decreases the efficiency of CNS insulin transport (136).

Furthermore, it is hypothesized that the metabolic actions of corticosteroids rely on concentration-dependent interactions with type I and type II glucocorticoid receptors (137).

The association of feeding and HPA axis activity has been studied in humans under physiological and pathological conditions. The demonstration of a large peak of plasma cortisol coinciding with the noon meal and a smaller peak after the evening meal gives evidence for the influence of meal timing on the daily plasma cortisol pattern (138-140). The mechanism by which ingestion of food stimulates cortisol secretion is unknown. Higher postprandial plasma ACTH and cortisol increments related to high-protein meals have been demonstrated (141,142) and a role of gut peptides and neurotransmitter substrates as neuroendocrine links between gut and brain has been proposed. The role played by these peptides in HPA axis activity is supported by the finding that parenteral feeding during a restricted time of day completely abolished blood corticosterone rhythm in rats (143). In humans, the parenteral nutritional support did not alter the circadian rhythm of cortisol as compared with enteral nutrition (144). Al-Damluji et al. (104) suggested a stimulatory effect of alpha-1 adrenoceptors on the ACTH and cortisol postprandial peak. However, the physiological mechanisms leading to postprandial ACTH and cortisol release remain to be determined. Corticosteroids appear to play an important role in regulating the circadian fluctuations of brain-gut peptides and cell cycle of the gastrointestinal mucosa (145).

Anorexia nervosa has long been known to be associated with hypothalamic-pituitary-adrenal axis abnormalities. Anorectic patients present elevated levels of plasma cortisol with the loss of normal daily rhythm, failure of suppression of plasma ACTH and cortisol levels by dexamethasone, a deficient response of plasma cortisol to insulin-induced hypoglycemia and blunted ACTH and cortisol responses to CRH (146-149). Although little is known about the pathophysiology of hypercortisolism of anorexia nervosa, evidence points to a disorder at or above the hypothalamus leading to hypersecretion of CRH (146,149-152). Since these abnormalities of cortisol secretion are reversed with improvement in nutrition and body weight, they could be regarded only as secondary to malnutrition. However, as pointed out by Gold et al. (149), CRH hypersecretion may be a defect associated with primary affective disorder, given the clinical and pathophysiologic similarities between anorexia nervosa and depression.

The investigation of HPA axis function in bulimia has revealed abnormalities that are independent of weight disturbances (153,154). Although the cortisol circadian variation appears to be normal, 24-h integrated plasma ACTH and cortisol levels are elevated and ACTH and cortisol responses to CRH are blunted (153). These findings are in disagreement with those of Gold et al. (149). A prominent finding in bulimia is the lack of cortisol suppression by dexamethasone (155). However, it is difficult to state if this abnormality is related to psychic distress or to eating behavior itself (154). Interestingly, bulimics do not present the usual cortisol increase in response to a mixed meal (153).

The changes of adrenal function in malnutrition include increased serum cortisol concentration, abolition of daily rhythm, decreased cortisol metabolic clearance, decreased cortisol responsiveness to CRH and incomplete dexamethasone suppression (156,157). This pattern of HPA axis activity has been attributed to endogenous CRH hypersecretion (158). These alterations are all reversible with refeeding. Some of these changes are also observed in normal men after fasting (159).

Although the mechanisms of the altered adrenal function common to fasting, malnutrition and eating disorders are not known, the role of corticosteroids may be considered to be an adaptive response important for the metabolic adjustments for fuel storage to assure survival (160,161).

There is evidence that HPA axis activity is altered by obesity. On the other hand, it is well known that HPA axis components, in particular CRH and corticosteroids, influence the patterns of calorie and nutrient intake. The control of food intake is complex and involves numerous brain neurotransmitters and central and peripheral neural structures. Glucocorticoids are believed to interact with hypothalamus neurotransmitters to mediate their effects on nutrient intake (108,109). Obese humans have normal plasma ACTH and cortisol circadian rhythm, higher cortisol production rate (162), normal cortisol response to hypothalamic-pituitary stimulation by hypoglycemia and direct adrenal stimulation by ACTH, and impaired cortisol response to pituitary stimulation by CRH (163). In addition, obese individuals may fail to suppress plasma cortisol following dexamethasone administration (164). The various animal models of obesity have provided important data to elucidate metabolic disorders in this human disease. Corticosterone has been shown to be necessary for the expression of genetic and hypothalamic lesion-induced obesity (165). The genetically obese fa/fa rat presents many metabolic and endocrine abnormalities that are dependent on adrenal glucocorticoids. Most of these metabolic impairments are reversed by adrenalectomy and restored by corticosterone treatment (166). Adrenalectomy, through the loss of corticosterone, may act on food intake, sympathetic activity and insulin (167) and NPY (3) secretion. In spite of controversial findings in the literature, studies of hypercorticism in genetically obese rats have suggested alterations in the central regulation of the HPA axis (168-171) by still unidentified mechanisms. A regulatory role of glucocorticoids in obese gene expression and leptin secretion has been indicated (172). An interaction between leptin and NPY has also been suggested (173), with inhibition of NPY synthesis and release by leptin.

In normal man, glucose tolerance varies with time of day. Plasma glucose responses to oral and intravenous glucose or meals are higher in the evening than in the morning (174,175). Van Cauter et al. (176) demonstrated that the daily variation in glucose levels during constant glucose infusion is paralleled by a similar variation in insulin secretion, which is inversely related to the circadian rhythm of cortisol secretion. Under controlled conditions, a similar result was obtained in response to mixed meal ingestion in the morning and in the evening. These studies suggest that factors other than cortisol and gastrointestinal hormones are implicated in the circadian changes in glucose tolerance. Such factors could affect the insulin response through changes in the pancreatic beta cell sensitivity to glucose (177). Additionally, in a recent study our group suggested a modulatory role of cortisol in the IGF-IGF binding protein system under physiological conditions, especially in situations of low insulin concentrations (178).

Finally, the study of hypothalamic-pituitary-adrenocortical activity in diabetic patients has revealed a state of hypercorticism (179,180). The origin of the increased activity of the HPA axis is not clear. It was suggested that fluctuations in blood sugar could be the cause (179). In addition, temporal and quantitative correlations between glucose and circadian cortisol variations were observed in patients with noninsulin-dependent diabetes and normal subjects submitted to fasting. Altogether, these findings indicate the role of glucocorticoids in the control of the daily variations in glucose levels and fuel availability (181,182) and, therefore, the importance of time of day in the diagnosis and treatment of diabetes mellitus.

Cushing's syndrome is characterized by, among other things, HPA rhythmicity abnormalities, insulin resistance and hyperglycemia secondary to hypercortisolism. Hypercortisolemia is associated with increased glucose production, decreased glucose transport and utilization, decreased protein synthesis and increased protein degradation in muscle. It was demonstrated that glucocorticoids may interfere with the early steps of insulin signal transduction in liver and muscle (183). Centrally localized adipose tissue is another feature of corticosteroid excess and this typical fat distribution has been attributed to elevated adipocyte lipoprotein lipase activity and low lipolytic activity (184). After the noon meal, the normal postprandial elevation in cortisol is depressed or absent in pituitary-dependent Cushing's syndrome patients (185).

Interestingly, two recent studies demonstrated that a rare pituitary-independent type of Cushing's syndrome can be food-dependent (186,187). In this uncommon case the development of abnormal adrenal sensitivity to the stimulatory action of secreted gastric inhibitory polypeptide (GIP) was possibly secondary to aberrant expression of GIP receptors on adrenal cells. Thus, in this newly described nodular adrenal hyperplasia cortisol production depends on how much and how often the patients eat.

In conclusion, the present review examined the role of food ingestion as an important synchronizing agent for HPA axis regulation. The modulation of the HPA axis by feeding is complex and may involve a neurohumoral circuitry with both central and peripheral components.

## REFERENCES

1. Aschoff J (1979). Circadian rhythms: general features and endocrinological aspects. In: Krieger DT (Editor), Endocrine Rhythms. Raven Press, New York.
2. Moore-Ede MC (1986). Physiology of the circadian timing system: predictive versus reactive homeostasis. American Journal of Physiology, 250: R737-R752.
3. Dallman MF, Strack AM, Akana SF, Bradbury MJ, Hanson ES, Scribner KA & Smith M (1993). Feast and famine: critical role of glucocorticoids with insulin in daily energy flow. Frontiers in Neuroendocrinology, 14: 303-347.
4. Menaker M, Takahashi JS & Eskin A (1978). The physiology of circadian pacemakers. Annual Review of Physiology, 40: 501-526.
5. Rusak B & Zucker I (1979). Neural regulation of circadian rhythms. Physiological Reviews, 59: 449-526.
6. Turek FW (1994). Circadian rhythms. Recent Progress in Hormone Research, 49: 43-90.
7. Minors DS (1985). Chronobiology: its importance in clinical medicine. Clinical Science, 69: 369-376.
8. Moore RY & Eichler VB (1972). Loss of a circadian adrenal corticosterone rhythm following suprachiasmatic lesions in the rat. Brain Research, 42: 201-206.

9. Stephan FK & Zucker I (1972). Circadian rhythms in drinking behavior and locomotor activity of rats are eliminated by hypothalamic lesions. Proceedings of the National Academy of Sciences, USA, 69: 1583-1586.

10. Ralph MR, Foster RG, Davis FC & Menaker M (1990). Transplanted suprachiasmatic nucleus determines circadian period. Science, 247: 975-978.

11. Krieger DT, Hauser H & Krey LC (1977). Suprachiasmatic nuclear lesions do not abolish food-shifted circadian adrenal and temperature rhythmicity. Science, 197: 398-399.

12. Moore-Ede MC, Schmelzer WS, Kass DA & Herd JA (1976). Internal organization of the circadian timing system in multicellular animals. Federation Proceedings, 35: 2333-2338.

13. Aronson BD, Bell-Pedersen D, Block GD, Bos NPA, Dunlap JC, Eskin A, Garceau NY, Geusz ME, Johnson KA, Khalsa SBS, Koster-Van Hoffen GC, Koumenis C, Lee TM, LeSauter J, Lindgren KM, Lin Q, Loros JJ, Michel SH, Mirmiran M, Moore RY, Ruby NF, Silver R, Turek FW, Zatz M & Zucker I (1993). Circadian rhythms. Brain Research Reviews, 18: 315-333.

14. Berk ML & Finkelstein JA (1981). An autoradiographic determination of the efferent projections of the suprachiasmatic nucleus of the hypothalamus. Brain Research, 226: 1-13.

15. Stephan FK, Berkley KJ & Moss RL (1981). Efferent connections of the rat suprachiasmatic nucleus. Neuroscience, 6: 2625-2641.

16. Dallman MF, Akana SF, Cascio CS, Darlington DN, Jacobson L & Levin N (1987). Regulation of ACTH secretion: variations on a theme of B. Recent Progress in Hormone Research, 43: 113-173.

17. Cascio CS, Shinsako J & Dallman MF (1987). The suprachiasmatic nuclei stimulate evening ACTH secretion in the rat. Brain Research, 423: 173-178.

18. Abe K, Kroning J, Greer MA & Critchlow V (1979). Effects of destruction of the suprachiasmatic nuclei on the circadian rhythms in plasma corticosterone, body temperature, feeding and plasma thyrotropin. Neuroendocrinology, 29: 119-131.

19. Bellinger LL, Bernardis LL & Mendel VE (1976). Effect of ventromedial and dorsomedial hypothalamic lesions on circadian corticosterone rhythms. Neuroendocrinology, 22: 216-225.

20. Slusher MA (1964). Effects of chronic hypothalamic lesions on daily and stress corticosteroid levels. American Journal of Physiology, 206: 1161-1164.

21. Kaneko M, Hiroshige T, Shinsako J & Dallman MF (1980). Daily changes in amplification of hormone rhythms in the adrenocortical system. American Journal of Physiology, 239: R309-R316.

22. Honma S, Honma K-I & Hiroshige T (1984). Dissociation of circadian rhythms in rats with a hypothalamic island. American Journal of Physiology, 246: R949-R954.

23. Szafarczyk A, Alonso G, Ixart G, Malaval F & Assenmacher I (1985). Daily-stimulated and stress-induced ACTH release in rats is mediated by ventral noradrenergic bundle. American Journal of Physiology, 249: E219-E226.

24. Szafarczyk A, Guillaume V, Conte-Devolx B, Alonso G, Malaval F, Pares-Herbute N, Oliver C & Assenmacher I (1988). Central catecholaminergic system stimulates secretion of CRH at different sites. American Journal of Physiology, 255: E463-E468.

25. Szafarczyk A, Ixart G, Malaval F, Nouguier-Soule J & Assenmacher I (1979). Effects of lesions of the suprachiasmatic nuclei and of p-chlorophenylalanine on the circadian rhythms of adrenocorticotrophic hormone and corticosterone in the plasma, and on locomotor activity of rats. Journal of Endocrinology, 83: 1-16.

26. Linkowski P, Van Onderbergen A, Kerkhafs M, Bosson D, Mendlewicz J & Van Cauter E (1993). Twin study of the 24-h cortisol profile: Evidence for genetic control of the human circadian clock. American Journal of Physiology, 264: E173-E181.

27. Ralph MR & Menaker M (1988). A mutation in the circadian system of the golden hamster. Science, 241: 1225-1227.

28. Hall JC (1990). Genetics of circadian rhythms. Annual Review of Genetics, 24: 659-697.

29. Konopka RJ & Benzer S (1971). Clock mutants of Drosophila melanogaster. Proceedings of the National Academy of Sciences, USA, 68: 2112-2116.

30. Krieger DT (1974). Food and water restriction shifts corticosterone, temperature, activity and brain amine periodicity. Endocrinology, 95: 1195-1201.

31. Hayden P & Lindberg RG (1969). Circadian rhythm in mammalian body temperature entrained by cyclic pressure changes. Science, 164: 1288-1289.

32. Gwinner E (1966). Periodicity of a circadian rhythm in birds by species-specific song cycles (Aves, Fringillidae: Carduelis spinus, Serinus serinus). Experientia, 22: 765-766.

33. McClintock MK (1971). Menstrual synchrony and suppression. Nature, 229: 244-245.

34. Earnest DJ, Iadarola M, Yeh HH & Olschowka JA (1990). Photic regulation of c-fos expression in neural components governing the entrainment of circadian rhythms. Experimental Neurology, 109: 353-361.

35. Kornhauser JM, Nelson DE, Mayo KE & Takahashi JS (1992). Regulation of jun-B messenger RNA and AP-1 activity by light and a circadian clock. Science, 255: 1581-1584.

36. Pincus G (1943). A daily rhythm in the excretion of urinary ketosteroids by young men. Journal of Clinical Endocrinology, 3: 195-199.

37. David-Nelson MA & Brodish A (1969). Evidence for a daily rhythm of corticotrophin-releasing factor (CRF) in the hypothalamus. Endocrinology, 85: 861-866.

38. Hiroshige T & Sakakura M (1971). Circadian rhythm of corticotropin-releasing activity in the hypothalamus of normal and adrenalectomized rats. Neuroendocrinology, 7: 25-36.

39. Takebe K, Sakakura M & Mashimo K (1972). Continuance of daily rhythmicity of CRF activity in hypophysectomized rats. Endocrinology, 90: 1515-1520.

40. Moldow RL & Fischman AJ (1982). Physiological changes in rat hypothalamic CRF: circadian, stress and steroid suppression. Peptides, 3: 837-840.

41. Owens MJ, Bartolome J, Schanberg SM & Nemeroff CB (1990). Corticotropin-releasing factor concentrations exhibit an apparent daily rhythm in hypothalamic and extrahypothalamic brain regions: differential sensitivity to corticosterone. Neuroendocrinology, 52: 626-631.

42. Honma K-I, Noe Y, Honma S, Katsuno Y & Hiroshige T (1992). Roles of paraventricular catecholamines in feeding-associated corticosterone rhythm in rats. American Journal of Physiology, 262: E948-E955.

43. Watabe T, Tanaka K, Kumagae M, Itoh S, Hasegawa M, Horiuchi T, Miyabe S, Ohno H & Shimizu N (1987). Daily rhythm of plasma immunoreactive corticotropin-releasing factor in normal subjects. Life Sciences, 40: 1651-1655.

44. Watts AG & Swanson LW (1989). Daily variations in the content of preprocorticotropin-releasing hormone messenger ribonucleic acids in the hypothalamic paraventricular nucleus of rats of both sexes as measured by in situ hybridization. Endocrinology, 125: 1734-1738.

45. Kwak SP, Young EA, Morano I, Watson SJ & Akil H (1992). Daily corticotropin-releasing hormone mRNA variation in the hypothalamus exhibits a rhythm distinct from that of plasma corticosterone. Neuroendocrinology, 55: 74-83.

46. Akana SF, Cascio CS, Du JZ, Levin N & Dallman MF (1986). Reset of feedback in the adrenocortical system: an apparent shift in sensitivity of adrenocorticotropin to inhibition by corticosterone between morning and evening. Endocrinology, 119: 2325-2332.

47. Leal AMO & Moreira AC (1996). Feeding and the daily variation of the hypothalamic-pituitary-adrenal axis and its responses to CRH and ACTH in rats. Neuroendocrinology, 64: 14-19.

48. Charlton BG, Leake A, Ferrier IN, Linton EA & Lowry PJ (1986). Corticotropin-releasing factor in plasma of depressed patients and controls. Lancet, i: 161-162.

49. Bagdy G, Chrousos GP & Calogero AE (1991). Circadian patterns of plasma immunoreactive corticotropin, beta-endorphin, corticosterone and prolactin after immunoneutralization of corticotropin-releasing hormone. Neuroendocrinology, 53: 573-578.

50. Avgerinos PC, Schurmeyer TH, Gold PW, Tomai TP, Loriaux DL, Sherins RJ, Cutler GB & Chrousos GP (1986). Administration of human corticotropin-releasing hormone in patients with secondary adrenal insufficiency: restoration of the normal cortisol secretory pattern. Journal of Clinical Endocrinology and Metabolism, 62: 816-821.

51. Nicholson S, Lin J-H, Mahmoud S, Campbel E, Gillham B & Jones M (1985). Daily variations in responsiveness of the hypothalamo-pituitary-adrenocortical axis of the rat. Neuroendocrinology, 40: 217-224.

52. DeCherney GS, Debold CR, Jackson RV, Sheldon WR, Island DP & Orth DN (1985). Daily variation in the response of plasma adrenocorticotropin and cortisol to intravenous ovine corticotropin-releasing hormone. Journal of Clinical Endocrinology and Metabolism, 61: 273-279.

53. Desir D, Van Cauter E, Beyloos M, Bosson D, Golstein J & Copinschi G (1986). Prolonged pulsatile administration of ovine corticotropin-releasing hormone in normal man. Journal of Clinical Endocrinology and Metabolism, 63: 1292-1299.

54. Shulte HM, Chrousos GP, Gold PW, Booth JD, Oldfield EH, Cutler GB & Loriaux DL (1985). Continuous administration of synthetic ovine corticotropin-releasing factor in man. Journal of Clinical Investigation, 75: 1781-1785.

55. Salata RA, Jarret DB, Verbalis JG & Robinson AG (1988). Vasopressin stimulation of adrenocorticotropin hormone (ACTH) in humans. Journal of Clinical Investigation, 81: 766-774.

56. Dallman MF, Engeland WC, Rose JC, Wilkinson CW, Shinsako J & Siedenburg F (1978). Nycthemeral rhythm in adrenal responsiveness to ACTH. American Journal of Physiology, 135: R210-R218.

57. Tanaka K, Nicholson WE & Orth DN (1978). Daily rhythm and disappearance half-time of endogenous plasma immunoreactive ß-MSH (LPH) and ACTH. Journal of Clinical Endocrinology and Metabolism, 46: 883-890.

58. Dent RRM, Guilleminault C, Albert LH, Posner BI, Cox BM & Goldstein A (1981). Daily rhythm of plasma immunoreactive ß-endorphin and its relationship to sleep stages and plasma rhythms of cortisol and prolactin. Journal of Clinical Endocrinology and Metabolism, 52: 942-947.

59. Veldhuis JD, Iranmanesh A, Johnson ML & Lizarralde G (1990). Amplitude, but not frequency, modulation of adrenocorticotropin secretory bursts gives rise to the nyctohemeral rhythm of the corticotropic axis in man. Journal of Clinical Endocrinology and Metabolism, 71: 452-463.

60. Veldhuis JD, Iranmanesh A, Johnson ML & Lizarralde G (1990). Twenty-four-hour rhythms in plasma concentrations of adenohypophyseal hormones are generated by distinct amplitude and/or frequency modulation of underlying pituitary secretory bursts. Journal of Clinical Endocrinology and Metabolism, 71: 1616-1623.

61. Kaneko M, Kaneko K, Shinsako J & Dallman MF (1981). Adrenal sensitivity to adrenocorticotropin varies daily. Endocrinology, 109: 70-75.

62. Fehm HL, Klein E, Holl R & Voigt KH (1984). Evidence for extrapituitary mechanisms mediating the morning peak of plasma cortisol in man. Journal of Clinical Endocrinology and Metabolism, 58: 410-414.

63. Dallman MF, Levin N, Cascio CS, Akana SF, Jacobson L & Kuhn RW (1989). Pharmacological evidence that the inhibition of daily corticotropin secretion by corticosteroids is mediated via type I, corticosterone-preferring receptors. Endocrinology, 124: 2844-2850.

64. Bradbury MJ, Akana SF & Dallman MF (1994). Roles of type I and II corticosteroid receptors in regulation of basal activity in the hypothalamo-pituitary-adrenal axis during the daily trough and the peak: Evidence for a nonadditive effect of combined receptor occupation. Endocrinology, 134: 1286-1296.

65. Andrews RV (1968). Temporal secretory responses of cultured hamster adrenals. Comparative Biochemistry and Physiology, 26: 179-193.

66. O'Hare MJ & Hornsby PJ (1975). Absence of a circadian rhythm of corticosterone secretion in monolayer cultures of adult rat adrenocortical cells. Experientia, 31: 378-380.

67. Meier AH (1976). Daily variation in concentrations of plasma corticosteroid in hypophysectomized rats. Endocrinology, 98: 1475-1479.

68. Cheifetz P, Gaffud N & Dingman JF (1968). Effects of bilateral adrenalectomy and continuous light on the circadian rhythm of corticotropin in female rats. Endocrinology, 82: 1117-1124.

69. Kwak SP, Morano MI, Young EA, Watson SJ & Akil H (1993). Daily CRH mRNA rhythm in the hypothalamus: decreased expression in the evening is not dependent on endogenous glucocorticoids. Neuroendocrinology, 57: 96-105.

70. Krieger DT & Gewirtz GP (1974). The nature of the circadian periodicity and suppressibility of immunoreactive ACTH levels in Addison's disease. Journal of Clinical Endocrinology and Metabolism, 39: 46-52.

71. Moreira AC, Leal AMO & Castro M (1990). Characterization of adrenocorticotropin secretion in a patient with 17 a-hydroxylase deficiency. Journal of Clinical Endocrinology and Metabolism, 71: 86-91.

72. Woodward CJH, Hervey GR, Oakey RE & Whitaker EM (1991). The effects of fasting on plasma corticosterone kinetics in rats. British Journal of Nutrition, 66: 117-127.

73. Marotta SF, Hiles LG, Lanuza DM & Boonayathap U (1975). The relation of hepatic in vitro inactivation of corticosteroids to the circadian rhythm of plasma corticosterone. Hormone and Metabolic Research, 7: 334-337.

74. Lacerda L, Kowarski A & Migeon CJ (1973). Daily variation of the metabolic clearance rate of cortisol. Effect on measurement of cortisol production rate. Journal of Clinical Endocrinology and Metabolism, 36: 1043-1049.

75. Krieger DT (1979). Rhythms in CRF, ACTH and corticosteroids. In: Krieger DT (Editor), Endocrine Rhythms. Raven Press, New York, 123-142.

76. Santiago LB, Jorge SM & Moreira AC (1996). Longitudinal evaluation of the development of salivary cortisol circadian rhythm in infancy. Clinical Endocrinology, 44: 157-161.

77. Spangler G (1991). The emergence of adrenocortical circadian function in newborns and infants and its relationship to sleep, feeding and maternal adrenocortical activity. Early Human Development, 25: 197-208.

78. Morimoto Y, Arisue K & Yamamura Y (1977). Relationship between circadian rhythm of food intake and that of plasma corticosterone and effect of food restriction on circadian adrenocortical rhythm in the rat. Neuroendocrinology, 23: 212-222.

79. Nelson W, Scheving L & Halberg F (1975). Circadian rhythms in mice fed a single daily meal at different stages of lighting regimen. Journal of Nutrition, 105: 171-184.

80. Gallo PV & Weinberg J (1981). Corticosterone rhythmicity in the rat: Interactive effects of dietary restriction and schedule of feeding. Journal of Nutrition, 111: 208-218.

81. Inouye ST (1982). Restricted daily feeding does not entrain circadian rhythms of the suprachiasmatic nucleus in the rat. Brain Research, 232: 194-199.

82. Shibata S, Liou SY, Ueki S & Oomura Y (1983). Effects of restricted feeding on single neuron activity of suprachiasmatic neurons in rat hypothalamus slice preparation. Physiology and Behavior, 31: 523-528.

83. Krieger DT (1980). Ventromedial hypothalamic lesions abolish food-shifted circadian adrenal and temperature rhythmicity. Endocrinology, 106: 649-654.

84. Inouye ST (1982). Ventromedial hypothalamic lesions eliminate anticipatory activities of restricted daily feeding schedules in the rat. Brain Research, 250: 183-187.

85. Honma K-I, Honma S & Hiroshige T (1983). Critical role of food amount for prefeeding corticosterone peak in rats. American Journal of Physiology, 245: R339-R344.

86. Wilkinson CW, Shinsako J & Dallman MF (1979). Daily rhythms in adrenal responsiveness to adrenocorticotropin are determined primarily by the time of feeding in the rat. Endocrinology, 104: 350-359.

87. Ottenweller JE & Meier A (1982). Adrenal innervation may be an extrapituitary mechanism able to regulate adrenocortical rhythmicity in rats. Endocrinology, 111: 1334-1338.

88. Holzwarth MA, Cunningham LA & Kleitman N (1987). The role of adrenal nerves in the regulation of adrenocortical functions. Annals of the New York Academy of Sciences, 512: 449-464.

89. Vinson GP, Hinson JP & Tóth IE (1994). The neuroendocrinology of the adrenal cortex. Journal of Neuroendocrinology, 6: 235-246.
90. Charlton BG (1989). Adrenal cortical innervation and glucocorticoid secretion. Journal of Endocrinology, 126: 5-8.
91. Engeland WC & Gann DS (1989). Splanchnic nerve stimulation modulates steroid secretion in hypophysectomized dogs. Neuroendocrinology, 50: 124-131.
92. Edwards AV, Jones CT & Bloom SR (1986). Reduced adrenal cortical sensitivity to ACTH in lambs with cut splanchnic nerves. Journal of Endocrinology, 110: 81-85.
93. Dunn J, Scheving L & Millet P (1972). Circadian variation in stress-evoked increases in plasma corticosterone. American Journal of Physiology, 222: 402-406.
94. Yasuda N, Takebe K & Greer MA (1976). Evidence of nycterohemeral periodicity in stress-induced pituitary-adrenal activation. Neuroendocrinology, 21: 214-224.
95. Bradbury MJ, Cascio CS, Scribner KA & Dallman MF (1991). Stress-induced adrenocorticotropin secretion: daily responses and decreases during stress in the evening are not dependent on corticosterone. Endocrinology, 128: 680-688.
96. Leal AMO, Forsling ML & Moreira AC (1995). Daily variation of the pituitary-adrenal and AVP responses to stress in rats under food restriction. Life Sciences, 56: 191-198.
97. Hanson ES, Bradbury MJ, Akana SF, Scribner KA, Strack AM & Dallman MF (1994). The daily rhythm in adrenocorticotropin responses to restraint in adrenalectomized rats is determined by caloric intake. Endocrinology, 134: 2214-2220.
98. Moreira AC & Krieger DT (1982). The effects of subdiaphragmatic vagotomy on circadian corticosterone rhythmicity in rats with continuous or restricted food access. Physiology and Behavior, 28: 787-790.
99. Leibowitz SF, Roland CR, Hor L & Schillari V (1984). Noradrenergic feeding elicited via the paraventricular nucleus is dependent upon circulating corticosterone. Physiology and Behavior, 32: 857-864.
100. Bhakthavatsalam P & Leibowitz SF (1986). a2-Noradrenergic feeding rhythm in paraventricular nucleus: relation to corticosterone. American Journal of Physiology, 250: R83-R88.
101. Mitome M, Honma S, Yoshihara T & Honma K-I (1994). Prefeeding increase in paraventricular NE release is regulated by a feeding-associated rhythm in rats. American Journal of Physiology, 226: E606-E611.
102. Stanley BG, Schwartz DH, Hernandez L, Hoebel BG & Leibowitz SF (1989). Patterns of extracellular norepinephrine in the paraventricular hypothalamus: relationship to circadian rhythm and deprivation-induced eating behavior. Life Sciences, 45: 275-282.
103. Shor-Posner G, Grinker JA, Marinescu C & Leibowitz SF (1985). Role of hypothalamic norepinephrine in control of meal patterns. Physiology and Behavior, 35: 209-214.
104. Al-Damluji S, Iveson T, Thomas JM, Pendlebury DJ, Rees LH & Besser GM (1987). Food-induced cortisol secretion is mediated by central alpha-1 adrenoceptor modulation of pituitary ACTH secretion. Clinical Endocrinology, 26: 629-636.
105. Morley JE (1987). Neuropeptide regulation of appetite and weight. Endocrine Reviews, 8: 256-287.
106. Nagai K & Nakagawa H (1992). Central Regulation of Energy Metabolism with Special Reference to Circadian Rhythm. CRC Press, Boca Raton.

107. Antoni FA (1986). Hypothalamic control of adrenocorticotropin secretion: advances since the discovery of 41-residue corticotropin-releasing factor. Endocrine Reviews, 7: 351-378.

108. Leibowitz SF (1987). Hypothalamic neurotransmitters in relation to normal and disturbed eating patterns. Annals of the New York Academy of Sciences, 499: 137-143.

109. Tataranni PA, Larson DE, Snitker S, Young JB, Flatt JP & Ravussin E (1996). Effects of glucocorticoids on energy metabolism and food intake in humans. American Journal of Physiology, 34: E317-E325.

110. Koenig JI (1990). Regulation of the hypothalamo-pituitary-adrenal axis by neuropeptide Y. Annals of the New York Academy of Sciences, 611: 317-328.

111. Brady LS, Smith MA, Gold PW & Herkenham M (1990). Altered expression of hypothalamic neuropeptide mRNAs in food-restricted and food deprived rats. Neuroendocrinology, 52: 441-447.

112. Dequidt ME & Emson PC (1986). Distribution of neuropeptide Y-like immunoreactivity in the rat central nervous system. II. Immunohistochemical analysis. Neuroscience, 18: 545-618.

113. Clark JT, Kalra PS & Kalra SP (1985). Neuropeptide Y stimulates feeding but inhibits sexual behavior in rats. Endocrinology, 117: 2435-2442.

114. Sahu A & Kalra SP (1993). Neuropeptidergic regulation of feeding behavior: neuropeptide Y. Trends in Endocrinology and Metabolism, 4: 217-224.

115. Jhanwar-Uniyal M, Beck B, Burlet C & Leibowltz SF (1990). Daily rhythm of neuropeptide Y-like immunoreactivity in the suprachiasmatic, arcuate and paraventricular nuclei and other hypothalamic sites. Brain Research, 536: 331-334.

116. Kalra SP, Dube MG, Sahu A, Phelps CP & Kalra PS (1991). Neuropeptide Y secretion increases in the paraventricular nucleus in association with increased appetite for food. Proceedings of the National Academy of Sciences, USA, 88: 10931-10935.

117. Wahlestedt C, Skagerberg G, Ekman R, Heilig M, Sundler F & Hakanson R (1987). Neuropeptide Y (NPY) in the area of the hypothalamic paraventricular nucleus activates the pituitary-adrenocortical axis in the rat. Brain Research, 417: 33-38.

118. Haas DA & George SR (1989). Neuropeptide Y-induced effects on hypothalamic corticotropin-releasing factor content and release are dependent on noradrenergic/ adrenergic neurotransmission. Brain Research, 498: 333-338.

119. Ponsalle P, Srivastava LS, Uht RM & White JD (1992). Glucocorticoids are required for food deprivation-induced increases in hypothalamic neuropeptide Y expression. Journal of Neuroendocrinology, 4: 585-591.

120. Stanley BG, Lanthier D, Chin AS & Leibowitz SF (1989). Suppression of neuropeptide Y-elicited eating by adrenalectomy or hypophysectomy: reversal with corticosterone. Brain Research, 501: 32-36.

121. Oliveira MHA, Antunes-Rodrigues J, Leal AMO, Elias LLK & Moreira AC (1993). Circadian variation of plasma atrial natriuretic peptide and corticosterone in rats with continuous or restricted access to food. Life Sciences, 53: 1795-1801.

122. Oliveira MHA, Antunes-Rodrigues J, Gutkowska J, Leal AMO, Elias LLK & Moreira AC (1997). Atrial natriuretic peptide and feeding activity patterns in rats. Brazilian Journal of Medical and Biological Research, 30: 1-5.

123. Dallman MF, Darlington DN, Suemaru S, Cascio CS & Levin N (1989). Corticosteroids in homeostasis. Acta Physiologica Scandinavica, 136: 227-234.

124. Leveille GA (1967). In vivo fatty acid synthesis in adipose tissue and liver of meal-fed rats. Proceedings of the Society for Experimental Biology and Medicine, 125: 85-88.
125. Leveille GA (1966). Glycogen metabolism in meal-fed rats and chicks and the time sequence of lipogenic and enzymatic adaptive changes. Journal of Nutrition, 90: 449-460.
126. Leveille GA & Chakrabarty K (1967). Daily variations in tissue glycogen and liver weight of meal-fed rats. Journal of Nutrition, 93: 546-554.
127. Stevenson JAF, Feleki V, Szlavko A & Beaton JR (1964). Food restriction and lipogenesis in the rat. Proceedings of the Society for Experimental Biology and Medicine, 116: 178-182.
128. Lima FB, Hell NS, Timo-Iaria C, Scivoletto R, Dolnikoff MS & Pupo AA (1981). Metabolic consequences of food restriction in rats. Physiology and Behavior, 27: 115-123.
129. Hell NS, Oliveira LBC, Dolnikoff MS, Scivoletto R & Timo-Iaria C (1980). Changes of carbohydrate metabolism caused by food restriction, as detected by insulin administration. Physiology and Behavior, 24: 473-477.
130. Curi R, Hell NS, Bazotte RB & Timo-Iaria C (1984). Metabolic performance of free fed rats subjected to prolonged fast as compared to the metabolic pattern in rats under long term food restriction. Physiology and Behavior, 33: 525-531.
131. Leveille GA & Chakrabarty K (1968). Absorption and utilization of glucose by meal-fed and nibbling rats. Journal of Nutrition, 96: 69-75.
132. Bazotte RB, Curi R & Hell NS (1989). Metabolic changes caused by irregular-feeding schedule as compared with meal-feeding. Physiology and Behavior, 46: 109-113.
133. Berdanier CD, Wurdeman R & Tobin RB (1976). Further studies on the role of the adrenal hormones in the responses of rats to meal-feeding. Journal of Nutrition, 106: 1791-1800.
134. Wiley JH & Leveille GA (1970). Significance of insulin in the metabolic adaptation of rats to meal ingestion. Journal of Nutrition, 100: 1073-1080.
135. Schwartz MW, Figlewicz DP, Baskin DG, Woods SC & Porte Jr D (1992). Insulin in the brain: A hormonal regulator of energy balance. Endocrine Reviews, 13: 387-414.
136. Baura GD, Foster DM, Kaiyala K, Porte D, Kahn SE & Schwartz MW (1996). Insulin transport from plasma into the central nervous system is inhibited by dexamethasone in dogs. Diabetes, 45: 86-90.
137. Devenport L, Knehans A, Sundstrom A & Thomas T (1989). Corticosterone's dual metabolic actions. Life Sciences, 45: 1389-1396.
138. Follenius M, Brandenberger G & Hietter B (1982). Daily cortisol peaks and their relationships to meals. Journal of Clinical Endocrinology and Metabolism, 55: 757-761.
139. Quigley ME & Yen SSC (1979). A mid-day surge in cortisol levels. Journal of Clinical Endocrinology and Metabolism, 49: 945-947.
140. Goldman J, Wajchenberg BL, Liberman B, Nery M, Achando S & Germek OA (1985). Contrast analysis for the evaluation of the circadian rhythms of plasma cortisol, androstenedione, and testosterone in normal men and the possible influence of meals. Journal of Clinical Endocrinology and Metabolism, 60: 164-167.
141. Slag MF, Ahmed M, Gannon MC & Nuttall FQ (1981). Meal stimulation of cortisol secretion: A protein induced effect. Metabolism, 30: 1104-1108.

142. Ishizuka B, Quigley ME & Yen SSC (1983). Pituitary hormone release in response to food ingestion: Evidence for neuroendocrine signals from gut to brain. Journal of Clinical Endocrinology and Metabolism, 57: 1111-1116.

143. Saito M, Kato H, Suda M & Yugari Y (1981). Parenteral feeding abolishes the circadian adrenocortical rhythm in rats. Experientia, 37: 754-755.

144. Marchini JS, Neto JB & Lara RS (1988). Ritmo nictêmero de cortisol e insulina em pacientes submetidos ao suporte nutricional enteral e parenteral. Revista do Hospital das Clínicas da Faculdade de Medicina de São Paulo, 43: 232-236.

145. Pasley JN, Burns ER & Rayford PL (1994). Circadian variations of gastrointestinal peptides and cell proliferation in rats: Effects of adrenalectomy. Recent Progress in Hormone Research, 49: 359-365.

146. Frankel RJ & Jenkins JS (1975). Hypothalamic-pituitary function in anorexia nervosa. Acta Endocrinologica, 78: 209-221.

147. Berger M, Pirke K, Doerr P, Krieg C & von Zerssen D (1983). Influence of weight loss on the dexamethasone suppression test. Archives of General Psychiatry, 40: 585-586.

148. Sirinathsinghyi DJS & Milles IH (1985). Concentration patterns of plasma dehydroepiandrosterone, D5-androstenediol and their sulphates, testosterone and cortisol in normal healthy women and in women with anorexia nervosa. Acta Endocrinologica, 108: 255-260.

149. Gold PW, Gwirtsman H, Avgerinos PC, Nieman LK, Gallucci WT, Kaye W, Jimerson D, Ebert M, Rittmaster R, Loriaux L & Chrousos GP (1986). Abnormal hypothalamic-pituitary-adrenal function in anorexia nervosa. New England Journal of Medicine, 314: 1335-1342.

150. Hotta M, Shibasaki T, Masuda A, Imaki T, Demura H, Ling N & Shizume K (1986). The response of plasma adrenocorticotropin and cortisol to corticotropin-releasing hormone (CRH) and cerebrospinal fluid immunoreactive CRH in anorexia nervosa patients. Journal of Clinical Endocrinology and Metabolism, 62: 319-324.

151. Kaye VH, Gwirtsman HE, George DT, Ebert MH, Jimerson DC, Tomai TP, Chrousos GP & Gold PW (1987). Elevated cerebrospinal fluid levels of immunoreactive corticotropin-releasing hormone in anorexia nervosa: relation to state of nutrition, adrenal function, and intensity of depression. Journal of Clinical Endocrinology and Metabolism, 64: 203-208.

152. Cavagnini F, Invitti C, Passamonti M & Polli EE (1986). Response of ACTH and cortisol to corticotropin-releasing hormone in anorexia nervosa. New England Journal of Medicine, 314: 184-185.

153. Mortola JF, Rasmussen DD & Yen SSC (1989). Alterations of the adrenocorticotropin-cortisol axis in normal weight bulimic women: Evidence for a central mechanism. Journal of Clinical Endocrinology and Metabolism, 68: 517-522.

154. Gwirtsman HE, Roy-Birne P, Yager J & Gerner RH (1983). Neuroendocrine abnormalities in bulimia. American Journal of Psychiatry, 140: 559-563.

155. Walsch BT, Lo SE, Cooper T, Lindy DC, Roose SP, Gladis M & Glassman AH (1987). Dexamethasone suppression test and plasma dexamethasone levels in bulimia. Archives of General Psychiatry, 44: 797-800.

156. Smith SR, Bledsoe T & Chhetri MK (1975). Cortisol metabolism and the pituitary-adrenal axis in adults with protein-calorie malnutrition. Journal of Clinical Endocrinology and Metabolism, 40: 43-52.

157. Malozowski S, Muzzo S, Burrows R, Leiva L, Loriaux L, Chrousos G, Winterer J & Cassorla F (1990). The hypothalamic-pituitary-adrenal axis in infantile malnutrition. Clinical Endocrinology, 32: 461-465.

158. Alleyne GAO & Young VH (1967). Adrenocortical function in children with severe protein-calorie malnutrition. Clinical Science, 33: 189-200.

159. Vance ML & Thorner MO (1989). Fasting alters pulsatile and rhythmic cortisol release in normal men. Journal of Clinical Endocrinology and Metabolism, 68: 1013-1018.

160. Eigler N, Sacca L & Sherwin R (1979). Synergistic interactions of physiologic increments of glucagon, epinephrine, and cortisol in the dog. Journal of Clinical Investigation, 63: 114-123.

161. Brasel JA (1980). Endocrine adaptation to malnutrition. Pediatric Research, 14: 1299-1303.

162. Streeten DHP, Stevenson CT, Dalakos TG, Nicholas JJ, Dennick LG & Fellerman H (1969). The diagnosis of hypercortisolism. Biochemical criteria differentiating patients from lean and obese normal subjects and from females on oral contraceptives. Journal of Clinical Endocrinology and Metabolism, 29: 1191-1211.

163. Kopelman PG, Grossman A, Lavender P, Besser GM, Rees LH & Coy D (1988). The cortisol response to corticotropin-releasing factor is blunted in obesity. Clinical Endocrinology, 28: 15-18.

164. Crapo L (1979). Cushing's syndrome: a review of diagnostic tests. Metabolism, 28: 955-977.

165. Dallman MF (1984). Viewing the ventromedial hypothalamus from the adrenal gland. American Journal of Physiology, 246: R1-R12.

166. Freedman MR, Horwitz BA & Stern JS (1986). Effect of adrenalectomy and glucocorticoid replacement on development of obesity. American Journal of Physiology, 250: R595-R607.

167. Bray GA, York DA & Fisler JS (1989). Experimental obesity: A homeostatic failure due to defective nutrient stimulation of the sympathetic nervous system. Vitamins and Hormones, 45: 1-125.

168. Guilhaume-Gentil C, Rohner-Jeanrenaud F, Abramo F, Bestetti GE, Rossi GL & Jeanrenaud B (1990). Abnormal regulation of the hypothalamo-pituitary-adrenal axis in the genetically obese fa/fa rat. Endocrinology, 126: 1873-1879.

169. Plotsky PM, Thrivikraman KV, Watts AG & Hauger RL (1992). Hypothalamic-pituitary-adrenal function in the zucker obese rat. Endocrinology, 130: 1931-1941.

170. Walker CD, Scribner KA, Stern JS & Dallman MF (1992). Obese zucker (fa/fa) rats exhibit normal target sensitivity to corticosterone and increased drive to adrenocorticotropin during the daily trough. Endocrinology, 131: 2629-2637.

171. Havel PJ, Busch BL, Curry DL, Johnson PR, Dallman MF & Stern JS (1996). Predominately glucocorticoid agonist actions of RU-486 in young specific-pathogen-free zucker rats. American Journal of Physiology, 271: R710-R717.

172. Slieker LJ, Sloop KW, Surface PL, Kriauciunas A, LaQuier F, Manetta J, Bue-Valleskey J & Stephens TW (1996). Regulation of expression of ob mRNA and protein by glucocorticoids and cAMP. Journal of Biological Chemistry, 271: 5301-5304.

173. Stephens TW, Basinsky M, Bristow PK, Bue-Valleskey JM, Burgett SG, Craft L, Hale J, Hoffmann J, Hsiung HM, Kriauciunas A, MacKellar W, Rosteck Jr PR,

Schoner B, Smith D, Tinsley FC, Zhang X & Heiman M (1995). The role of neuro-peptide Y in the antiobesity action of the obese gene product. Nature, 377: 530-532.

174. Carrol K & Nestel P (1973). Daily variation in glucose tolerance and in insulin se-cretion in man. Diabetes, 22: 333-348.

175. Van Cauter E, Shapiro ET, Tillil H & Polonsky KS (1992). Circadian modulation of glucose and insulin responses to meals: relationship to cortisol rhythm. American Journal of Physiology, 262: E467-E475.

176. Van Cauter E, Blackman JD, Roland D, Spire JP, Refetoff S & Polonsky KS (1991). Modulation of glucose regulation and insulin secretion by circadian rhythmicity and sleep. Journal of Clinical Investigation, 88: 934-942.

177. Aparício NJ, Puchulu FE, Gagliardino JJ, Ruiz M, Llorens JM, Ruiz J, Lamas A & Miguel R (1974). Circadian variation of the blood glucose, plasma insulin and hu-man growth hormone level in response to an oral glucose load in normal subjects. Diabetes, 23: 132-137.

178. Martinelli C, Yateman M, Cotterril A, Moreira A & Camacho-Hubner C (1997). Interaction between the GH-IGF system and spontaneous cortisol secretion in chil-dren. Growth Hormone Research Society Conference 96. Endocrinology and Me-tabolism, 4 (Suppl A): 85 (Abstract).

179. Asfeldt VH (1972). Hypophyseo-adrenocortical function in diabetes mellitus. Acta Medica Scandinavica, 191: 349-354.

180. Cameron OG, Kronfol Z, Greden JF & Carrol BJ (1984). Hypothalamic-pituitary-adrenocortical activity in patients with diabetes mellitus. Archives of General Psy-chiatry, 41: 1090-1095.

181. Shapiro ET, Polonsky KS, Copinschi G, Bosson D, Tillil H, Blackman J, Lewis G & Van Cauter E (1991). Nocturnal elevation of glucose levels during fasting in noninsulin-dependent diabetes. Journal of Clinical Endocrinology and Metabolism, 72: 444-454.

182. Faiman C & Moorhouse JA (1967). Daily variation in the levels of glucose and related sub-stances in healthy and diabetic subjects during starvation. Clinical Science, 32: 111-126.

183. Saad MJ, Folli F, Kalin JA & Kahn CR (1993). Modulation of insulin receptor, in-sulin receptor substrate-1, and phosphatidylinositol 3-kinase in liver and muscle of dexamethasone-treated rats. Journal of Clinical Investigation, 92: 2065-2072.

184. Rebuffé-Scrive M, Krotkiewski M, Elfverson J & Björntorp P (1988). Muscle and adipose tissue morphology and metabolism in Cushing's syndrome. Journal of Clini-cal Endocrinology and Metabolism, 67: 1122-1127.

185. Liu LH, Kazer RR & Rasmussen DD (1987). Characterization of the twenty-four hour secretion patterns of adrenocorticotropin and cortisol in normal women and patients with Cushing's disease. Journal of Clinical Endocrinology and Metabolism, 64: 1027-1035.

186. Lacroix A, Bolté E, Tremblay J, Dupré J, Poitras P, Fournier H, Garon J, Garrel D, Bayard F, Taillefer R, Flanagan RJ & Hamet P (1992). Gastric inhibitory polypep-tide-dependent cortisol hypersecretion - a new case of Cushing's syndrome. New England Journal of Medicine, 327: 974-980.

187. Reznik Y, Allali-Zerah V, Chayvialle JA, Leroyer R, Leymare P, Travert G, Lebre-thon M-E, Budi I, Balliere A-M & Maloudeau J (1992). Food-dependent Cushing's syndrome mediated by aberrant adrenal sensitivity to gastric inhibitory polypeptide. New England Journal of Medicine, 327: 981-986.

# CHAPTER 7

# CIRCADIAN AND DARK-PULSE ACTIVATION OF OREXIN/ HYPOCRETIN NEURONS

OLIVER J. MARSTON, RHOANNAN H. WILLIAMS, MARIA M. CANAL, RAYNA E. SAMUELS, NEIL UPTON, AND HUGH D. PIGGINS

Temporal control of brain and behavioral states emerges as a consequence of the interaction between circadian and homeostatic neural circuits. This interaction permits the daily rhythm of sleep and wake, regulated in parallel by circadian cues originating from the suprachiasmatic nuclei (SCN) and arousal-promoting signals arising from the orexin-containing neurons in the tuberal hypothalamus (TH). Intriguingly, the SCN circadian clock can be reset by arousal-promoting stimuli while activation of orexin/hypocretin neurons is believed to be under circadian control, suggesting the existence of a reciprocal relationship. Unfortunately, since orexin neurons are themselves activated by locomotor promoting cues, it is unclear how these two systems interact to regulate behavioral rhythms. Here mice were placed in conditions of constant light, which suppressed locomotor activ-

*This chapter was originally published under the Creative Commons Attribution License. Marston OJ, Williams RH, Canal MM, Samuels RE, Upton N, and Piggin HD. Circadian and Dark-Pulse Activation of Orexin/Hypocretin Neurons. Molecular Brain 1,19 (2008). doi:10.1186/1756-6606-1-19.*

ity, but also revealed a highly pronounced circadian pattern in orexin neuronal activation. Significantly, activation of orexin neurons in the medial and lateral TH occurred prior to the onset of sustained wheel-running activity. Moreover, exposure to a 6 h dark pulse during the subjective day, a stimulus that promotes arousal and phase advances behavioral rhythms, activated neurons in the medial and lateral TH including those containing orexin. Concurrently, this stimulus suppressed SCN activity while activating cells in the median raphe. In contrast, dark pulse exposure during the subjective night did not reset SCN-controlled behavioral rhythms and caused a transient suppression of neuronal activation in the TH. Collectively these results demonstrate, for the first time, pronounced circadian control of orexin neuron activation and implicate recruitment of orexin cells in dark pulse resetting of the SCN circadian clock.

## 7.1 BACKGROUND

The mammalian hypothalamus plays a fundamental role in the control of numerous critical brain and behavior states. For example, within the suprachiasmatic nuclei (SCN), site of the brain's dominant circadian clock, neurons orchestrate daily rhythms responsible for a wide range of physiological and neural processes [1,2]. This SCN circadian clock is synchronized (entrained) by exogenous time cues (zeitgebers) such as varying levels of environmental light (photic stimuli), as well as by so-called nonphotic cues that promote behavioral arousal [3,4]. Photic information is conveyed to the SCN via the retinohypothalamic tract [5,6], while nonphotic stimuli activate pathways originating in the thalamic intergeniculate leaflet (IGL) and the median raphe (MRN) of the brain stem [7,8]. Unfortunately, our understanding of how neural substrates integrate circadian and arousal information is far from complete.

Recently, significant progress was made in identifying the neurochemical basis of arousal with the isolation and characterization of the orexin/

hypocretin neuropeptides (referred to as orexins in this study) [9,10]. There are two bioactive forms, orexin-A (OXA) and orexin-B, which are cleaved from the common precursor prepro-orexin. The orexins are mainly excitatory and mediate their biological actions through two G-protein coupled receptors, OXR1 and OXR2. In mammals, neurons expressing orexins are mostly limited to the lateral hypothalamic area and dorsomedial nucleus of the tuberal hypothalamus (TH). Immunohistochemical studies have established that these orexin-containing neurons have extensive neuronal projections and innervate key circadian structures including the SCN, IGL and MRN [11-13].

SCN efferents project to the TH [14] and may directly contact orexin-containing cells [15]. Transgenic and pharmacological impairment of orexin-OXR1/R2 signaling implicates this neuropeptide system in the promotion of arousal and wakefulness [16]. Indeed, orexin neurons demonstrate diurnal variation in activity/activation, with highest levels in nocturnal animals occurring during the night [17,18]. Since orexin neuronal activation corresponds with forward locomotor activity [19,20], and because such behavior increases at night, it is unclear whether SCN-derived signals regulate the nighttime activation of orexin neurons.

In this study, using c-Fos as a marker of cellular activation, we demonstrate that under constant light (LL), a condition that suppresses the amplitude of wheel-running rhythms, TH cells including OXA-immunoreactive (OXA-ir) neurons are much more active during the subjective night than the subjective day. We also show that activation of OXA-ir neurons in the medial TH occurs prior to the nocturnal onset of vigorous wheel-running. Transient exposure to 6 h of darkness during the subjective day promotes arousal, suppresses c-Fos expression in the SCN and activates OXA-ir neurons, particularly those in the medial TH. Such changes in arousal and cellular activity accompany the resetting actions of this dark pulse stimulus at this time. These results implicate SCN-derived signals in exerting temporal control over TH cells including OXA-ir neurons and highlight extra-SCN actions of an arousal-promoting phase-resetting stimulus.

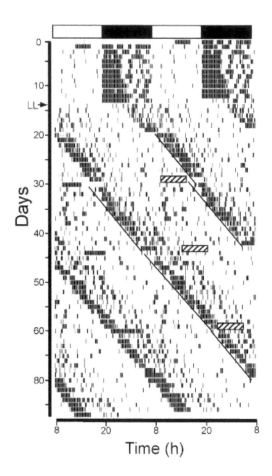

**FIGURE 1:** Dark pulses phase-dependently phase-reset murine wheel-running rhythms. Double-plotted wheel-running actogram showing the effects of diurnal (LD) and constant light (LL) lighting regimes and 6 h dark pulses (hatched boxes) on the behavioral activity of a C57BL/6J mouse. Horizontal bar at the top of the actogram depicts the lights-on (unfilled) and lights-off (filled) cycle. Arrow indicates the transfer from LD to LL and black bars indicate locomotion in a running-wheel equipped cage. The solid black lines indicate the onset of the main bout of wheel-running activity (in LL; CT12 convention). The first dark pulse was centered at ~CT6 and elicited a 1.27h phase advance. Subsequent dark pulses delivered at ~CT22 and ~CT13 had negligible phase-shifting effects.

## 7.2 RESULTS

### 7.2.1 BEHAVIORAL RESULTS

#### 7.2.1.1 EFFECTS OF CONSTANT LIGHT (LL)

Under LD conditions, all singly housed male C57BL/6J mice (n = 92) showed robust diurnal rhythms in wheel-running activity with most of their locomotor activity occurring during the lights-off phase (Figure 1). With the transition from LD to LL, all mice demonstrated an immediate suppression of wheel-running activity. Under LD conditions the average number of wheel revolutions in the 24 h preceding this transition was $15193 \pm 109$ (mean ± SEM), and this was significantly reduced by 81% to $2839 \pm 43$ revolutions during the first 24 h in LL ($p < 0.001$). With prolonged exposure to LL, the period of wheel-running (tau) significantly lengthened from ~24 h to ~24.8 h ($p < 0.001$) and the duration of the active phase (alpha) also significantly increased from ~11.8 h to ~13.1 h ($p < 0.05$) (Table 1). The intensity of wheel-running during alpha was greatly suppressed from ~19.7 in LD to ~5.3 revolutions/min in LL ($p < 0.001$) and the percentage of variance explained by the dominant period of the running-wheel rhythm (PVE) was also significantly reduced from ~67% in LD to ~27% in LL ($p < 0.001$), indicating that the strength of the locomotor rhythm diminished in these conditions (Table 1).

#### 7.2.1.2 DARK PULSE PHASE-RESPONSE CURVE

Twenty-five mice, from the above 92, received dark pulses of 6 h duration at various points in the circadian cycle. Dark pulses centred between mid-subjective day and early subjective night significantly advanced circadian phase (Figures 1, 2). More specifically, pulses initiated between CT3–7 (n = 16) elicited phase shifts with an average magnitude of ~6.17 h. Dark pulses starting between CT7–11 (n = 9) elicited smaller but still significant phase shifts with an average magnitude of ~1.38 h (mean ± 95% confidence intervals (CI) values did not overlap zero). Dark pulses applied at other circadian times, failed to elicit significant phase shifts (mean ± CI values overlapped zero) (Figure 2). In addition to the resetting actions, dark pulse exposure acutely increased wheel-running by ~2.3 km on the day of the pulse. However, this induced activity did not correlate with the resultant phase shift magnitude (Pearson correlation, $p > 0.05$; data not shown), suggesting that the dark pulse elicited increase in wheel-running is not a key factor influencing phase shift magnitude to this stimulus. Interestingly, on the days following the dark pulse, the strength of the wheel-running rhythm was significantly reduced (PVE reduced from 31.1% to 28.6%; $p < 0.05$). Further, although tau and the duration of alpha were not affected by the dark pulse, the intensity of wheel-running during alpha was significantly reduced from ~5.7 to ~4.7 revolutions/min ($p < 0.05$). Taken together, these data (Table 2) indicate that in addition to phasic resetting, dark pulses have prolonged effects on murine behavioral rhythms.

**TABLE 1:** Effects of transition from light-dark to constant light on properties of Murine wheel-running rhythms

| Circadian Parameter | Light-Dark (LD) | Constant Light (LL) |
|---|---|---|
| tau (h) | 24.08 ± 0.03 h | 24.84 ± 0.04 h* |
| Percentage of Variance Explained by the Dominant Rhythmic Component (PV%) | 66.6 ± 1.47 | 26.6 ± 0.98*** |
| Alpha Duration (h) | 11.8 ± 0.15 | 13.1 ± 0.27* |
| Motor Activity (RPM) | 19.7 ± 1.19 | 5.3 ± 0.51*** |

*\*\*\*P < 0.001; \*P < 0.05*

**TABLE 2:** Effects of dark pulses on murine wheel-running rhythms

| Circadian Parameter | Pre-Dark Pulse | Post-Dark Pulse |
|---|---|---|
| tau (h) | 24.77 ± 0.05 | 24.67 ± 0.04 |
| Percentage of Variance Explained by the Dominant Rhythmic Component (PV%) | 31.1 ± 1.6 | 28.6 ± 1.6* |
| Alpha Duration (h) | 12.6 ± 0.5 | 12.4 ± 0.4 |
| Motor Activity (RPM) | 5.71 ± 0.9 | 4.7 ± 0.73* |

*\*p < 0.05*

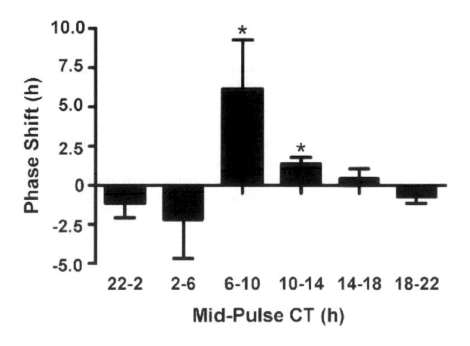

**FIGURE 2:** Phase-response curve to 6 h dark pulses of mouse wheel-running rhythms. Histograms represent mean ± 95% CI. Significant advances were elicited by dark pulses centered between CT6-10 and CT10-14, while pulses centered on the late subjective night/ early subjective day had inconsistent resetting actions.

## 7.2.2 IMMUNOHISTOCHEMISTRY

### 7.2.2.1 CIRCADIAN VARIATION IN EXPRESSION AND ACTIVATION OF OXA NEURONS

Consistent with previous reports in other rodent species [11-13,20,21], OXA-ir was detected within the cytoplasm and processes of a population of hypothalamic neurons. OXA-ir neurons were mostly restricted to the TH, with the lateral TH containing more immunopositive cells than the medial TH. OXA-ir fibres and terminals were found in many brain areas including the PeriSCN region and within the IGL, MRN, and dorsal raphe (DRN) (Additional file 1). Using c-Fos-ir as a marker of neuronal activation, we assessed the numbers of activated cells in the medial and lateral TH as well as within key structures of the neural circadian system. Sections from animals under the LL condition were used as controls against those examined during and after dark pulse exposure. Single-labeled OXA-containing neurons, single-labeled c-Fos-ir, and those OXA-ir neurons double-labeled with c-Fos-ir were counted. In the medial TH, one-way ANOVA indicated a highly significant effect of circadian time on neuronal activation ($F_{6,23} = 8.47$, $p < 0.001$). Planned contrast comparison of the mean c-Fos-ir expression level during subjective day (collapsed across CT5, 6, and 9), with the mean c-Fos-ir expression during subjective night (collapsed across CT16, 17, and 20), revealed a highly significant increase in c-Fos-ir during subjective night ($p < 0.001$; Figure 3A). The number of OXA-ir neurons did not vary as a function of circadian time ($p > 0.05$; Figure 3C), but there was a highly significant effect of circadian time on the number of OXA-ir cells that co-expressed c-Fos-ir ($F6,23 = 4.63$, $p < 0.01$); with more OXA-ir neurons activated during the subjective night than the subjective day ($p < 0.0001$; Figure 3E). A separate comparison of the number of c-Fos-ir OXA neurons at CT9 ($1.2 \pm 0.5$) and CT12 ($7.4 \pm 2.3$) revealed a significant increase ($p < 0.05$) at the transition to subjective night, indicating that activation of OXA cells in the medial TH begins prior to the onset of vigorous wheel-running. c-Fos-ir in non-OXA neurons did not show this pattern of activation ($p > 0.05$).

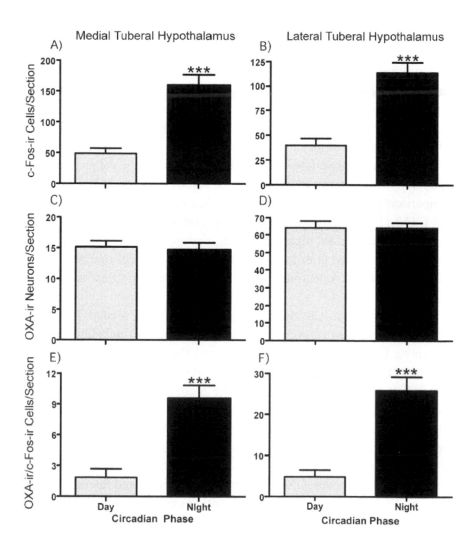

**FIGURE 3:** Circadian day-night profiles of c-Fos and orexin-A expression in the tuberal hypothalamus. The expression of c-Fos-ir was significantly higher during the subjective night (dark filled histograms) compared with the subjective day (gray filled histograms) in both the medial (A) and lateral (B) tuberal hypothalamus. Co-expression of c-Fos with OXA neurons showed a similar temporal relationship in medial (E) and lateral (F) tuberal hypothalamus. The numbers of OXA neurons did not vary from subjective day to night in either the medial (C) or lateral (D) tuberal hypothalamus. Histograms show mean ± SEM. ***p < 0.001.

Similar trends were observed in the lateral TH. Here c-Fos-ir expression varied significantly across the circadian cycle ($F_{6,23}$ = 4.44, p < 0.01) with substantially more activated cells visualized from subjective night time points than from the subjective day (p < 0.001; Figure 3B). The number of OXA-ir neurons did not vary across the circadian cycle in LL (p > 0.05; Figure 3D). However, the number of OXA-ir neurons co-expressing c-Fos-ir varied across the circadian cycle ($F_{6,23}$ = 4.91, p < 0.01), with significantly more double-labeled cells detected during the subjective night compared with the subjective day (p < 0.0001; Figure 3F). A separate comparison of the number of c-Fos-ir OXA neurons at CT9 (4.6 ± 2.5) and CT12 (19.7 ± 5.1) revealed a significant increase (p < 0.05) at the transition to subjective night, indicating that activation of OXA cells in the lateral TH begins prior to the onset of vigorous wheel-running. Again, c-Fos-ir in non-OXA neurons did not show this pattern of activation (p > 0.05).

From these data, it is clear that in the lateral and medial TH, cellular activation displays a pronounced circadian profile (including neurons containing OXA). Parametrically, it appears that the lateral TH has more activated OXA-ir neurons at subjective night than in the medial TH. However, when the data are normalized, the medial TH OXA-ir population shows the greater activation, with double-labeled OXA-ir cells rising from ~9.5% during the subjective day to ~60% during the subjective night. In the lateral TH, activated OXA-ir cells rose less dramatically, from ~6.4% of OXA-ir neurons during the subjective day to ~37% during the subjective night. Moreover, OXA neurons in the medial and lateral TH (but not non-OXA neurons) express significantly more c-Fos-ir at CT12. Since detection of c-Fos-ir in neurons typically occurs >60 min following an appropriate stimulus [22], these increases cannot be attributable to the commencement of wheel-running at CT12 and instead must be due to a circadian signal. Activity in the SCN of nocturnal mice is high during the behaviorally quiescent subjective day and low during the active subjective night. Available data indicate that SCN output signals suppress locomotor activity during the day, with the decline of this output at late day/early subjective night permitting locomotor activity. Therefore, the maximal levels of c-Fos/OXA co-expression seen around the mid-subjective night are presumably due to the combined actions of circadian disinhibition and feedback from behavioral arousal including forward locomotion.

## 7.2.3 DO DARK PULSES ACTIVATE OREXIN NEURONS?

We examined whether a stimulus, which promotes arousal and phase-dependent SCN resetting, could alter cellular activation within the medial and/or lateral TH. This was established by administering a 6 h dark pulse, initiated at either CT5 or 16, and determining the expression of c-Fos-ir in both OXA-ir positive and negative cells. At these timepoints, the SCN is most and least responsive respectively, to the phase-resetting actions of a dark pulse (see dark pulse PRC above). Mice dark pulsed at CT5 were sampled 1 h (CT6) and 4 h (CT9) following pulse onset, and 1 h after reinstatement of light (CT12). Animals dark pulsed at CT16 were sampled 1 h (CT17) and 4 h (CT20) following the onset of dark. All sets of tissue were compared to time-matched unpulsed LL controls. Representative photomicrographs showing c-Fos-ir and OXA-ir the medial and lateral TH at CT6 and CT9 under unpulsed and pulsed conditions are shown in Figure 4. In all samples, the number of detectable OXA-ir cells did not change significantly between animals or lighting condition (data not shown).

In the medial TH, dark pulse exposure at CT5, significantly elevated c-Fos-ir 4 h (CT9) into the pulse ($p < 0.05$; Figure 5A), but not at other timepoints (CT6 and CT12) examined. In the lateral TH, dark pulse exposure had no significant effects on c-Fos-ir at these timepoints (Figure 5B). In comparison, in medial and lateral TH, the number of OXA-ir neurons expressing c-Fos increased significantly at both the CT6 and CT9 analysis time-points (medial TH: $p < 0.01$ and $p < 0.05$ respectively and lateral TH: both $p < 0.05$ respectively; Figures. 4C–J and 5C, D). Further, the extent of co-localization differed modestly between areas. More than half the total medial OXA-ir cells (~58%) became activated during the pulse, whereas ~40% of lateral TH OXA-ir cells were activated. Additionally, the finding that non-OXA-ir cells in medial TH become activated by this stimulus, establishes that dark pulse activation is a feature exhibited by many cells types in this part of the hypothalamus.

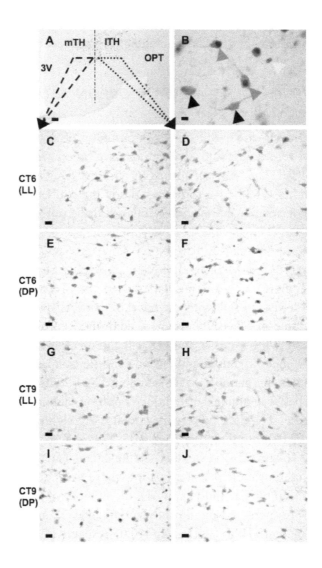

**FIGURE 4:** Mid-subjective day dark pulses activate orexin-A neurons in the tuberal hypothalamus. Photomicrographs illustrating c-Fos-ir and OXA-ir cells as well as c-Fos/OXA double-labeled cells within the TH. Panel (A) shows a low magnification representation of the regions shown in subsequent panels. Panel (B) shows OXA-ir cells (black arrows), a c-Fos-ir nucleus (light gray arrow) and c-Fos/OXA double-labeled cells (red arrows) within the TH at high magnification. 3 V = third ventricle; lTH = lateral tuberal hypothalamus; mTH = medial tuberal hypothalamus; OPT = optic tract. Calibration bars = 100 μm (A), 10 μm (B), 25 μm (C-J).

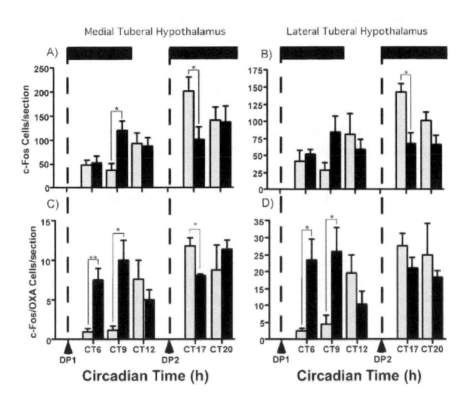

**FIGURE 5:** Circadian and dark pulse regulation of orexin-A and non-orexin-A neuronal activation in the tuberal hypothalamus. c-Fos expression (A) and c-Fos co-expression in OXA neurons (C) are increased in the medial TH by a dark pulse (DP1; onset indicated by the left vertical broken line at DP1 arrowhead, while the 6 h duration of DP1 is shown as the filled horizontal bar top left) beginning at CT5, while after 1 h exposure to a 6 h dark pulse (DP2; beginning at the right broken vertical line and arrowhead at CT16 with the 6 h duration, depicted by the filed horizontal bar top right) suppresses c-Fos and c-Fos/OXA co-expression. In the lateral TH c-Fos expression is not altered by the subjective day dark pulse (B), but co-expression of c-Fos with OXA neurons is elevated 1 h and 4 h into the pulse (D). By contrast, c-Fos expression in the subjective night in the lateral TH is suppressed within 2 h (B); co-expression of c-Fos with OXA was unaffected. Histograms show mean ± SEM. **p < 0.01, *p < 0.05.

For animals that were exposed to a dark pulse beginning at CT16, no significant change in total c-Fos-ir was detected in the medial TH at any time-point sampled. However, there was a significant suppression of OXA-ir activated cells at 1 h (CT17) after pulse initiation (p < 0.01; Figure 5C) with the proportion of activated OXA-ir cells reducing from ~60% to ~52%. Conversely, lateral TH expression of c-Fos-ir was significantly reduced 1 h (CT17) but not 4 h (CT20) into the pulse (p < 0.05; Figure 5B). There was no effect on activated OXA cells at either CT (Figure 5D). Overall, a dark pulse centered around the end of the subjective night modestly, and transiently, suppressed OXA activation in the medial TH, while reducing non-OXA cell activation levels in the lateral TH.

## 7.2.4 EFFECT OF A DARK PULSE ON C-FOS-IR WITHIN THE SCN, IGL, MRN AND DRN STRUCTURES

Since OXA-ir neurons of the TH are anatomically linked to many components of the neural circadian system, including the SCN, IGL, MRN, and DRN, we assessed if the activational state of cells in these regions varied in response to a dark pulse beginning at CT5. In unpulsed LL controls at CT6 and CT9, c-Fos-ir was spontaneously expressed throughout all levels of the SCN. At 4 h, but not 1 h, into the 6 h dark pulse, c-Fos-ir in the SCN was significantly reduced (unpaired t-test, p < 0.01 Figure 6A). Qualitatively, the area most prominently suppressed by the dark pulse appeared to be the rostral SCN and preliminary inspections indicated both 'core' and 'shell' regions [23] of the mid-rostrocaudal SCN were similarly affected by the dark pulse (data not shown). In both the IGL and DRN, small but non-significant increases in c-Fos-ir were coincident with dark pulse exposure (Figure 6B, C). More robust changes in cellular activation were observed within the MRN, where the number of c-Fos-ir cells became significantly elevated 4 h into the dark pulse (unpaired t-test, p < 0.01; Figure 6D). Collectively, these data indicate that a dark pulse given during the subjective day significantly and differentially affects cell activation in the neural circadian system, specifically suppressing SCN cells while activating MRN cells.

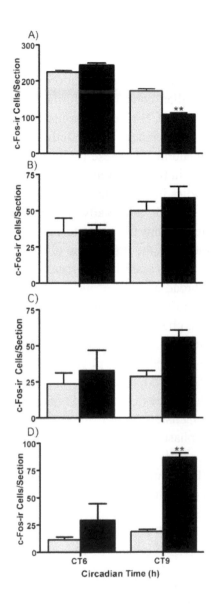

**FIGURE 6:** Mid-subjective day dark pulses suppress the suprachiasmatic nuclei and activate the median raphe. Histograms show expression of c-Fos (mean ± SEM) at CT6 and CT9 in constant light (gray-filled histograms) and 1 h and 4 h into a 6 h dark pulse beginning at CT5 (black-filled histograms) in the SCN (A), IGL (B), DRN (C), and MRN (D). **p < 0.01.

## 7.3 DISCUSSION

This study demonstrates unequivocally that orexin neuronal activation is under pronounced circadian control and further that orexin neurons are selectively activated by an SCN-resetting arousal-promoting stimulus. We also highlight potential differences in the activation state of orexin neurons in the medial and lateral TH. These findings reveal new complexities of SCN-TH interactions in the regulation of brain states and behavior.

Consistent with studies in Syrian hamster and Swiss mouse, we found that a 6 h dark pulse robustly phase-advances C57BL/6J wheel-running rhythms when initiated during the mid- to late subjective day [24-30]. Further, our observation that the magnitude of dark pulse-evoked wheel-running activity does not necessarily correlate with the magnitude of the phase shift is also in broad agreement with other studies [31-33]. Previously, dark pulses given during the late subjective night/early subjective day were found to elicit phase-delays in Syrian hamster and Swiss mouse wheel-running rhythms [24-26]. Although we did observe that some C57BL/6J mice phase-delayed to dark pulses given at this time of the circadian cycle (see Figures 2 and 3), delays were not consistently evoked. This discrepancy is likely to be due to a bona fide species-related difference, as we found that Syrian hamsters housed under identical conditions invariably show significant phase-delays to 6 h dark pulses beginning around CT16 and extending to early subjective day [26]. Collectively, these data suggest that the C57BL/6J mouse is more readily phase-advanced than phase-delayed by 6 h dark pulses.

Our study complements and extends earlier research in which temporal variation in orexin cell activation was determined primarily under diurnal conditions [20,34,35] or limited (two time points) circadian sampling frequencies [17]. Under LL conditions in which the amplitude and intensity of murine wheel-running are greatly suppressed, we detected a highly significant circadian profile in the levels of activated of OXA-ir and non-OXA-ir neurons in the medial and lateral TH. Here, neurons demonstrated substantially higher levels of c-Fos-ir during the subjective night phase. Interestingly, we detected significant (but sub-maximal) increases in OXA-ir/c-Fos-ir double-labeled neurons in both the medial and lateral

TH at CT12 compared to CT9. Because detection of c-Fos-ir in neurons typically occurs ~60 min following an appropriate stimulus, this is evidence that OXA cells are not simply reactive to the initiation of locomotor activity at CT12 and are subject to genuine circadian control. However, because maximal levels of OXA activation are not seen until the mid subjective night (when locomotor activity is well established) (see Figure 5C, D) it is likely that behavioral feedback mechanisms further activate OXA cells. This circadian pattern of orexin neuron activation is consistent with the circadian profile of orexin detected in the cerebrospinal fluid of nocturnal rodents; the amplitude of which is suppressed by exposure to LL and abolished in SCN-lesioned animals [36,37]. This indicates that c-Fos-labelling as a marker of neuronal activation corresponds with the release of OXA.

The effects of dark exposure during the mid-subjective day on c-Fos-ir expression in the circadian system support earlier findings from Syrian hamster [27]. A significant suppression of c-Fos-ir in the SCN was detected during the daytime dark pulse. This was accompanied by activation of MRN neurons, OXA-ir and non-OXA-ir neurons in the medial TH, and OXA-ir neurons in the lateral TH. Projections from cells in the IGL and MRN to the SCN are both important for the phase-advancing actions of various non-photic stimuli [3,8,38]. However, we observed that unlike the MRN, daytime dark pulses did not robustly activate neurons in the IGL and DRN. This suggests that cells in MRN are more involved in dark pulse evoked phase shifts than those of the IGL or DRN. Consistent with this interpretation, Coogan and Piggins [27] did not observe significant increases in c-Fos-ir labeling in the hamster IGL following a daytime dark pulse. Similarly, Harrington and Rusak [28] found that IGL lesions do not abolish the resetting actions of dark pulses in Syrian hamsters. Although other non-photic stimuli, such as running in a novel wheel, can induce c-Fos-ir in the hamster IGL [39,40], activation of the geniculo-hypothalamic tract (GHT) does not appear to be critical for dark-pulse evoked phase advances. Electrical stimulation of GABA and serotonin containing-neurons in the MRN reduces light-evoked c-Fos-ir in the SCN and similar effects have been documented with exogenous application of serotonergic or GABAergic agonists into the SCN [8,41-43]. Moreover, analogous to daytime dark pulses, serotonergic agonists given during the subjective day phase advance rodent wheel-running rhythms and suppress clock gene expression in the rodent SCN [44,45]. Further, serotonergic agonists given during the subjective day can potentiate dark pulse evoked phase advances, supporting the contention that the MRN-SCN pathway is involved dark pulse resetting of circadian rhythms [45].

Within the TH, our results suggest functional differences in the circadian and photic regulation of both orexin and non-orexin neuronal groups. Cells in the TH demonstrated circadian variation in c-Fos-ir expression, and in the degree of activated OXA-ir neurons. In the medial and lateral TH, the basal level of OXA-ir activation during the subjective day is similar (~10% and ~7% respectively), but across subjective night, the medial TH OXA-ir cells show a larger activation, with ~60% containing c-Fos-ir while ~42% of lateral OXA are activated. When exposed to a 6 h dark pulse during the subjective day, it is also the medial TH that expresses the largest increase in the proportion of OXA-ir neurons co-expressing c-Fos-ir. Complementary findings have been published recently by Webb et al. [40] who report that hamsters confined to running wheels (an arousal-inducing procedure) demonstrate a greater proportion of OXA-ir/c-Fos-ir double-labeled cells in medial TH areas compared with lateral TH areas.

Intriguingly, dark pulse exposure at subjective night causes a small but significant decrease in OXA-ir/c-Fos-ir co-localization in the medial TH, without affecting the activational state of non-OXA-ir cells. A different pattern is seen in the lateral TH; here it is the non-OXA-ir cells whose activation is suppressed, while the OXA-ir neurons are not significantly affected. These data support suggestions that different populations of orexin neurons undergo differential tonic regulation and respond differently to various stimuli [17,46,47]. Here, activation of OXA neurons in the medial TH appears more tightly linked to circadian regulation of behavioral arousal than those located laterally. This may be a reflection of the extensive innervation of medial hypothalamic sites by SCN efferents and/or their proximity to the third ventricle, in which cerebrospinal fluid borne SCN-derived signals can be communicated [48]. Additionally, SCN-controlled peripheral signals such as corticosterone can potentially alter orexin cellular activity [49].

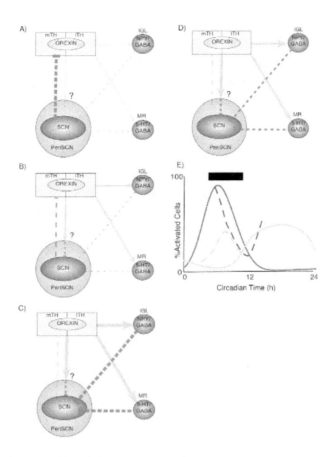

**Figure 7.** Circadian and dark pulse regulation of orexin cellular activation. (A) Mid-subjective day: inhibitory output (broken red lines) from the SCN is high, with cells in the medial (mTH) and lateral tuberal hypothalamus (lTH), including orexin neurons, minimally active with little/no excitatory outputs (green arrows) to the IGL and median raphe (MR) whose cellular activity/output is also low. Orexin efferents may (?) act via the PeriSCN to suppress SCN activity [53]. (B) Late subjective day: SCN inhibitory output reduced, orexin cells submaximally activated, with increased excitatory output to the PeriSCN, IGL, and MR. (C) Mid-subjective night: SCN inhibitory output minimal, orexin cellular activation maximal. Increased excitatory input to the PeriSCN, IGL and MR increases inhibitory outputs to the SCN. (D) Dark pulse at mid-subjective day interrupts retinal input, reducing SCN activity and its inhibition of the mTH and lTH. Disinhibited orexin cells excite PeriSCN, IGL and MR neurons whose outputs suppress the SCN. (E) Circadian variation in SCN (blue line) and orexin (green line) activation and the effects of a daytime dark pulse (timing and duration indicated by filled horizontal box) on this activation (broken lines). In (A-D), the width of the lines indicates the level of excitatory or inhibitory signal. NPY = neuropeptide Y; 5-HT = serotonin; GABA = γ-aminobutyric acid.

Orexin neurons are ideally positioned to integrate arousal and circadian cues. The results of the present study, as well as those of other researchers, indicates that the pronounced difference in the activation state of orexin neurons from the quiescent subjective day to the behaviorally active night, is likely caused by both circadian influences and arousal/behavioral feedback. During the subjective day, SCN neuronal activity is maximal and, as the SCN output signal is believed to be predominantly inhibitory, acts to suppress other brain areas including the TH (Figure 7A, E). When neuronal activity in the SCN declines, as seen before subjective night, there is a significant rise in c-fos expression in orexin cells which occurs at least 1 h prior to the onset of vigorous subjective nighttime wheel-running (Figure 7B, E). Together, the alteration in SCN input results in a disinhibition of orexin neurons leading to arousal and priming of the animals behavior for waking. Further sustained activation of orexin neurons during the subjective night arises through behavioral feedback and activation of IGL-SCN and MRN-SCN pathways, which in turn, facilitate sustained suppression of the SCN (Figure 7C, E). Accordingly, the cessation of subjective night develops through increased SCN neuronal output through the late night and early subjective day.

Phase-shifting actions of dark pulses can also be explained by similar mechanisms. Application of a daytime dark pulse causes an interruption of the excitatory photic input to the SCN, which results in reduced inhibitory output drive from the SCN. The consequence of this is disinhibition and activation of the orexin cells, and other neuronal populations, to promote arousal and behavioral feedback (Figure 7D, E). The latter effect activates the MRN-SCN pathway, leading to further suppression of SCN neurons. Termination of the dark pulse restores the excitatory light input to the SCN, activating SCN cells and elevating inhibitory output signals to many brain regions, ending neuronal activation in orexin and non-orexin cells. Based on our present data, we predict that MRN-SCN projections are more important than IGL-SCN projections under these conditions. This is in contrast to other arousal promoting non-photic stimuli, such as novelty induced locomotion, for which the GHT projection between the IGL and the SCN appears critical for clock resetting [32].

An additional contributing factor to the phase resetting actions of daytime dark pulses is sleep deprivation. In Syrian hamsters, it is reported that it is sleep deprivation occurring during the dark pulse rather than wheel-running activity that determines phase-resetting to this stimulus [33]. Here, in our study on mice, wheel-running activity during the pulse does not correlate with the magnitude of the phase shift. However, in a small cohort of mice (n = 4) visually monitored with infra-red goggles during the dark pulse given CT5–11, we found that the mice rested a lot less and engaged in many more active behaviors (general exploration, cage-top climbing, etc) than had been recorded in these same animals over CT5–11 in LL conditions (Marston and Piggins, unpublished observations). Since orexin release is enhanced by sleep deprivation [50], this indicates another mechanism via which dark pulses can regulate these and other TH cells.

OXA may also have other direct and indirect effects on SCN neuronal activity. For example, in addition to innervating the IGL and MRN, OXA-ir fibres project to the Peri-SCN region [12,51] and OX1R protein is detectable within the rat SCN [52]. This raises the possibility that locally released OXA may act on the SCN. Indeed, we recently showed that OXA and OXB can alter rat SCN neuronal activity in vitro, with some actions involving recruitment of GABAergic mechanisms [53]. Such actions of locally released orexins on the SCN may feedback to modulate TH cellular activity since one study has described SCN projections to OXA neurons [15].

## 7.4 CONCLUSION

Collectively, our findings raise the possibility that activation of OXA neurons is involved in resetting of the SCN circadian clock and further allude to the pathway from the MRN to the SCN being functionally more important than the GHT for dark pulse-induced phase-shifting. Moreover, our findings identify at least two separate populations of OXA neurons that are differentially activated by endogenous and exogenous cues, thereby enabling the orexin system to collectively 'multitask' and coordinate appropriate physiological and behavioral states.

## 7.5 METHODS

Adult male C57BL/6J mice were purchased from Harlan (Loughborough, UK). All procedures were carried out in accordance the Animal (Scientific Procedures) act, 1986 (UK). Animals were initially group housed (6–8 animals per cage) for 1–2 weeks under a 12 h:12 h light/dark cycle (LD; lights-on 07:00) before being individually housed in running wheel-equipped (stainless steel, 16 cm diameter, North Kent Plastics, Kent, UK) polycarbon cages (overall dimensions 45 cm × 21 cm × 19 cm). Individually housed mice were kept under 12 h:12 h LD cycle for a further 10 days and then released into constant light (LL; light intensity at cage level ~100 lux) to establish stable free-running activity rhythms for at least 10 circadian cycles prior to experimental procedures. Food (B&K Universal, Hull, UK) and water were available ad libitum in all conditions.

Each revolution of the running wheel depressed an externally mounted microswitch, the activation of which was recorded and counted via a PC using the collect module of the Chronobiology Kit software suite (Stanford Software Systems, Santa Cruz, CA, USA). Actograms of wheel-running rhythms and wheel revolution counts were produced with the Analyze 9 module (Stanford Software Systems). Changes in endogenous period (tau) under LD and LL conditions were estimated by the chi-square periodogram. Wheel-running activity rhythms were visualized offline as double-plotted actograms. The El Temps programme (Dr. Noguerra, University of Barcelona, Barcelona, Spain) was used to measure a number of key properties of the wheel-running rhythm and to determine the effects of exposure to LL and dark pulses (see [26] for further details).

### 7.5.1 DARK PULSE PHASE-RESPONSE CURVE

To generate a phase-response curve (PRC) to dark pulses, mice (n = 25) were given a 6 h dark pulse every 10–16 days at various points across the circadian cycle. Dark pulses were initiated by turning off the room lights for 6 h and terminated by reinstatement of light. Animals remained undisturbed in their home cages throughout the dark pulse. All animals received at least one dark pulse, with some animals receiving up to 3 pulses over 60 circadian cycles.

Steady state phase shifts were independently assessed by three experienced researchers (two blind to experimental conditions) using the line of best-fit method [25,27,54]. Briefly, two lines of best fit were drawn through the onsets of wheel-running activity (CT12 by convention). The first line delineated activity onset (CT12) over the 7 cycles prior to the dark pulse. This line was extrapolated to predict CT12 on the first cycle following the pulse. The second line identified activity onset over the 7–10 cycles following the dark pulse (for the purposes of line-fitting, circadian cycles containing transients were discounted from this process). Interpolation of the second line also allowed CT12 to be predicted on the first cycle following the dark pulse. The difference (in min) between the CT12 values obtained by extrapolation and interpolation was taken to be the steady state phase shift elicited by the dark pulse. Animals with unstable behavioral rhythms were excluded from analysis.

Steady state phase shifts in response to dark pulses across the circadian cycle were initially graphed on a scatterplot to aid visualization. For analysis, phase shift data were grouped into 4 h bins (e.g. dark pulses centered between CT2–6, 6–10 etc). Each bin contained at least 6 data points (range n = 6–16) with no animal contributing more than a single data point to any individual CT bin. Where an animal received more than a single pulse within a specific 4 h period the values were averaged to provide a single value. The relationship between intensity of wheel-running activity induced by a subjective day dark pulse and the magnitude of resulting phase shifts was examined by parametric correlation.

## 7.5.2 IMMUNOHISTOCHEMISTRY

In the immunolabeling experiment, mice (n = 67) were sampled either in LL (for use as time-matched unpulsed controls), or at 1 h or 4 h into a 6 h dark pulse (initiated at either CT5 or CT16). In addition, some mice were sampled 1 h after cessation of the CT5 dark pulse (CT12). Animals were culled by cervical dislocation and decapitation under halothane anesthesia.

Brains were carefully removed from the skull and placed in fixative [4% paraformaldehyde in 0.1 M phosphate buffer (PB)] for 4 days at 4°C. Following cryoprotection (30% sucrose in 0.1 M PB solution), brains were rapidly frozen with crushed dry ice and mounted onto the cryostage of a sledge microtome (Series 8000, Bright Instruments Ltd., Huntingdon, UK) and cut into 30 μm thick coronal sections (four serial sets of sections per brain).

Free-floating sections were washed 3 × 10 min in 0.1 M PB then incubated for 20 min in 1.5% hydrogen peroxide made in 0.1 M PB (Sigma, Poole, UK) to remove endogenous peroxidase activity. Sections were washed (3 × 10 min in 0.1 M PB) and subsequently incubated for 60 min in a blocking solution of 5% normal donkey serum (NDS; Sigma, Poole, UK) in 0.1 M PB; then transferred into the primary antibody (made up in 5% NDS) for 36–48 h at 4°C. The primary antibodies used were polyclonal goat anti-orexin-A (1:1000; Santa Cruz Biotechnology, Santa Cruz, CA, USA) and polyclonal rabbit anti-c-Fos (1:8000; Santa Cruz Biotechnology).

After incubation the sections were returned to room temperature (22°C) and washed in 0.1 M PB (3 × 10 min) before addition for 90 min in an appropriate biotinylated IgG secondary antibody (1:400 donkey anti-goat or 1:400 donkey anti-rabbit in 0.1 M PB; Jackson Immunoresearch, West Grove, PA, USA). Sections were washed (3 × 10 min in 0.1 M PB) then transferred to avidin-biotin complex (ABC) solution (1:200; Vector Laboratories, Peterborough, UK) for 90 min. Slices were then prepared for enzymatic detection after two further 10 min 0.1 M PB washes. For c-Fos-ir development, sections were placed for 10 min in a 0.1 M sodium acetate solution (pH 6.0) and then exposed to a nickel-intensified diaminobenzidine chromagen (NiDAB). The reaction was catalyzed with 0.015% glucose oxidase (Sigma), yielding a blue/black reaction stain. For OXA-ir double-labeling, sections were returned to 1.5% hydrogen peroxide before being rerun in the previous steps with the corresponding primary and secondary antibody until enzymatic detection. Diaminobenzidine chromagen without nickel intensification (DAB), catalyzed with 0.015% hydrogen peroxide produced a red/brown reaction product indicating OXA detection. The reaction was quenched in dH$_2$O. Stained sections were rinsed in ~0.005 M PB and mounted onto gelatin coated slides and air-dried. They were then dehydrated through a series of graded ethanol baths (70%, 95% and 2 × 100%), cleared in Histoclear (National Diagnostics, Hull, UK) and air-dried before coverslipping.

Sections were visually inspected under an Olympus BX-50 microscope and photographed with an attached digital camera (Olympus c-4000 z). High resolution digital images of representative rostral, intermediate and caudal SCN, IGL, MRN and DRN sections were taken and imported into Microsoft PowerPoint (XP edition; Microsoft, Seattle, WA, USA). The SCN, IGL, MRN and DRN were delineated from adjacent neuroanatomical structures with reference to a stereotaxic atlas [55] and a series of cresyl violet stained C57BL/6J brain sections (provided by Dr David Cutler). Another experienced researcher confirmed accuracy of neuroanatomical delineation. OXA-ir neurons and c-Fos-ir nuclei were counted directly under microscope examination. Two sections (both hemispheres) per rostral, mid- and caudal level of the TH were analyzed from each animal (6 sections/animal). Using a modification of the medial/lateral subdivisions described by other researchers [17,46], we divided the TH into two major divisions, medial and lateral, defined by two counting boxes (each 1.05 mm in height × 0.7 mm in width) corresponding to stereotaxic coordinates from [55] with the medial box: ~4.7—~5.75 mm height × ~0.7 mm from midline; and the lateral box: ~4.7—~5.75 mm height × ~0.7—~1.4 mm from midline) single-labeled and co-localized cells were counted (See additional file 2). All counts were conducted blind to experimental conditions and verified by an independent researcher experienced in cellular and nuclear counting techniques. Immunostaining is expressed as average values/animal/timepoint.

## 7.5.3 STATISTICAL ANALYSIS

To evaluate the effects of constant light on key features of the wheel-running rhythms we used paired t-tests. To determine the significance of phase shifts to dark pulses, we collapsed the data into 4 h circadian time bins and compared the mean ± 95% confidence interval with 0 min shift and interpreted the absence of an overlap as significant. One way analysis of variance was used for evaluating the significance of circadian time on c-

Fos and OXA cellular labeling, with planned comparisons of mean levels at day-night phases. Unpaired t-tests were used as described. The JMP version 6 (SAS Institute, Cary, NC) and Prism Graphpad version 4 (Graphpad Software Inc. San Diego, CA) software packages were used for statistics and construction of graphs.

## REFERENCES

1.  Morin LP, Allen CN: The circadian visual system, 2005. Brain Res Rev 2006, 51(1):1-60.
2.  Rusak B, Zucker I: Neural regulation of circadian rhythms. Physiol Rev 1979, 59(3):449-526.
3.  Mrosovsky N: Locomotor activity and non-photic influences on circadian clocks. Biol Rev Camb Philos Soc 1996, 71(3):343-372.
4.  Mistlberger RE, Skene DJ: Nonphotic entrainment in humans? J Biol Rhythms 2005, 20(4):339-352.
5.  Hannibal J: Neurotransmitters of the retino-hypothalamic tract. Cell Tissue Res 2002, 309(1):73-88.
6.  Berson DM: Strange vision: ganglion cells as circadian photoreceptors. Trends Neurosci 2003, 26(6):314-320.
7.  Harrington ME: The ventral lateral geniculate nucleus and the intergeniculate leaflet: interrelated structures in the visual and circadian systems. Neurosci Biobehav Rev 1997, 21(5):705-727.
8.  Morin LP: Serotonin and the regulation of mammalian circadian rhythmicity. Ann Med 1999, 31(1):12-33.
9.  de Lecea L, Kilduff TS, Peyron C, Gao X, Foye PE, Danielson PE, Fukuhara C, Battenberg EL, Gautvik VT, Bartlett FS 2nd, et al.: The hypocretins: hypothalamus-specific peptides with neuroexcitatory activity. Proc Natl Acad Sci USA 1998, 95(1):322-327.
10. Sakurai T, Amemiya A, Ishii M, Matsuzaki I, Chemelli RM, Tanaka H, Williams SC, Richardson JA, Kozlowski GP, Wilson S, et al.: Orexins and orexin receptors: a family of hypothalamic neuropeptides and G protein-coupled receptors that regulate feeding behavior. Cell 1998, 92(4):573-585.
11. Cutler DJ, Morris R, Sheridhar V, Wattam TA, Holmes S, Patel S, Arch JR, Wilson S, Buckingham RE, Evans ML, et al.: Differential distribution of orexin-A and orexin-B immunoreactivity in the rat brain and spinal cord. Peptides 1999, 20(12):1455-1470.
12. McGranaghan PA, Piggins HD: Orexin A-like immunoreactivity in the hypothalamus and thalamus of the Syrian hamster (Mesocricetus auratus) and Siberian hamster (Phodopus sungorus), with special reference to circadian structures. Brain Res 2001, 904(2):234-244.

13. Peyron C, Tighe DK, Pol AN, de Lecea L, Heller HC, Sutcliffe JG, Kilduff TS: Neurons containing hypocretin (orexin) project to multiple neuronal systems. J Neurosci 1998, 18(23):9996-10015.
14. Deurveilher S, Semba K: Indirect projections from the suprachiasmatic nucleus to major arousal-promoting cell groups in rat: Implications for the circadian control of behavioural state. Neuroscience 2005, 130(1):165-183.
15. Abrahamson EE, Leak RK, Moore RY: The suprachiasmatic nucleus projects to posterior hypothalamic arousal systems. Neuroreport 2001, 12(2):435-440.
16. Nishino S, Sakarai T, Eds.: The orexin/hypocretin system: Physiology and pathophysiology. Totowa, New Jersey: Humana Press; 2006.
17. Estabrooke IV, McCarthy MT, Ko E, Chou TC, Chemelli RM, Yanagisawa M, Saper CB, Scammell TE: Fos expression in orexin neurons varies with behavioral state. J Neurosci 2001, 21(5):1656-1662.
18. Espana RA, Scammell TE: Orexin and hypothalamic control of sleeping and waking. In The Orexin/hypocretin system: Physiology and and pathophysiology. Edited by Nishino S, Sakurai T. Totowa, New Jersey: Humana Press; 2006:189-207.
19. Mileykovskiy BY, Kiyashchenko LI, Siegel JM: Behavioral correlates of activity in identified hypocretin/orexin neurons. Neuron 2005, 46(5):787-798.
20. Nixon JP, Smale L: Individual differences in wheel-running rhythms are related to temporal and spatial patterns of activation of orexin A and B cells in a diurnal rodent (Arvicanthis niloticus). Neuroscience 2004, 127(1):25-34.
21. Mintz EM, Pol AN, Casano AA, Albers HE: Distribution of hypocretin-(orexin) immunoreactivity in the central nervous system of Syrian hamsters (Mesocricetus auratus). J Chem Neuroanat 2001, 21(3):225-238.
22. Sharp FR, Sagar SM, Hicks K, Lowenstein D, Hisanaga K: c-fos mRNA, Fos, and Fos-related antigen induction by hypertonic saline and stress. J Neurosci 1991, 11(8):2321-2331.
23. Yan L, Silver R: Differential induction and localization of mPer1 and mPer2 during advancing and delaying phase shifts. Eur J Neurosci 2002, 16(8):1531-1540.
24. Barbacka-Surowiak G: Is the PRC for dark pulses in LL a mirror image of light pulses in DD in mice? Biol Rhythm Res 2000, 31:531-544.
25. Boulos Z, Rusak B: Circadian phase response curve for dark pulses in hamsters. J Comp Physiol [A] 1982, 146:411-417.
26. Canal MM, Piggins HD: Resetting of the hamster circadian system by dark pulses. Am J Physiol Regul Integr Comp Physiol 2006, 290(3):R785-792.
27. Coogan AN, Piggins HD: Dark pulse suppression of P-ERK and c-Fos in the hamster suprachiasmatic nuclei. Eur J Neurosci 2005, 22(1):158-168.
28. Harrington ME, Rusak B: Lesions of the thalamic intergeniculate leaflet alter hamster circadian rhythms. J Biol Rhythms 1986, 1(4):309-325.
29. Ellis GB, McKlveen RE, Turek FW: Dark pulses affect the circadian rhythm of activity in hamsters kept in constant light. Am J Physiol 1982, 242(1):R44-50.
30. Mendoza JY, Dardente H, Escobar C, Pevet P, Challet E: Dark pulse resetting of the suprachiasmatic clock in Syrian hamsters: behavioral phase-shifts and clock gene expression. Neuroscience 2004, 127(2):529-537.

31. Antle MC, Mistlberger RE: Circadian clock resetting by sleep deprivation without exercise in the Syrian hamster. J Neurosci 2000, 20(24):9326-9332.

32. Biello SM, Janik D, Mrosovsky N: Neuropeptide Y and behaviorally induced phase shifts. Neuroscience 1994, 62(1):273-279.

33. Mistlberger RE, Belcourt J, Antle MC: Circadian clock resetting by sleep deprivation without exercise in Syrian hamsters: dark pulses revisited. J Biol Rhythms 2002, 17(3):227-237.

34. Espana RA, Valentino RJ, Berridge CW: Fos immunoreactivity in hypocretin-synthesizing and hypocretin-1 receptor-expressing neurons: effects of diurnal and nocturnal spontaneous waking, stress and hypocretin-1 administration. Neuroscience 2003, 121(1):201-217.

35. Martinez GS, Smale L, Nunez AA: Diurnal and nocturnal rodents show rhythms in orexinergic neurons. Brain Res 2002, 955(1–2):1-7.

36. Deboer T, Overeem S, Visser NA, Duindam H, Frolich M, Lammers GJ, Meijer JH: Convergence of circadian and sleep regulatory mechanisms on hypocretin-1. Neuroscience 2004, 129(3):727-732.

37. Zhang S, Zeitzer JM, Yoshida Y, Wisor JP, Nishino S, Edgar DM, Mignot E: Lesions of the suprachiasmatic nucleus eliminate the daily rhythm of hypocretin-1 release. Sleep 2004, 27(4):619-627.

38. Marchant EG, Watson NV, Mistlberger RE: Both neuropeptide Y and serotonin are necessary for entrainment of circadian rhythms in mice by daily treadmill running schedules. J Neurosci 1997, 17(20):7974-7987.

39. Mikkelsen JD, Vrang N, Mrosovsky N: Expression of Fos in the circadian system following nonphotic stimulation. Brain Res Bull 1998, 47(4):367-376.

40. Webb IC, Patton DF, Hamson DK, Mistlberger RE: Neural correlates of arousal-induced circadian clock resetting: hypocretin/orexin and the intergeniculate leaflet. Eur J Neurosci 2008, 27(4):828-835.

41. Gillespie CF, Beek EM, Mintz EM, Mickley NC, Jasnow AM, Huhman KL, Albers HE: GABAergic regulation of light-induced c-Fos immunoreactivity within the suprachiasmatic nucleus. J Comp Neurol 1999, 411(4):683-692.

42. Morin LP, Meyer-Bernstein EL: The ascending serotonergic system in the hamster: comparison with projections of the dorsal and median raphe nuclei. Neuroscience 1999, 91(1):81-105.

43. Pickard GE, Rea MA: Serotonergic innervation of the hypothalamic suprachiasmatic nucleus and photic regulation of circadian rhythms. Biol Cell 1997, 89(8):513-523.

44. Horikawa K, Yokota S, Fuji K, Akiyama M, Moriya T, Okamura H, Shibata S: Nonphotic entrainment by 5-HT1A/7 receptor agonists accompanied by reduced Per1 and Per2 mRNA levels in the suprachiasmatic nuclei. J Neurosci 2000, 20(15):5867-5873.

45. Mendoza J, Clesse D, Pevet P, Challet E: Serotonergic potentiation of dark pulse-induced phase-shifting effects at midday in hamsters. J Neurochem 2008, 106(3):1404-1414.

46. Fadel J, Bubser M, Deutch AY: Differential activation of orexin neurons by antipsychotic drugs associated with weight gain. J Neurosci 2002, 22(15):6742-6746.

47. Satoh S, Matsumura H, Nakajima T, Nakahama K, Kanbayashi T, Nishino S, Yoneda H, Shigeyoshi Y: Inhibition of rostral basal forebrain neurons promotes wakefulness and induces FOS in orexin neurons. Eur J Neurosci 2003, 17(8):1635-1645.

48. Silver R, LeSauter J, Tresco PA, Lehman MN: A diffusible coupling signal from the transplanted suprachiasmatic nucleus controlling circadian locomotor rhythms. Nature 1996, 382(6594):810-813.

49. Ford GK, Al-Barazanji KA, Wilson S, Jones DN, Harbuz MS, Jessop DS: Orexin expression and function: glucocorticoid manipulation, stress, and feeding studies. Endocrinology 2005, 146(9):3724-3731.

50. Yoshida Y, Fujiki N, Nakajima T, Ripley B, Matsumura H, Yoneda H, Mignot E, Nishino S: Fluctuation of extracellular hypocretin-1 (orexin A) levels in the rat in relation to the light-dark cycle and sleep-wake activities. Eur J Neurosci 2001, 14(7):1075-1081.

51. Date Y, Ueta Y, Yamashita H, Yamaguchi H, Matsukura S, Kangawa K, Sakurai T, Yanagisawa M, Nakazato M: Orexins, orexigenic hypothalamic peptides, interact with autonomic, neuroendocrine and neuroregulatory systems. Proc Natl Acad Sci USA 1999, 96(2):748-753.

52. Backberg M, Hervieu G, Wilson S, Meister B: Orexin receptor-1 (OX-R1) immu-noreactivity in chemically identified neurons of the hypothalamus: focus on orexin targets involved in control of food and water intake. Eur J Neurosci 2002, 15(2):315-328.

53. Brown TM, Coogan AN, Cutler DJ, Hughes AT, Piggins HD: Electrophysiologi-cal actions of orexins on rat suprachiasmatic neurons in vitro. Neurosci Lett 2008, 448:273-278.

54. Daan S, Pittendrigh CS: A functional analysis of circadian pacemakers in nocturnal rodents. II. The variability of phase response curves. J Comp Physiol [A] 1976, 106:253-266.

55. Paxinos G, Franklin KB: The mouse brain in stereotaxic coordinates. San Diego: Academic Press; 2001.

*There are several supplemental files that are not available in this version of the article. To view this additional information, please use the citation information cited on the first page of this chapter.*

# CHAPTER 8

# MEAL TIME SHIFT DISTURBS CIRCADIAN RHYTHMICITY ALONG WITH METABOLIC AND BEHAVIORAL ALTERATIONS IN MICE

JI-AE YOON, DONG-HEE HAN, JONG-YUN NOH, MI-HEE KIM, GI HOON SON, KYUNGJIN KIM, CHANG-JU KIM, YOUNGMI KIM PAK, AND SEHYUNG CHO

## 8.1 INTRODUCTION

Life on this rotating planet is confronted with periodic changes in environmental conditions. Yet, some of the environmental changes, such as environmental illumination, temperature, food/predator availability, are quite predictable throughout a day/night cycle. Thus, virtually all organisms on Earth have successfully evolved endogenous mechanisms that allow organisms to harmonize their behavioral and physiological processes according to time of day. The resulting circadian rhythms are believed to optimize energy utilization, reproduction and survival [1], [2].

The importance of endogenous circadian rhythms becomes evident when they are disrupted. For example, genetic defects within the core clock genes or circadian disturbances has been linked to various patholo-

*This chapter was originally published under the Creative Commons Attribution License. Yoon J-A, Han D-H, Noh J-Y, Kim M-H, Son GH, Kim K, Kim C-J, Pak YK, and Cho S. Meal Time Shift Disturbs Circadian Rhythmicity along with Metabolic and Behavioral Alterations in Mice. PLoS ONE 7,8 (2012). doi:10.1371/journal.pone.0044053.*

gies including obesity, metabolic syndrome, cancer, cardiovascular diseases, gastric disorders, and other physical and mental problems [3]–[5].

Humans have evolved to be active predominately during the light phase [6], [7]. In modern society, however, more and more workers are involved in various kinds of shift works. Shift work forces people to be active in a phase of the light-dark cycle during which normally they would be resting. Epidemiological evidence also indicates that shift works are closely associated with increased risk for obesity, type 2 diabetes, cardio-metabolic consequences, and sleep disturbances [5]. Yet, the precise mechanism(s) underlying these pathological changes needs to be resolved. To this end, however, proper animal models are necessary to delineate the specific aspects of circadian disruptions.

Some investigators have already utilized animal models for 'shift works (night work)' [8]–[10]. However, these models have their own advantages and limitations, and fall short of mimicking important aspects of circadian disruption in human. Specifically, mimicking shifts in usual meal time under a given day/night cycle may reveal important aspects of circadian disturbances that lead to metabolic consequences, as the feeding/fasting cycle plays a crucial role in metabolic homeostasis. Actually, eating at unusual times of the day has been suspected to cause metabolic disturbances and gastrointestinal symptoms in shift workers [11]–[13].

Previously, it was demonstrated that one week of daytime feeding in nocturnal mice shifts the phases of core clock genes expression in the peripheral oscillators but not in the SCN central clock [14]. However, the physiological or pathological consequences of the uncoupling between central and peripheral clocks have yet to be determined.

Nocturnal mice are known to consume most of daily food intake during the early half of their scotophase [3]. So, an interesting question arises what would happen to their behavioral and metabolic rhythms when their usual meal time is significantly advanced or delayed. Also interesting will be whether chronic shifts in their usual meal time lead to any metabolic anomalies. In the present study, the effects of 6 h advance or 6 h delay of meal time was investigated by feeding young adult male mice in a time-restrictive manner. Using a computerized monitoring system, the effects of time-restrictive feeding on body temperature and home cage activity were continuously monitored. In addition, the effects on cholesterol and glucose homeostasis were also explored.

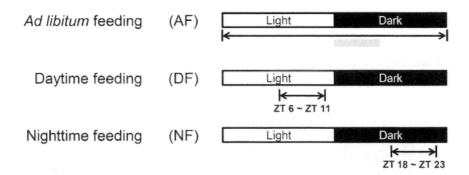

**FIGURE 1:** Experimental scheme. Young adult C57BL/6J male mice (8 weeks old) were first entrained to a 12:12 LD photoperiodic cycle for two weeks with food and water available ad libitum. Then mice were randomly divided into three groups: food available ad libitum (AF), food available during the late day (ZT 6 to 11) (DF), and food available during the late night (ZT 18 to 23) (NF) with water available all the time. This time-restrictive feeding regimen was maintained either up to the end of each experiment or for 4 weeks and then returned to ad libitum feeding (Figure 2 and 3). Gray bar indicates major meal time of normal adult mouse (Figure S1A).

## 8.2 RESULTS

### 8.2.1 TIME-RESTRICTIVE FEEDING DRAMATICALLY BUT REVERSIBLY ALTERS BODY TEMPERATURE AND HOME CAGE ACTIVITY RHYTHMS IN YOUNG ADULT MALE MICE

As reported previously [3], adult C57BL/6J male mice consumed most of their food during the early scotophase when fed ad libitum (Figure S1A). To see whether 6 h advance or 6 h delay of their usual meal time affects diurnal rhythms in physiology and metabolism, three experimental groups were adopted (Figure 1). Young adult male mice, surgically implanted with E-mitter probes, were entrained for two weeks to a 12:12 LD photo-periodic cycle with food and water available ad libitum. Then mice were

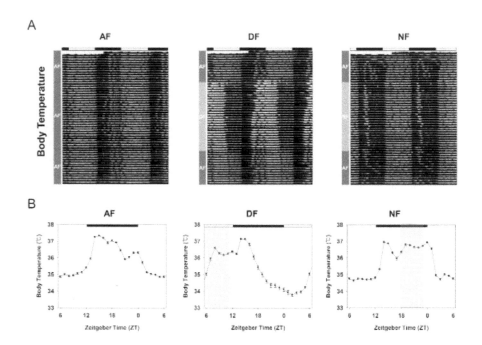

**FIGURE 2:** Daily rhythms of body temperature in young adult male mice under time-restrictive feeding regimen. Young adult male mice, surgically implanted with E-mitter probes, were first entrained to a 12:12 LD photoperiodic cycle for two weeks with food and water available ad libitum. Then mice were fed time-restrictively as schematized in Figure 1 for 4 weeks and returned to being fed ad libitum. Body temperature (BT) was continuously recorded for 7 subsequent weeks (See M&M). (A) Representative double-plot actograms of BT in AF, DF, and NF mice. Dark rectangles above the actograms indicate the 12 h scotophase maintained throughout the experiment. (B) Daily patterns of BT during the time-restrictive feeding. To generate the daily pattern of BT, monitoring results for the whole time-restrictive period were averaged as 1 h bins and the resulting 28 day profiles were pooled according to the indicated ZT to generate the averaged daily pattern (mean ± S.E.M.). Statistical analyses are summarized in Table 1.

randomly divided into three groups. First group of mice (AF) were continuously fed ad libitum throughout the whole experimental period. The other two groups were fed either during the late day (DF group: ZT06~ZT11) or during the late night (NF group: ZT18~ZT23) for 4 weeks with water available all the time. Under the condition adopted, we confirmed that the amount of food intake in DF and NF groups was lower for the first 3~4 days upon initiating time-restrictive feeding, but comparable amount of food were consumed within 4–5 days and thereafter as in AF group (Fig S1B). After 4 weeks of time-restrictive feeding, all the mice returned to being fed ad libitum. Their body temperature (BT) and home cage activity (HCA) were continuously recorded at 6 min intervals, and their representative actograms are shown in Figure 2A & 3A. As expected, distinct daily patterns of BT and HCA were evident in AF mice with rapid increase of BT and HCA at dusk, moderate dipping during the late night, and smaller but clear peak of BT and HCA at dawn (Figure 2B & 3B). In contrast, both BT and HCA rhythms were dramatically altered by time-restrictive feeding regimens (Figure 2 & 3), and two-way ANOVA revealed that these altered daily rhythms of BT and HCA are the results of interactions between the feeding schedule and zeitgeber time (Table 1). Interestingly, rapid increases of BT and HCA at dusk were preserved regardless of feeding time, indicating that the peaking of BT and HCA at the start of scotophase is driven by the central clock set by the imposed LD cycle. However, this elevated BT and HCA in DF and NF mice were not sustained as much as in AF mice (Figure 2B & 3B), suggesting that the prolongation of elevated BT and HCA is dependent upon the food availability. Moreover, meal time clearly affected the shape of BT and HCA rhythms. In contrast to AF mice, food-anticipatory increases of BT and HCA were clearly seen in both DF and NF mice. In addition, the elevated BT during the meal time was sustained throughout the 5 h of feeding period while HCA was not much so. This suggests that the sustained increment of BT during the meal time is attributable to the food intake, but not to the increased activity. Another interesting point is that feeding during the late day caused torpor-like symptoms during the late night (Figure 2B, middle panel; see also Figure S2 for individual profiles), indicating that a prolonged absence of food when it is most expected makes the animals enter energy-saving mode by lowering their BT. Importantly, the changes in BT and HCA rhythms induced by time-restrictive feeding seemed quite reversible as normal BT and HCA rhythms were recovered within a week when they returned to being fed ad libitum (Figure 2A & 3A). Intriguingly, 6 h delay of usual meal time caused hyperactivity in some animals. Of 12 NF animals recorded, five mice showed increased daily activity during the restrictive feeding period (Figure 3). Moreover, the NF-induced hyperactivity was sustained even when they were fed ad libitum again (Figure 3C).

**TABLE 1:** ANOVA F and p values for BT and HCA rhythms.

| Physiological Indices | Factors | | |
|---|---|---|---|
| | Feeding Schedule | Zeitgeber Time | Interaction |
| Body Temperature | $F_{(2, 1944)} = 364.85$; ****$p < 0.0001$ | $F_{(23, 1944)} = 363.98$; ****$p < 0.0001$ | $F_{(46, 1944)} = 150.34$; ****$p < 0.0001$ |
| Home Cage Activity | $F_{(2, 1944)} = 381.29$; ****$p < 0.0001$ | $F_{(23, 1944)} = 420.83$; ****$p < 0.0001$ | $F_{(46, 1944)} = 71.36$; ****$p < 0.0001$ |

*Significant differences (****$P<0.001$) are indicated in bold type. ANOVA = analysis of variance*

## 8.2.2 FOOD AND WATER INTAKES ARE MARGINALLY AFFECTED BY TIME-RESTRICTIVE FEEDING REGIMEN

To examine whether time-restrictive feeding affects the amount of food and water intakes, weekly food and water consumptions were measured throughout the whole experimental period. As shown in Figure 4A, food intakes were significantly lower during the first week of restrictive feeding, especially in DF mice, but comparable food consumption was recovered by the second week and thereafter. Total food consumption during the 4 weeks of time-restrictive feeding was marginally but significantly lower in DF group than in other groups (Figure 4A, right panel). Weekly water intakes were also reduced by daytime feeding regimen especially at the third and fourth weeks of restrictive feeding, which were progressively recovered by returning to ad libitum feeding (Figure 4B, left panel). Yet,

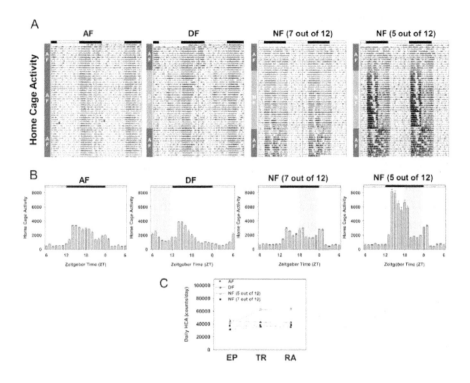

**FIGURE 3:** Daily rhythms of home cage activity in young adult male mice under time-restrictive feeding regimen. Young adult male mice, surgically implanted with E-mitter probes, were first entrained to a 12:12 LD photoperiodic cycle for two weeks with food and water available ad libitum. Then mice were fed time-restrictively as schematized in Figure 1 for 4 weeks and returned to being fed ad libitum. Home cage activity (HCA) was continuously recorded for 7 subsequent weeks (See M&M). (A) Representative double-plot actograms of HCA in AF, DF, and NF mice. Dark rectangles above the actograms indicate the 12 h scotophase maintained throughout the experiment. (B) Daily patterns of HCA during the time-restrictive feeding. To generate the daily pattern of HCA, monitoring results for the whole time-restrictive period were summed up as 1 h bins and the resulting 28 day profiles were pooled according to the indicated ZT to generate the averaged daily pattern (mean ± S.E.M.). Statistical analyses are summarized in Table 1. (C) Changes in daily HCA during the weeks of entrainment period (EP), 4 weeks of time-restrictive feeding (TR) and when returned to ad libitum feeding for 2 weeks (RA).

the total water intakes during the 4 weeks of time-restrictive feeding were statistically indistinguishable among the three groups (Figure 4B, right panel). Thus, it can be concluded that nighttime feeding does not affect weekly food and water intakes while daytime feeding marginally reduces the weekly food and water consumption.

## 8.2.3 ONE WEEK OF TIME-RESTRICTIVE FEEDING DRAMATICALLY ALTERS THE DAILY RHYTHMS OF METABOLIC PARAMETERS

Recent studies indicate that circadian disruption may potentiate the onset of metabolic disorders. For example, genetic defects within the core clock genes *Clock* and *Bmal1* have been associated with obesity, metabolic phenotypes, hypertension, and type 2 diabetes [15]–[17]. To test whether the altered BT and HCA rhythms induced by time-restrictive feeding regimen are also associated with disturbances in metabolic rhythms, daily variation in the levels of total cholesterol, high-density lipoprotein (HDL) cholesterol, triglyceride, and blood glucose were determined after a week of time-restrictive feeding (Figure 5). When nocturnal mice were fed ad libitum, total cholesterol levels remained fairly stable throughout a circadian cycle but slightly decreased at the time of light-dark transition. HDL cholesterol remained rather stable throughout a day. Blood triglyceride levels seemed to be mainly affected by the meal time, since they reached the highest level after the usual meal time and progressively declined thereafter. Blood glucose levels were fairly stable when mice were fed ad libitum. When mice were fed time-restrictively, however, these metabolic rhythms were differentially affected. In case of total cholesterol and HDL, the effects were rather moderate (Figure 5A&B). Once again, blood triglyceride levels seemed to be mainly affected by the meal time. As shown in Figure 5C, blood triglyceride levels reached the maximum after the meal time (ZT12 in DF and ZT00 in NF mice) and progressively declined thereafter. On the other hand, blood glucose reached the minimum before the meal time (ZT6 in DF and ZT18 in NF mice) and elevated after the foraging (Figure 5D). Also notable is the sharp increase of blood glucose in NF mice at the light/dark transition. When combined with the activity onset observed in

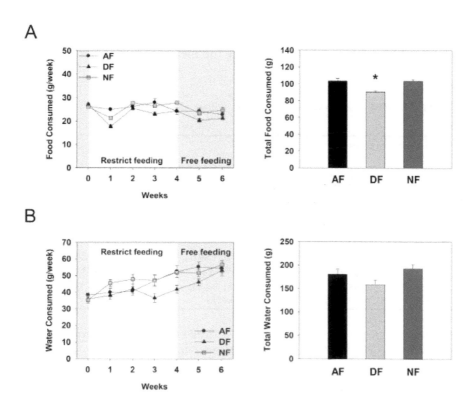

**FIGURE 4:** Weekly food and water consumption profiles. Young adult male mice were first entrained to a 12:12 LD photoperiodic cycle for 1 week, fed time-restrictively for 4 weeks, and then fed ad libitum for 2 weeks as described in Figure 1. Weekly consumption of food and water measured regularly at the end of each week. (A) Weekly food consumption profiles during the whole experimental period (left) and total food consumption during the 4 weeks of time restrictive feeding period (right). (B) Weekly water consumption profiles during the whole experimental period (left) and total water consumption during the 4 weeks of time restrictive feeding period (right). Data are expressed as mean ± S.E.M. (n = 4), *p<0.05 vs. other groups.

these mice (Figure 2 & 3), it is probable that this rise in blood glucose may reflect the metabolic needs required for the activity onset. Two-way ANOVA revealed that these altered daily rhythms of total cholesterol, triglyceride, and glucose are the results of interactions between the feeding schedule and zeitgeber time (Table 2). Thus, we conclude that just a week of time-restrictive feeding differentially affects the metabolic rhythms, thereby destroying the harmony among the metabolic parameters.

**TABLE 2:** ANOVA F and p values for each physiological index.

| Physiological Indices | Factors | | |
|---|---|---|---|
| | Feeding Schedule | Zeitgeber Time | Interaction |
| Total Cholesterol | $F_{(2, 44)} = 8.84$; ***$p = 0.0006$ | $F_{(3, 44)} = 4.47$; **$p < 0.0080$ | $F_{(6, 44)} = 2.45$; *$p < 0.0393$ |
| HDL | $F_{(2, 43)} = 6.46$; **$p = 0.0035$ | $F_{(3, 43)} = 0.15$; ns$p = 0.9259$ | $F_{(6, 43)} = 0.62$; ns$p = 0.7125$ |
| Triglyceride | $F_{(2, 43)} = 3.03$; ns$p = 0.0589$ | $F_{(3, 43)} = 3.21$; *$p = 0.0324$ | $F_{(6, 43)} = 6.55$; ****$p < 0.0001$ |
| Blood Glucose | $F_{(2, 48)} = 8.23$; ***$p = 0.0008$ | $F_{(3, 48)} = 4.83$; **$p = 0.0051$ | $F_{(6, 48)} = 5.75$; ***$p = 0.0001$ |

*Significant differences (*$P < 0.05$, **$P < 0.01$, ***$P < 0.001$, and ****$P < 0.0001$) are indicated in bold type. ANOVA = analysis of variance; ns = not significant*

## 8.2.4 LDLR, SREBP1C AND SCAP MRNAS OSCILLATE IN THE MOUSE LIVER

Daily variation of metabolic parameters related to cholesterol metabolism was altered by time-restrictive feeding (Figure 5A-C). Cholesterol metabolism is controlled by various factors including low density lipoprotein receptor (LDLR), sterol regulatory element-binding protein-1 (SREBP-1), sterol regulatory element-binding protein-2 (SREBP-2), SREBP-cleavage activating protein (SCAP), insulin-induced gene-1 (INSIG-1), site-1 protease (S1P), and site-1 protease (S2P) [18]–[20]. Previously, LDLR has

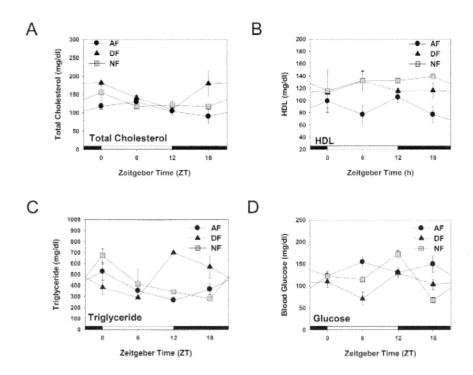

**FIGURE 5:** Daily rhythms of blood glucose and some metabolic parameters related to cholesterol homeostasis in mice fed time-restrictively. Young adult male C57BL/6J mice were first entrained to a 12:12 LD photoperiodic cycle for two weeks. Then mice were fed time-restrictively for seven consecutive days as denoted in Figure 1. Mice were sacrificed by cervical dislocation at the indicated ZT and whole blood samples were collected. Total cholesterol (A), HDL cholesterol (B), plasma triglyceride (C), blood glucose (D) levels were determined by specific kits obtained from Callegari™. All data are expressed as mean ± S.E.M. (n = 4–8). Statistical analyses are summarized in Table 2.

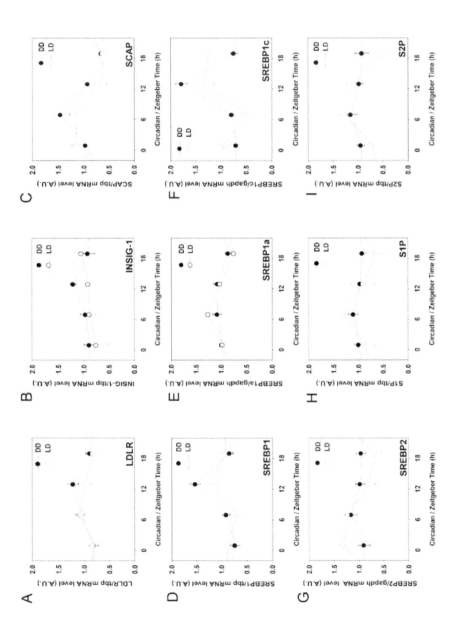

**FIGURE 6:** Daily and circadian expressions of LDLR and some LDLR regulatory factors in the mouse liver. To determine daily expression patterns, young adult C57BL/6J male mice were entrained to a 12L:12D cycle for two weeks and liver samples were quickly obtained at the indicated ZT. For circadian sampling, mice were entrained to a 12L:12D cycle for two weeks and released to constant darkness (DD). On the second day after light-off, liver samples were obtained at the indicated circadian time (CT). RNA isolation, reverse transcription, and real-time polymerase chain reaction to measure specific messages for mouse ldlr, and LDLR regulatory factors. All mRNA levels were normalized to tbp mRNA levels. Data are expressed as mean ± S.E.M. (n = 8).

been shown to have a circadian rhythm in the rat [21]. To examine whether the LDLR and LDLR regulatory factors expressions exhibit daily and/or circadian rhythms in the mouse liver, young adult male mice were first entrained to a 12:12 LD photoperiodic cycle for two weeks. Then, mice liver samples were obtained throughout a day in the presence of LD cycle, or throughout a circadian cycle under DD condition on the second day after light-off. As shown in Figure 6, *ldlr* and some LDLR regulatory factors expression oscillated in the mouse liver in the presence or absence of exogenous light cues. Notably, the *ldlr, srebp1* and *srebp1c* mRNA levels peaked at ZT13 or CT13, while *scap* mRNA levels reached the maximum at ZT07 and CT07. The *insig, srebp-1a, srebp2, s1p,* and *s2p* mRNA levels did not exhibit any significant circadian variations.

## 8.2.5 ONE WEEK OF TIME-RESTRICTIVE FEEDING DRAMATICALLY ALTERS THE DAILY EXPRESSION OF LDLR AND LDLR REGULATORY FACTORS

Previously, it has been shown that one week of daytime feeding shifts the phase of circadian genes expression in the peripheral oscillators like liver [11], [22]. With the circadian oscillation of LDLR and some LDLR regulatory factors expression in hands (Figure 6), next question was whether these oscillations would be affected by time-restrictive feeding regimen. Young adult male mice were entrained to a 12:12 photoperiodic cycle for two weeks and fed either during the late day (DF group: ZT06~ZT11) or during the late night (NF group: ZT18~ZT23) for 7 consecutive days with

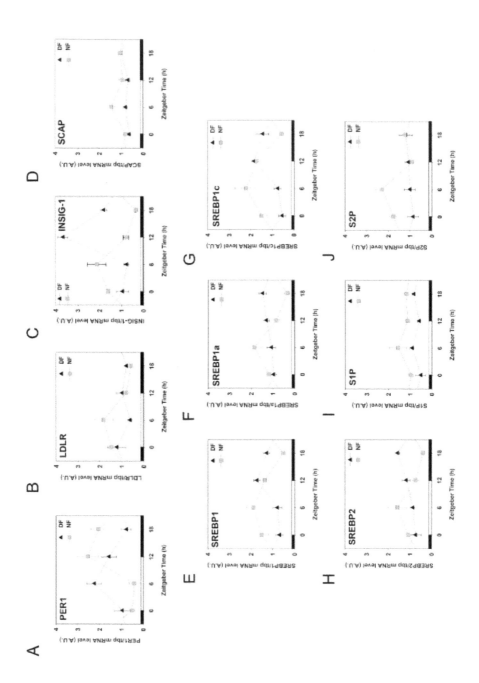

**FIGURE 7:** Effects of one week of time-restrictive feeding on the phases of Per1, LDLR, and LDLR regulatory factors gene expression in the mouse liver. Young adult male mice, entrained to a 12:12 photoperiodic cycle, were fed time-restrictively for seven consecutive days as described in Figure 1. On the 8th day, mice were sacrificed at the indicated zeitgeber time (ZT) and liver samples were obtained. RNA isolation, reverse transcription, and real-time polymerase chain reaction were performed to measure specific messages for mouse Per1, ldlr, and LDLR regulatory factors. All mRNA levels were normalized to tbp mRNA levels. Data are expressed as mean ± S.E.M. (n = 4).

water available all the time. On the eighth day, mice were sacrificed at 6 h intervals, liver samples were obtained, and messages for the ldlr and LDLR regulatory factors were analyzed using real-time PCR. As shown in Figure 7A, the expression of a core clock gene, per1, clearly phase-shifted by time restrictive feeding regimen. Moreover, the phases of the ldlr and most LDLR regulatory factors expression were significantly altered by time-restrictive feeding regimen. Specifically, all mRNA except s1p reached the maximum at ZT06 in NF mice, while *insig-1, scap, srebp1, srebp1a, srebp1c,* and *srebp2* reached the highest level at ZT 12–18 in DF mice. Interestingly, the phases of all mRNA accumulation profiles differed by 6–12 h between DF and NF mice. These results indicate that the daily expression of LDLR and LDLR regulatory factors are severely affected by time-restrictive feeding regimen in the mouse liver.

## 8.2.6 CHRONIC TIME-RESTRICTIVE FEEDING SIGNIFICANTLY AFFECTS GLUCOSE HOMEOSTASIS IN YOUNG ADULT MALE MICE

Since daily patterns of blood glucose levels were significantly altered by time-restrictive feeding regimen (Figure 5D), it was tempting to examine whether these changes lead to any metabolic consequences. Thus, young adult male mice were first entrained to a 12:12 LD photoperiodic cycle for two weeks. Then, mice were fed time-restrictively for 9 consecutive weeks. Changes in body weight, fasting blood glucose, tolerance to the oral glucose load, and response to the insulin challenge were determined weekly from the 5th week of restrictive feeding and thereafter. As shown in Figure 8A, fasting body weights were slightly but significantly reduced in DF mice compared to other groups, probably reflecting the reduced food intake in these mice (Figure 4A). More significant impacts were observed in fasting glucose levels. As shown in Figure 8B, fasting glucose levels were significantly higher in mice fed time-restrictively, especially in NF mice. These elevations of fasting glucose levels were observed from the 5th week of time-restrictive feeding to the end of experiment at the 9th week. However, the responses to the oral glucose load were almost indistinguishable among the three groups, not only at the 5th week (Figure 8C&D) but to the end of experiment (data not shown). Importantly, responses to the insulin challenge exacerbated as the daytime feeding regimen continued. Specifically, altered responses to insulin were already notable from the 6th week of time-restrictive feeding (data not shown) and insulin resistances were evident at the 9th week (Figure 8E&F). Thus, it can be concluded that homeostatic regulation of blood glucose are significantly and progressively affected by shift in usual meal time.

## 8.3 DISCUSSION

The present study explored the effects of 6 h advance or 6 h delay of usual meal time in young adult male mice, and found that both BT and HCA rhythms were significantly altered by shifts in meal time with concurrent pathological changes in metabolic rhythms. Since shift workers are known to be exposed to high risks of metabolic problems [23], the observation that time-restrictive feeding alters daily variation of factors regulating glucose and cholesterol homeostasis poses great implications that necessitate future works.

Previously, Damiola et al. [14] observed that daytime-restrictive feeding alters the phases of core clock genes expression in the peripheral tissues, but not in the central clock SCN. In the present study, rapid elevations of both BT and HCA at the early scotophase were preserved regardless of feeding regimens, indicating that these increases are mainly controlled by the central clock set by the imposed LD cycle. Accordingly, *mPer1⁻/⁻mCry2⁻/⁻* $mPer1^{-/-}mCry2^{-/-}$ clock mutant mice did not exhibit these peaks [24], [25], supporting the dominant role of central clock machinery in the activity onset. Nevertheless, the prolongation of elevated BT and HCA seems to be dependent upon food availability, because they were not sustained as much in the absence of food. Moreover, food availability significantly affected the BT and HCA rhythms. Interestingly, a prolonged absence of food when it is most expected induced the regulated hypothermia in DF animals (Figure 2B and individual profiles in Figure S2B). Torpor has been believed to be an energy-saving mode that enables the small animals to endure prolonged food-deficient period [26], [27]. Yet, torpor-like symptom was observed only in DF mice, but not in NF mice with the same 19 h fasting period a day, suggesting an unexpected role of circadian clock in the physiological regulation of torpor-like symptoms. Leptin and ghrelin, which are known to affect torpor [28], [29], exhibit daily variations in rodents [30]. Recently, Crispim et al. [31] observed that leptin and ghrelin levels showed significant differences from the day shift subjects in human. Thus, time-restrictive feeding may alter daily patterns of leptin and ghrelin, leading to a torpor-like symptom. This possibility needs to be addressed in the future works.

Another interesting point found in this work is that hyperactivity was observed in a significant portion of NF animals (42%, 5 out of 12 animals; Figure 3A, far right panel). Surprisingly, the NF-induced hyperactivity was continued even when they were fed ad libitum again, indicating a sustained aftereffect of 6 h delay of meal time on behavioral phenotypes. In this context, it is noteworthy that clinical evidence suggests a role of circadian time-keeping system in the etiology of attention-deficit/hyperactivity disorders (ADHD) [32]–[34]. Moreover, circadian rhythm disturbance has been linked to bipolar depression [35] one of whose symptom is hyperactivity [36]. Taken together, hyperactivity observed in NF animals can be associated with mental illnesses. Further works are needed to confirm this issue.

The present work demonstrated that chronic time-restrictive feeding induces differential metabolic changes along with the alteration in BT and HCA rhythms, which is in good agreement with the recent studies suggesting that circadian rhythm disturbances are linked to obesity, type 2 diabetes, and metabolic phenotypes [15], [17]. The present results showing the disturbed metabolic rhythms also correspond with previous reports in rodents and human studies that eating during the normal rest phase lead to a loss of blood glucose and triglyceride rhythms [10], [37]–[39].

**TABLE 3:** Primer sequences used in real-time PCR.

| Gene | | Sequence | NCBI ID |
|---|---|---|---|
| LDLR | Forward | 5'-GAA CTC AGG GCC TCT GTC TG-3' | NM_010700 |
| | Reverse | 5'-AGC AGG CTG GAT GTC TCT GT-3' | |
| SREBP1 | Forward | 5'-GTG AGC CTG ACA AGC AAT CA-3' | NM_011480 |
| | Reverse | 5'-GGT GCC TAC AGA GCA AGA GG-3' | |
| SREBP1a | Forward | 5'-AAG TCA CTG TCT TGG TTG TTG-3' | NM_011480 |
| | Reverse | 5'-AAG TCA CTG TCT TGG TTG TTG-3' | |
| SREBP1c | Forward | 5'ATC GGC GCG GAA GCT GTC GG-3' | NM_011480 |
| | Reverse | 5'-AAG TCA CTG TCT TGG TTG TTG-3' | |
| SREBP2 | Forward | 5'-GTG GAG CAG TCT CAA CGT CA-3' | NM_033218 |
| | Reverse | 5'-TGG TAG GTC TCA CCC AGG AG-3' | |
| SCAP | Forward | 5'-GAT GTG TTC CGG TCA CCT CT-3' | NM_001103162 |
| | Reverse | 5'-TTG GTC CCT GAG CTGTCT CT-3' | |
| INSIG-1 | Forward | 5'-ACA CGTGGG ACC TAA CTTT GC-3' | NM_153526 |
| | Reverse | 5'-CTT CTC CGG AAT AGC TCG TG-3' | |
| S1P | Forward | 5'-TCC CCA GCA GAG ACA GAG TT-3' | NM_019709 |
| | Reverse | 5'-GAG GTA CTG GTC CCA GAG GA-3' | |
| S2P | Forward | 5'-CAC TGG GAC TCT GGA TGG TT-3' | NM_172307 |
| | Reverse | 5'-TTG GCC AAG GTG TTT TAA GG-3' | |
| PER1 | Forward | 5'-GTG TCG TGA TTA AAT TAG TCA G-3' | NM_011065 |
| | Reverse | 5' ACC ACT CAT GTC GTC TGG GCC-3' | |

Cholesterol is an important source of bile acid, biological membrane, and steroid hormones [18], and increased plasma cholesterol has been associated with an increased risk of coronary heart disease and atherosclerosis [40]. LDLR is known to play a key role in cholesterol metabolism. The transcription of the LDLR is regulated by SREBP pathway. SREBP pathway is composed of various factors including SREBP-1a, SREBP-1c, SREBP-2, INSIG-1, SCAP, S1P, and S2P [19], [20], [41], [42]. The present study examined whether mRNA expressions of these factors oscillate in the mouse liver and found that LDLR, SREBP1, and SREBP1c expressions oscillated in the mouse liver under free-running condition that is in good agreement with previous reports [21], [43]. Moreover, it was also found that scap mRNA oscillates with maximum peak at CT07 (Figure 6C), suggesting that LDLR and some LDLR regulatory factors are clock-controlled genes.

More importantly, the present study revealed that just a week of meal time shift disturbed the daily patterns of LDLR and most of LDLR regulatory factors expressions (Figure 7). Severe impacts of time-restrictive feeding on the daily expression of genes regulating cholesterol homeostasis may have critical implications for shift workers, since they are known to be more vulnerable to cardiovascular diseases [44]–[46]. However, chronic effects of time-restrictive feeding on cholesterol homeostasis and related pathologies need to be addressed by the future works. In this respect, a recent observation that interaction between temporal feeding and circadian clock determines the hepatic circadian transcriptome [22] provides a valuable clue. Future works addressing which genes are driven by feeding only, circadian clock only, or interaction of both would help understand the pathophysiology related to chronic shift of meal time.

Blood glucose levels are controlled by many factors such as leptin, insulin, and corticosterone [47], [48]. In particular, altered responses to insulin or to glucose load indicate disturbances in glucose homeostasis [49]. Since daily variations in circulating glucose levels were significantly influenced by time-restrictive feeding regimens (Figure 5D), the present work implies that metabolic syndrome can ensue with significant shifts in meal time. Yet, the direction of shifts seemed to make a difference. In the present study, fasting glucose levels were most severely affected by 6 h delay in meal time (NF mice; Figure 8), while altered response to insulin were observed only by 6 h advance (DF mice; Figure 8E&F) without altering the serum insulin levels (data not shown). At present, it is unclear what made such differences. One possibility is that, as mice are born to be predominantly active during the scotophase, 6 h advance of meal time makes them active during their usual rest phase, imposing more severe stress in these animals, while 6 h delay causes prolonged activities during the night with increased metabolic needs. Alternatively, the direction of shifts causes differential influences on the hormonal secretion and insulin signaling. As insulin signaling pathways involve insulin receptor, phosphatidylinostiol-3kinase (PI3K), phosphatidylinositol-4,5-bisphosphte ($PIP_2$), and $PIP_3$-dependent protein kinase (PDK1) [50], [51] and virtually all hormones display diurnal variations [52], [53], future works are needed to address this issue.

In conclusion, the present study demonstrated that shifts in usual meal time greatly affects daily rhythms of HCA and BT, along with the alterations in daily rhythms of blood glucose and triglyceride levels, leading to some metabolic consequences. These data pose critical implications for the health and diseases of shift workers that are ever increasing in the modern society.

## 8.4 MATERIALS AND METHODS

### 8.4.1 ETHICS STATEMENT

All animal experiments were approved by the Kyung Hee University Institutional Animal Care and Use Committee (Permit number: KHUASP(SE)-11-035) and performed under the guidelines of the Committee. All the animals were treated to minimize suffering.

### 8.4.2 ANIMALS CARE AND HANDLING

C57BL/6J male mice were purchased from DBL (Seoul, Korea). Upon arrival, mice were acclimatized to a temperature-controlled room (23±1°C) with a 12:12 light-dark (LD) photoperiodic cycle. Food and water were provided all the time. For experimental settings, mice were individually housed in a light-proof clean animal rack cabinet (Shin Biotech, Seoul, Korea) with light intensity during the light phase maintained at 350~450 lux at the bottom of cage. Mice were continuously fed with normal food chows ad libitum until the start of time-restrictive feeding.

## 8.4.3 ACTIVITY MONITORING, RESTRICTIVE FEEDING SCHEDULE AND SAMPLING

For activity monitoring, mice were surgically implanted with a G2 E-mitter probe (Mini Mitter, Oregon, USA) on the dorsal neck under the skin [54], [55], and their HCA and BT were continuously monitored using Activity Monitoring System (Mini Mitter, Oregon, USA). Specifically, data were continuously recorded at 6 min intervals using the VitalView® Data Acquisition System. Individual actograms were obtained using the ActiView® software. To generate the daily pattern, monitoring results retrieved as a Microsoft® Excel file for the whole time-restrictive period were either averaged (in case of BT) or summed up (in case of HCA) as 1 h bins and the resulting 28 day profiles were pooled according to the indicated ZT. Time-restrictive feeding was applied two weeks after E-mitter implantation surgery. After a week of recovery, mice were further entrained for another week to a 12:12 LD photoperiodic cycle with food and water available ad libitum. Then mice were randomly divided into three groups (Figure 1). First group of mice (AF) were continuously fed ad libitum throughout the whole experimental period. The other two groups were fed either during the late day (DF group: ZT6~ZT11) or during the late night (NF group: ZT18~ZT23) for weeks as indicated in the Figure legends. In case of Figure 2 and 3, all the mice returned to being fed ad libitum after 4 weeks of time-restrictive feeding. For circadian sampling (Figure 6), mice were first entrained for two weeks to a 12:12 LD photoperiodic cycle with food and water available ad libitum. Then mice were released to constant darkness. On the second day after light-off, mice were sacrificed by cervical dislocation under the dim red light and liver samples were quickly obtained. To examine the effect of restrictive feeding on genes expression (Figure 7), mice were first entrained for two weeks to a 12:12 LD photoperiodic cycle, fed either during the late day (DF group) or during the late night (NF group) for seven consecutive days, and liver samples were obtained at the indicated ZT.

## 8.4.4 MEASUREMENT OF METABOLIC PARAMETERS

Blood samples were collected from the retro-orbital plexus at the time of sacrifice. Blood glucose levels were determined using the Accu-Chek® Performa kit (Roche, Seoul, Korea). After 30 min incubation at room termperature, blood samples were centrifuged at 3,000 rpm at 4°C for 10 min, and resulting serum was collected. Total cholesterol, HDL (high density lipoprotein) cholesterol, and triglyceride levels were determined using specific assay kits and CR-3000 apparatus obtained from CallegrariTM (Parma, Italy).

## 8.4.5 ORAL GLUCOSE TOLERANCE TEST (OGTT) AND INSULIN TOLERANCE TEST (ITT)

In a control experiment, we found that time-of-day has little impact on OGTT and ITT results (Figure S3). Thus, we performed OGTT and ITT after 16 h fasting since the last scheduled meal. For OGTT, D-glucose (Sigma, G5767; 2 g/kg body weight) was delivered using oral zonde. For ITT, insulin (0.5 U/kg body weight) was injected intraperitoneally after 16 h fasting. Blood samples were collected at 0, 15, 30, 60, and 120 min for determination of blood glucose levels.

## 8.4.6 RNA ISOLATION, REVERSE TRANSCRIPTION, AND REAL-TIME PCR

Total RNA was isolated from the mouse liver using single-step acid guanidinium thiocyanate-phenol-chloroform (AGPC) extraction method as described previously [56]. Concentration of RNA was determined using ND-1000 (Nanodrop Technologies, Wilmington, USA). RNA samples diluted to 1 μg /10 μl were incubated with 200 ng of random hexamer (Takara,

3801) at 65°C for 5 min, and rapidly cooled down on ice for 2 min. Then each sample was incubated with 9 μl of reverse transcription mixture (4 μl of RT buffer, 0.5 μl of RNase inhibitor, 4 μl of 2.5 mM ea of dNTPs and 0.5 μl of RTase M-MLV) at 37°C for 1 h and subsequently heated at 70°C for 10 min. The procedure for real-time PCR using LightCycler has been described [57]. The standards were prepared by pooling 5-fold diluted RT samples in 1 mM Tris. The templates for real-time PCR were prepared by diluting 75-fold from RT samples. 2X SYBR Premix EX Taq (Takara, RR041A) and LightCycler Version 1.5 (Roche, Salt Lake City, USA) were used for the real-time PCR. Primer sequences used for real-time PCR are shown in Table 3.

## 8.4.7 STATISTICAL ANALYSIS

Data were classified by group and time and were expressed as mean ± S.E.M. Statistical analyses were performed with GraphPad PRISM software (GraphPad Prism Software, Inc., LA Jolla, CA, USA). The factor analysis between groups was carried out using 2-way analysis of variance (ANOVA) with Bonferroni posttests. Food intake, water intake, fasting glucose, fasting body weight, AUC-OGTT, and AUC-ITT were statistically analyzed by ANOVA. Statistical significance was set at $p < 0.05$.

## REFERENCES

1. Dunlap JC, Loros JJ, DeCoursey PJ (2004) Chronobiology: Biological Timekeeping. Sinanuer Associates Inc, Sunderland, 406p.
2. Refinetti R (2006) Circadian Physiology, 2nd ed. Taylor & Francis, Boca Raton, 667p.
3. Sanchez-Alavez M, Klein I, Brownell SE, Tabarean IV, Davis CN, et al. (2007) Night eating and obesity in the EP3R-deficient mouse. PNAS USA 104: 3009–3014. doi: 10.1073/pnas.0611209104
4. Arble DM, Ramsey KM, Bass J, Turek FW (2010) Circadian disruption and metabolic disease: findings from animal models. Best Pract Res Clin Endocrinol Metab 24: 785–800. doi: 10.1016/j.beem.2010.08.003
5. Szosland D (2010) Shift work and metabolic syndrome, diabetes mellitus and ischaemic heart disease. Int J Occup Med Environ Health 23: 287–291. doi: 10.2478/v10001-010-0032-5

6.  Gutman R, Barnea M, Haviv L, Chapnik N, Froy O (2011) Peroxisome proliferator activated receptor α (PPARα) activation advances locomotor activity and feeding daily rhythms in mice. Int J Obes 10.1038/ijo.2011.215.

7.  Mieda M, Sakurai T (2011) Bmal1 in the nervous system is essential for normal adaptation of circadian locomotor activity and food intake to periodic feeding. J Neurosci 31: 15391–15396. doi: 10.1523/JNEUROSCI.2801-11.2011

8.  Désir D, Van Cauter E, Fang VS, Martino E, Jadot C, et al. (1981) Effects of "jet lag" on hormonal patterns. I. Procedures, variations in total plasma proteins, and disruption of adrenocorticotropin-cortisol periodicity. J Clin Endocrinol Metab 52: 628–641. doi: 10.1210/jcem-52-4-628

9.  Davidson AJ, Sellix MT, Daniel J, Yamazaki S, Menaker M, et al. (2006) Chronic jet-lag increases mortality in aged mice. Curr Biol 16: R914–916. doi: 10.1016/j.cub.2006.09.058

10. Salgado-Delgado R, Angeles-Castellanos M, Saderi N, Buijs RM, Escorba C (2010) Food intake during the normal activity phase prevents obesity and circadian desynchrony in a rat model of night work. Endocrinology 151: 1019–1029. doi: 10.1210/en.2009-0864

11. Habbal OA, Al-Jabri AA (2009) Circadian rhythm and the immune response: a review. Int Rev Immunol 28: 93–108. doi: 10.1080/08830180802645050

12. Culpepper L (2010) The social and economic burden of shift-work disorder. J Fam Pract 59: S3–S11.

13. Lowden A, Moreno C, Holmbäck U, Lennernäs M, Tucker P (2010) Eating and shift work – effects on habits, metabolism and performance. Scand J Work Environ Health 36: 150–162. doi: 10.5271/sjweh.2898

14. Damiola F, Le Minh N, Preitner N, Kornmann B, Fleury-Olela F, et al. (2000) Restricted feeding uncouples circadian oscillators in peripheral tissues from the central pacemaker in the suprachiasmatic nucleus. Genes Dev 14: 2950–2961. doi: 10.1101/gad.183500

15. Scott EM, Carter AM, Grant PJ (2008) Association between polymorphisms in the Clock gene, obesity and the metabolic syndrome in man. International Journal of Obesity 32: 658–662. doi: 10.1038/sj.ijo.0803778

16. Sookoian S, Castaño G, Gemma C, Gianotti TF, Pirola CJ (2007) Common genetic variations in CLOCK transcription factor are associated with nonalcoholic fatty liver disease. World J Gastroenterol 13: 4242–4248.

17. Woon PY, Kaisaki PJ, Bragança J, Bihoreau MT, Levy JC, et al. (2007) Aryl hydrocarbon receptor nuclear translocator-like (BMAL1) is associated with susceptibility to hypertension and type 2 diabetes. PNAS USA 104: 14412–14417. doi: 10.1073/pnas.0703247104

18. Goldstein JL, Brown MS (2009) The LDL receptor. Arterioscler Thromb Vasc Biol. 29: 431–438.

19. Dong XY, Tang SQ (2010) Insulin-induced gene: a new regulator in lipid metabolism. Peptides 31: 2145–2150. doi: 10.1016/j.peptides.2010.07.020

20. Sato R (2010) Sterol metabolism and SREBP activation. Arch Biochem Biophys 501: 177–181. doi: 10.1016/j.abb.2010.06.004

21. Balasubramaniam S, Szanto A, Roach PD (1994) Circadian rhythm in hepatic low-density-lipoprotein (LDL)-receptor expression and plasma LDL levels. Biochem J 298: 39–43.

22. Vollmers C, Gill S, DiTacchio L, Pulivarthy SR, Le HD, et al. (2009) Time of feeding and the intrinsic circadian clock drive rhythms in hepatic gene expression. PNAS USA 106: 21453–21458. doi: 10.1073/pnas.0909591106

23. Foster RG, Wulff K (2005) The rhythm of rest and excess. Nat Rev Neurosci 6: 407–414. doi: 10.1038/nrn1670

24. Oster H, Baeriswyl S, van der Horst GT, Albrecht U (2003) Loss of circadian rhythmicity in aging mPer1–/–mCyr2–/– mutant mice. Genes Dev. 17: 1366–1379. doi: 10.1101/gad.256103

25. Turek FW, Joshu C, Kohsaka A, Lin E, Ivanova G, et al. (2005) Obesity and metabolic syndrome in circadian Clock mutant mice. Science 308: 1043–1045. doi: 10.1126/science.1108750

26. Geiser F (2004) Metabolic rate and body temperature reduction during hibernation and daily torpor. Annu Rev Physiol 66: 239–274. doi: 10.1146/annurev.physiol.66.032102.115105

27. Swoap SJ (2008) The pharmacology and molecular mechanisms underlying temperature regulation and torpor. Biochem Pharmacol 76: 817–824. doi: 10.1016/j.bcp.2008.06.017

28. Nelson RJ (2004) Leptin: the "skinny" on torpor. Am J Physiol Regul Integr Comp Physiol 287: R6–R7. doi: 10.1152/ajpregu.00164.2004

29. Gluck EF, Stephens N, Swoap SJ (2006) Peripheral ghrelin deepens torpor bouts in mice through the arcuate nucleus neuropeptide Y signaling pathway. Am J Physiol Regul Integr Comp Physiol 291: R1303–R1309. doi: 10.1152/ajpregu.00232.2006

30. Kalra SP, Bagnasco M, Otukonyong EE, Dube MG, Kalra PS (2003) Rhythmic, reciprocal ghrelin and leptin signaling: new insight in the development of obesity. Regul Pept 111: 1–11. doi: 10.1016/S0167-0115(02)00305-1

31. Crispim CA, Waterhouse J, Dâmaso AR, Zimberg IZ, Padilha HG, et al. (2011) Hormonal appetite control is altered by shift work: a preliminary study. Metabolism 60: 1726–1735. doi: 10.1016/j.metabol.2011.04.014

32. Walters AS, Silvestri R, Zucconi M, Chandrashekariah R, Konofal E (2008) Review of the possible relationship and hypothetical links between attention deficit hyperactivity disorder (ADHD) and the simple sleep related movement disorders, parasomnias, hypersomnias, and circadian rhythm disorders. J Clin Sleep Med 4: 591–600.

33. Van Veen MM, Kooij JJ, Boonstra AM, Gordijn MC, Van Someren EJ (2010) Delayed circadian rhythm in adults with attention-deficit/hyperactivity disorder and chronic sleep-onset insomnia. Biol Psychiatry 67: 1091–1096. doi: 10.1016/j.biopsych.2009.12.032

34. Nováková M, Paclt I, Ptáček R, Kuželová H, Hájek I, et al. (2011) Salivary melatonin rhythm as a marker of the circadian system in healthy children and those with attention-deficit/hyperactivity disorder. Chronobiol Int. 28: 630–637. doi: 10.3109/07420528.2011.596983

35. Murray G, Harvey A (2010) Circadian rhythms and sleep in bipolar disorder. Bipolar Disord 12: 459–472. doi: 10.1111/j.1399-5618.2010.00843.x

36. Treuer T, Tohen M (2010) Predicting the course and outcome of bipolar disorder: a review. Eur Psychiatry 25: 328–333. doi: 10.1016/j.eurpsy.2009.11.012

37. Liu C, Li S, Liu T, Borjigin J, Lin JD (2007) Transcriptional coactivator PGC-1 alpha integrates the mammalian clock and energy metabolism. Nature 447: 477–481. doi: 10.1038/nature05767

38. Van Cauter E, Holmback U, Knutson K, Leproult R, Miller A, et al. (2007) Impact of sleep and sleep loss on neuroendocrine and metabolic function. Horm Res 1: 2–9. doi: 10.1159/000097543

39. Berg C, Lappas G, Wolk A, Strandhagen E, Torén K, et al. (2009) Eating patterns and portion size associated with obesity in a Swedish population. Appetite 52: 21–26. doi: 10.1016/j.appet.2008.07.008

40. Brown MS, Goldstein JL (1986) A receptor-mediated pathway for cholesterol homeostasis. Science 232: 34–47. doi: 10.1126/science.3513311

41. Horton JD, Goldstein JL, Brown MS (2002) SREBPs: activators of the complete program of cholesterol and fatty acid synthesis in the liver. J Clin Invest 109: 1125–1131. doi: 10.1172/JCI15593

42. Yokoyama C, Wang X, Briggs MR, Admon A, Wu J, et al. (1993) SREBP-1, a basic-helix-loop-helix-leucine zipper protein that controls transcription of the low density lipoprotein receptor gene. Cell 75: 187–197. doi: 10.1016/0092-8674(93)90690-r

43. Matsumoto E, Ishihara A, Tamai S, Nemoto A, Iwase K, et al. (2010) Time of day and nutrients in feeding govern daily expression rhythms of the gene for sterol regulatory element-binding protein (SREBP)-1 in the mouse liver. J Biol Chem 285: 33028–33036. doi: 10.1074/jbc.M109.089391

44. Bøggild H, Knutsson A (1999) Shift work, risk factors and cardiovascular disease. Scand J Work Environ Health 25: 85–99. doi: 10.5271/sjweh.410

45. Foster RG, Wulff K (2005) The rhythm of rest and excess. Nat Rev Neurosci 6: 407–414. doi: 10.1038/nrn1670

46. Esquirol Y, Bongard V, Mabile L, Jonnier B, Soulat JM, et al. (2009) Shift work and metabolic syndrome: respective impacts of job strain, physical activity, and dietary rhythms. Chronobiol Int 26: 544–559. doi: 10.1080/07420520902821176

47. Andrews RC, Walker BR (1999) Glucocorticoids and insulin resistance: old hormones, new targets. Clin Sci 96: 513–523. doi: 10.1042/CS19980388

48. Saltiel AR, Kahn CR (2001) Insulin signalling and the regulation of glucose and lipid metabolism. Nature 414: 799–806. doi: 10.1038/414799a

49. Fortes PC, de Moraes TP, Mendes JG, Stinghen AE, Ribeiro SC, et al. (2009) Insulin resistance and glucose homeostasis in peritoneal dialysis. Perit Dial Int 2: S145–148.

50. Lizcano JM, Alessi DR (2002) The insulin signalling pathway. Curr Biol 12: R236–R238. doi: 10.1016/S0960-9822(02)00777-7

51. Saltiel AR, Pessin JE (2002) Insulin signaling pathways in time and space. Trends Cell Biol 12: 65–71. doi: 10.1016/S0962-8924(01)02207-3

52. Marino JS, Xu Y, Hill JW (2011) Central insulin and leptin-mediated autonomic control of glucose homeostasis. Trends Endocrinol Metab 22: 275–285. doi: 10.1016/j.tem.2011.03.001

53. La Fleur SE, Kalsbeek A, Wortel J, Buijs RM (1999) A suprachiasmatic nucleus generated rhythm in basal glucose concentrations. J Neuroendocrinol 11: 643–652. doi: 10.1046/j.1365-2826.1999.00373.x

54. Son GH, Chung S, Choe HK, Kim HD, Baik SM, et al. (2008) Adrenal peripheral clock controls the autonomous circadian rhythm of glucocorticoid by causing rhythmic steroid production. PNAS USA 105: 20970–20975. doi: 10.1073/pnas.0806962106

55. Park N, Cheon S, Son GH, Cho S, Kim K (2012) Chronic circadian disturbance by a shortened light-dark cycle increases mortality. Neurobiol Aging 33: 1122.e11–e22. doi: 10.1016/j.neurobiolaging.2011.11.005

56. Cho S, Cho H, Geum D, Kim K (1998) Retinoic acid regulates gonadotropin-releasing hormone (GnRH) release and gene expression in the rat hypothalamic fragments and GT1-1 neuronal cells in vitro. Mol Brain Res 54: 74–84. doi: 10.1016/S0169-328X(97)00325-2

57. Doi M, Cho S, Yujnovsky I, Hirayama J, Cermakian N, et al. (2007) Light-inducible and clock-controlled expression of MAP kinase phosphatase 1 in mouse central pacemaker neurons. J Biol Rhythms 22: 127–139. doi: 10.1177/0748730406298332

*There are several supplemental files that are not available in this version of the article. To view this additional information, please use the citation information cited on the first page of this chapter.*

# CHAPTER 9

# A METABOLIC–TRANSCRIPTIONAL NETWORK LINKS SLEEP AND CELLULAR ENERGETICS IN THE BRAIN

JONATHAN P. WISOR

## 9.1 INTRODUCTION

The field of sleep research has gained profound insights from molecular genetic and classical genetic studies over the past decade (reviewed in Refs. [22, 67, 86]). Sleep loss triggers a large scale change in transcriptional regulatory networks [19, 50], including the circadian clock genes [28, 88]. However, a link between these transcriptional changes and the restorative function of sleep remains elusive. Published studies document that sleep/wake cycles are sensitive to, and paralleled by, changes in cellular metabolic status in the brain (reviewed in Refs. [10, 19, 71]). Others demonstrate that cellular metabolic sensors regulate circadian clock gene function (reviewed in Refs. [5, 9, 39]). Still others demonstrate that circadian clock genes regulate sleep/wake cycles and molecular responses

*With kind permission from Springer Science+Business Media: Pflügers Archiv:* European Journal of Physiology, *A Metabolic–Transcriptional Network Links Sleep and Cellular Energetics in the Brain, 463(1), 2012, 15–22, Jonathan P. Wisor, Figure 1,* © *Springer-Verlag 2011.*

to sleep loss in a manner that extends beyond their role in the generation of 24-hour rhythms (reviewed in Ref. [27] and Landgraf et al., this issue). This article seeks to unite these three themes in a unitary conceptual framework. The three themes converge to provide a framework whereby the interrelations of cellular metabolism, transcriptional regulatory events and sleep/wake-related changes in neuronal activity are united as a functional entity within the brain (Fig. 1). By this proposed mechanism, the detection of cellular metabolic status by the transcriptional network centered around circadian clock genes regulates sleep states to maintain metabolic homeostasis in the brain. Future efforts might exploit the interrelationship of circadian clock genes, sleep and cellular energetics for therapeutic benefit.

Sleep–wake cycles are accompanied by profound shifts in cerebral metabolism (reviewed in Ref. [51]). A reduction in the rate of cerebral glucose metabolism during nonrapid eye movement sleep (NREMS) relative to wakefulness is a reliable finding in positron emission tomography studies on human subjects. Estimates of the reduction in cerebral glucose metabolism during NREMS relative to wakefulness range from 12% [35] to 30% [44] to 44% [51]. This relationship does not apply for rapid eye movement sleep, a state in which the cerebral cortex is as active as it is during wake both electroencephalographically and metabolically [14, 52]. Since the majority of time spent asleep is in NREMS, the overall conclusion stands that sleep is a state of reduced metabolic demand in the brain.

What is the electrophysiological basis for the reduction in cerebral metabolism during sleep relative to wakefulness? Slow oscillations in the electroencephalogram (EEG) during NREMS are accompanied by oscillations in cerebral cortical neurons between an up (depolarized) state in which the cell is excitable and engages in burst firing, and a down (hyperpolarized) state in which the cell is silent. The cooccurrence of slow ($\leq 1$ Hz) waves and down state/up state alternations during NREMS is now a well-documented feature of NREMS in rodents [41, 81], cats [24, 56] and humans [61]. The alternation of firing between up and down states during NREMS contrasts with the tonic up states that occur during wakefulness. These silent down states may in fact be critical to the reduced metabolism that occurs during NREMS. Action potentials necessitate energy expenditure, as ion fluxes must be countered by energy efficient [4] but nonetheless energy-consuming [8, 15] mechanisms that repolarize the cell.

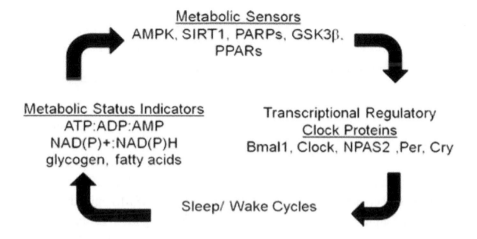

**Metabolic Sensors**
AMPK, SIRT1, PARPs, GSK3β,
PPARs

**Metabolic Status Indicators**
ATP:ADP:AMP
NAD(P)+:NAD(P)H
glycogen, fatty acids

**Transcriptional Regulatory**
**Clock Proteins**
Bmal1, Clock, NPAS2 ,Per, Cry

Sleep/ Wake Cycles

**FIGURE 1:** Proposed interrelationships of metabolic status, cellular metabolic sensors, transcriptional regulatory circadian clock genes, and the sleep–wake cycle. Intensive use of neuronal circuits during wakefulness poses a metabolic challenge that is manifested by changes in the relative concentrations of metabolic status indicators in the cell. Metabolic sensor proteins react to these changes by altering the concentrations or activities of transcriptional regulatory clock proteins. Changes in transcriptional regulatory clock protein levels or their functional activities alter the propensity for sleep. Sleep alters the metabolic status of the cell in a manner that reverses the metabolic challenge posed by wakefulness

There are caveats to this conceptual model of sleep as a mediator of cellular energetic functions. The model focuses largely on cerebral cortical EEG dynamics as a key readout for understanding sleep function. EEG dynamics are influenced by a complex system of subcortical regulatory centers. Some of these centers promote, and others inhibit, slow EEG activity (reviewed in Refs. [42, 75]). Still others serve REM sleep regulatory functions (reviewed in Ref. [72]). In accordance with their roles, these subcortical regulatory centers have their own state-specific activity patterns. These subcortical centers are likely to contribute to sleep-related changes in brain metabolic status, both through their effects on the cortical EEG, and changes in their own metabolic demand. Additionally, the ≤1-Hz slow waves associated with alternating up and down states should not be confused with what has traditionally been thought of as the EEG marker for sleep homeostasis, delta (0.5–4 Hz) activity [12], Slow waves and delta activity are concordant in at least two senses. First, both are prominent in NREMS and rare during wake and REMS. Second, slow waves are most likely to occur on a large spatial scale early in the sleep period, when delta activity and sleep need are highest [61]. Just as delta power dissipates across a night's sleep, the global span [61] and amplitude [1] of up/down states (also described as on/off states [61]) decreases with the discharge of sleep need. Nonetheless, there is evidence that these two types of NREMS-related activity are the products of distinct neuronal events. Whereas the decline in delta power across a night's sleep, presumed to reflect the discharge of sleep need, occurs incrementally across NREMS episodes, EEG power at frequencies below 1 Hz exhibits a distinct pattern of decline [1]. Therefore, it should not be assumed that any function attributed to ≤1 Hz up/down oscillations, including possibly a cellular energetic function, is in a 1:1 relationship with 0.5–4 Hz EEG power dynamics, the traditional and widely applied measure of sleep homeostasis.

The regulatory mechanisms that enforce the relationship between sleep and cellular metabolism are not fully characterized, but are likely to be related to the synthesis and use of adenosine triphosphate (ATP), an essential energy source for maintaining the cell membrane ionic concentration gradients critical for neuronal excitability. Down states during NREMS are defined by a precipitous decline in the occurrence of action potentials. The decline in the number of action potentials curtails demand for ATP-dependent membrane repolarization mechanisms [8]. There is thus considerable appeal to the notion that sleep serves an essential function for brain metabolism. However, what is the evidence that metabolic demand is a driving force in the regulation of sleep, as opposed to an epiphenomenon coincident to but independent of sleep regulation? There is evidence, reviewed below, that a number of metabolic status indicators vary across sleep states within the brain, and that these metabolic status indicators regulate sleep via their effects on cellular metabolic sensors. The mechanisms that mediate the relationship between molecular sensors of cellular metabolic status and sleep are ill-defined. While changes in the cellular metabolic status of neurons can occur on a timescale of seconds, regulatory changes in EEG-defined sleep occur on the scale of minutes to hours. Metabolically-induced transcriptional changes may bridge these timescales, transducing short-term cellular changes to long-term changes in sleep states. Beginning from this assumption, one can inquire about the effects of metabolic changes on transcriptional regulation. The circadian transcriptional regulatory machinery is well-positioned to transduce short-term metabolic changes into longer-term changes in the macromolecular composition of the cell. We now consider the relationships of a panel of cellular metabolic sensors to sleep/wake cycles and how the relationships between these sensors and sleep might be mediated by clock genes.

## 9.2 AMPK: A METABOLIC INDICATOR FOR CELLULAR ENERGY CHARGE

ATP is the primary energy currency of the cell. It is the cellular fuel that offers the greatest amount of potential energy in the oxidative metabolic chain [54, 58]. In the production of ATP, adenosine is the backbone for a series of energy transfer reactions. Consumption of glucose, fatty acid, or amino acid-derived fuels by the citric acid cycle results in the sequential attachment of phosphate groups to this adenosine backbone to form adenosine monophosphate (AMP), adenosine diphosphate (ADP) and ATP. Subsequent reversal of this set of reactions removes these phosphate groups, yielding energy to perform work such as the operation of ion pumps that produce the ion concentration gradients necessary for action potentials. NREMS is paralleled by a reduced ATP flux relative to wakefulness [25, 78]. Sleep loss, by contrast, causes in the brain an increase in the expression of the mitochondrial genome [20], an indication that the requirement for ATP use is increased during wake relative to sleep.

The regulation of ATP metabolism is highly tuned by an elaborate set of regulatory mechanisms [59], including the activity of the adenosine monophosphate-activated protein kinase (AMPK; reviewed in Ref. [32]). When the AMP/ATP ratio increases due to consumption of ATP (a decrease in cellular "energy charge"), AMPK is phosphorylated by upstream kinases and initiates changes in the cell that slow ATP consumption. This mechanism appears to be at work in the brain in association with sleep; temporal patterns of AMPK phosphorylation provide evidence that this metabolic sensor reacts to changes in sleep/wake states. AMPK phosphorylation in the brain is reduced during times of day when sleep predominates [25]. Enforced wake caused an increase in phosphorylated AMPK (pAMPK) [18, 25].

With its wide-ranging impact on cellular regulatory pathways [32], it is hard to imagine that sleep/wake-related changes in AMPK activity would not impact on sleep physiology. Indeed, AMPK does appear to affect sleep physiology. An AMPK inhibitor attenuated NREMS slow wave activity (SWA) during spontaneous sleep, while an activator enhanced it [18]. These data demonstrate that AMPK is a driver of sleep need. How are the effects of AMPK activation mediated? Multiple mechanisms may be at play, but one may involve the product of the canonical clock gene cryptochrome 1 (*cry1*). It is a target for phosphorylation by AMPK. Phosphorylation by AMPK destabilizes Cry1 protein [48], preventing it from performing its transcriptional inhibitory function. The effect of AMPK activation on sleep [18] is similar to *cry1/cry2* double gene knockout, which increases time spent in NREMS, NREMS consolidation and NREMS SWA [87]. The degradation of Cry proteins, analogous to gene knockout, may contribute to the SWA-promoting effect of pharmacological activation of AMPK [18].

## 9.3 NAD(P)H:NAD(P)$^+$: A METABOLIC INDICATOR FOR REDOX STATUS

The synthesis of ATP requires oxidation–reduction reactions at several stages of carbohydrate metabolism and during the citric acid cycle. As intermediates are oxidized, a pool of cellular nicotine adenine dinucleotides (NAD) undergoes reduction. NAD harboring an additional phosphate group (NADP) also serves as a reducing agent; NAD and NAD(P) are collectively labeled as NAD(P). A high rate of ATP production will alter the NAD(P)H:NAD(P)+ratio. This ratio, therefore, provides a metabolic indicator of changes in cellular redox status in parallel with metabolic load. Given the sleep state-dependence of ATP production in the brain, it seems likely that the ratios of NAD(P)H:NAD(P)$^+$ should also vary with sleep states.

So what evidence indicates that cellular redox status, and with it the ratio of NAD(P)H:NAD(P)$^+$, varies across sleep cycles? Several papers have found evidence of oxidative stress occurring after sleep loss. Upregulation of gluthathione and glutathione peroxidase occurs in the rat brain as a consequence of sleep deprivation [68]. Upregulation of this antioxidant pathway presumably serves to counteract the oxidative load associated with the SD-related increase in glycolytic enzyme activity (documented by both Refs. [68] and [76]). Increased lipid peroxidation and oxidized glutathione, additional measures of oxidative stress, have also been observed in the brains of sleep deprived mice [73]. That sleep loss accelerates metabolic pathways involving oxidation reactions can be inferred based on the effects of SD on transcripts related to oxidant defenses [50, 71]. These data are compatible with the concept that cellular oxidative stress is a consequence of sleep loss.

Oxidative stress caused by sleep loss may feed into cellular metabolic regulation through NAD(P)-sensing proteins. The positive transcriptional regulator of clock-related transcripts, NPAS2, is impacted by oxidative stress and the NAD(P)H:NAD(P)$^+$ ratio [70]. The molecular basis for effects of redox status on the clock mechanism was not clear at the time of its discovery, but latter observations on the effect of the NAD-sensing histone deacetylase SIRT1 on transcriptional regulatory clock genes [6] may be relevant to the matter. SIRT1 protein undergoes circadian oscillations and is necessary for high amplitude oscillations in *bmal1, dbp and period2 (per2)* gene expression in an in vitro fibroblast model of circadian clock function. In SIRT1-deficient mice, positive regulators Bmal1 and Clock are downregulated at the protein level and the negative regulators Per2 and Cry1 are upregulated. SIRT1 protein binds to Per2, Bmal1 and Clock and deacetylates Per2 protein, resulting in a reduction of the half-life of Per2 protein [6]. Collectively, these results demonstrate that SIRT1 deacetylation of Per2 is required for the timely degradation of Per2 protein and subsequent derepression of per and cry transcripts. In the absence of SIRT1-dependent deacetylation, Per2 protein remains in the cell longer, decreasing the amplitude and increasing the period of circadian oscillations. All of these effects occur in interaction with the transcriptional regulator, Clock, which is a histone acetyltransferase (HAT; [36]). SIRT1, as a histone deacetylase (HDAC) counteracts the enzymatic activity of Clock.

Being NAD+–sensitive [79], SIRT1 is positioned to modulate the clock gene network in concert with cellular redox state. Also, given the previously cited evidence that cellular redox status varies with sleep state, SIRT1 might be expected to contribute to sleep regulation. Data from SIRT1-deficient mice support this notion. SIRT1-deficient mice exhibit a failure to sustain state consolidation, characterized by reductions in time awake, wake episode duration and NREMS SWA [65]. That said, histochemical data reported in the same study document degeneration of wake-promoting subcortical nuclei in SIRT1-deficient mice. Whether the sleep phenotype is secondary to the degeneration, as opposed to an acute consequence of SIRT1-deficiency, cannot be determined based on these data alone. Studies on the acute effects of SIRT1 inhibitors (a number of which are available [3]) on sleep might advance this line of work.

## 9.4 POLY ADP-RIBOSE POLYMERASE (PARP): A SECONDARY SENSOR OF BOTH CELLULAR ENERGY CHARGE AND REDOX STATUS

ADP-ribosylation is a posttranslational modification that regulates the activities of dynamic proteins in the cell. PARPs are a family of enzymes capable of ADP ribosylation of target proteins [38]. PARPs exert some of their influence on cellular function as transcriptional regulatory proteins. PARP activity is regulated by both AMPK-dependent phosphorylation [82] and SIRT1 [33, 46], the potential clock gene- and sleep-regulatory functions which are mentioned above. So as a potential mediator of the cellular response to changes in both energy charge and redox status, PARPs have the potential to modulate cellular physiology in accordance with sleep state.

Indeed, there is evidence that PARP activity regulates sleep state. The acute response to the PARP inhibitor minocycline includes a period of insomnia lasting hours [89]. Additionally, minocycline strongly suppresses EEG slow wave activity in the cerebral cortex both after sleep deprivation [89] and in spontaneous sleep conditions in humans [62] and mice [85]. The somnolytic effect of this PARP inhibitor is indicative of a potential sleep-promoting role for PARP activity. It is possible that SIRT1 and PARP act antagonistically in sleep/wake regulation. SIRT1 activation, in association with a shift in redox status, inhibits PARP and (whether through this mechanism or independently) supports wake-promoting mechanisms. Reduced SIRT1 activity occurring as a consequence of a wake-dependent increase in oxidative stress, liberates PARP-1, and consequent PARP enzymatic/transcriptional activity that promote sleep. This argument hinges on the assumption that the sleep-suppressing effect of minocycline is mediated by PARP inhibition. It is a significant caveat, however, that the effects of minocycline may be mediated through other mechanisms (such as the antibiotic effect of this tetracycline derivative). Given this caveat, it would be very informative to study the sleep phenotype of PARP-1 deficient mice, and its modulation (or lack thereof) by minocycline.

Like other metabolically driven enzymes, PARP activity regulates the circadian clock proteins [7]. In the liver, at least, PARP activity (as measured by protein ADP-ribosylation) is circadian. PARP-1 binds to, and ADP-ribosylates, the Clock protein. Genetic deficiency for PARP-1 depresses Clock/Bmal1-dependent transcription and, thereby, alters the daily cycle of gene expression in the liver and its entrainment by restricted feeding.

## 9.5 GLYCOGEN METABOLISM: AVAILABILITY OF SUBSTRATES FOR THE CITRIC ACID CYCLE

The citric acid cycle, a source of ATP needed for cellular work, is initiated with the consumption of an energy substrate, which in the brain is typically derived from glycolytic processing of a glucose-derived substrate. Benington and Heller proposed that the energy challenge posed by wakefulness obligates the depletion of glycogen stores, which in turn obligates the replenishment of those glycogen stores through sleep [10]. Some earlier observations indicated that sleep facilitated the synthesis of glycogen within the brain [43]. Glycogen levels are, however, inconsistently affected by short-term sleep loss (reviewed in Ref. [71]). It may not be the concentration of glycogen, but rather its rate of turnover, which increases and decreases in concert with wake and sleep, respectively [55, 66].

Glycogen synthase kinases, including glycogen synthase kinase 3β (GSK3β), are essential to the regulation of cellular glycogen stores. GSK3β provides negative feedback to prevent the synthesis of glycogen when glycogen stores are sufficient or glucose supplies must be diverted to other uses [60]; it phosphorylates glycogen synthase, thereby suppressing the synthesis of glycogen. GSK3β, like AMPK, is sensitive to cellular metabolic status and enforced wakefulness, and affects sleep. The phosphorylation of GSK3β increases in synaptosomes during enforced wakefulness [80]. GSK3β overexpression in mice disrupts the consolidation of NREMS [2]. The role of GSK3β as a kinase extends beyond regulation of glycogen synthase into the realm of clock genes. It was first implicated in circadian rhythmicity through fruit fly studies. The Drosophila orthologue of GSK3β phosphorylates the Clock protein TIMELESS, and overexpression of GSK3β shortens circadian period in *Drosophila* [53]. Similar observations were subsequently made in studies on mammalian tissues [40]. Overexpression of GSK3β shortens circadian period in cultured mammalian cells while pharmacological inhibition lengthens it. These effects of GSK3β manipulations on the clock may be mediated by phosphorylation of Period proteins; the same study demonstrated direct interactions of mammalian GSK3β with Per2, GSK3β-dependent phosphorylation of Per2 and GSK3β-dependent nuclear entry of Per2 [40].

## 9.6 PEROXISOME PROLIFERATOR-ACTIVATED RECEPTORS (PPARS): SENSORS OF LIPID METABOLISM

Fatty acids, like glucose derivatives, can fuel the production of ATP through the citric acid cycle. Lipids endogenous to the central nervous system are known regulators of sleep [11] and lipid species have been demonstrated to vary in cerebrospinal fluid in association with sleep loss [21, 45]. PPARs, a family of transcriptional regulatory nuclear receptors, are sensitive to the endogenous sleep-promoting lipids anandamide [13] and oleylethanolamide [29], and therefore, mediate transcriptional responses related to fatty acid metabolism [74]. Two members of the PPAR family of receptors, PPARs α and γ, share in common with the above described metabolic sensors the ability to influence both the circadian clock and sleep–wake cycles. Chronic administration of dietary bezafibrate, the antihyperlipidemic PPARα agonist, increases NREMS SWA during the light phase in rodents [17]. This effect, which is phenomenologically similar to sleep deprivation, is compatible with a role for this transcriptional regulator in the sleep homeostat. However, the effect cannot be attributed to the brain with certainty as the treatment was systemic. The effects of PPARα agonist administration on sleep might be mediated by changes in the circadian clock gene network. PPARα binds to the bmal1 promoter, and its binding is necessary for the circadian expression of bmal1 in the rodent liver (though not in the suprachiasmatic nucleus). Fenofibrate, another PPARα agonist, upregulates clock gene expression in vitro [16]. PPARγ is also a positive regulator of bmal1 transcription [83] and may contribute to the sleep/wake effects of PPAR agonists.

## 9.7 A MISSING LINK: HOW MIGHT A TRANSCRIPTIONAL FEEDBACK LOOP MODULATE NEURONAL EXCITABILITY IN ASSOCIATION WITH SLEEP/WAKE STATES?

One missing link in this story is embodied by the question: are the effects of metabolic sensors on sleep/wake regulation mediated by their effects on circadian clock protein function, or by other means? If the effects are mediated by clock mechanisms, then how does a molecular feedback loop of the clock regulate neuronal excitability, the final common path of sleep regulation? We know from the data reviewed in this volume [49] and elsewhere [27] that spontaneous and experimentally induced genetic variations in circadian clock gene loci impact sleep homeostasis. However, the molecular and electrophysiological mechanisms by which the clock component proteins affect changes in sleep is a crucial gap in the current state of knowledge. The circadian clock, in its simplest most fundamental form, is a negative feedback loop consisting of a network of transcriptional regulatory proteins that regulate the transcription of their own genetic loci. Clock output pathways driven by the positive regulators of this feedback loop are a potential source of insight. Genetic disruption of the positive transcriptional components of the feedback loop present obvious circadian phenotypes, but additionally exhibit alterations in EEG measures associated with sleep homeostasis. Both NPAS2-deficient and Clock mutant mice exhibit reduced time in NREMS. The sleep phenotype of Bmal1-deficient mice increased NREMS bout duration and EEG delta activity relative to controls is, on its face, opposite those of NPAS2-deficient and Clock mutant mice. This discrepancy might reflect the fact that Clock and NPAS2, unlike Bmal1, overlap functionally. Loss of functional clock alleles can be compensated by NPAS2 expression [23, 31], and vice versa, whereas there is no compensatory change (at least in terms of circadian behavior) in response to the loss of *bmal1*. Therefore, the sleep phenotypes associated with Clock and NPAS2 mutations represent perturbed transcriptional networks, whereas that of bmal1 deficiency represents total disruption of the network.

So which clock outputs are relevant to sleep phenotypes? The fact that a significant portion of the genome is regulated by the circadian clock [63, 64] is at once a testament to the importance of this regulatory regime and a curse to those who seek a mechanistic link between the molecular clock components and sleep homeostasis. The identification of sleep regulatory loci extends beyond the core clock components to at least one transcriptional target of Clock and Bmal1, DEC2. A point mutation of the DEC2 gene identified in humans and subsequently engineered into mice confers reduced time asleep relative to the wild type allele [34]. Still, it will be a challenge to trace a path from these molecular events associated with the clock to the excitability of the cerebral cortex at the EEG level. Evidence that the clock can regulate neuronal excitability is rare but present. For instance, neuropeptide-induced *period1* expression drives an increase in the excitability of suprachiasmatic neurons in vitro [30] albeit through a still uncertain mechanism. Based on this observation, it can be hypothesized that clock genes regulate sleep state-specific changes in excitability in a cell-endogenous manner. The details of this regulatory path await characterization.

## 9.8 SYNTHESIS AND OUTLOOK

Sleep has long been posited to have a function in regulating brain metabolic status. Given the restorative effects on brain function that are attributed to sleep, there is considerable intellectual appeal to this line of reasoning. This review has described the evidence that metabolic indicators vary within the brain across sleep/wake cycles. It has identified metabolic sensors in the cell that mediate the effects of these indicators on cell function. It has described, for each such sensor, the evidence that the sensor affects sleep. Additionally, it has described the effects of these metabolic sensors on circadian clock protein function.

Segregation of enzymatic processes is necessary to prevent futile cycles of production and consumption and to generate the concentration gradients that build potential energy in the cell [60]. When spatial segregation is not possible, temporal segregation may suffice [77]. The transcriptional–translational loop that composes the circadian clock may have been adapted for this purpose in areas of the brain outside the SCN to enforce the temporal segregation of distinct metabolic processes into sleep and wake. It is a challenge to identify a cellular metabolic substrate for "sleep" if one defines sleep as a property of cell networks, which even the most reductionist models of sleep do [47, 69]. However, inasmuch as these network properties are influenced by metabolically responsive clock molecules, it should be possible to do so.

The availability of tools to study cellular metabolic status in brain-derived tissues and in the brain itself with increasing temporal and spatial resolution (for example, Refs. [25, 57, 84]) will continue to drive inquiries within this conceptual framework. These technological improvements can be coupled with the increasingly elegant genetic manipulations that characterize studies of clock gene function (for example, Refs. [26, 37]). From a biomarker discovery standpoint, the regulatory networks described in this review may contribute to the tremendous interindividual variability in sleep need in the general population. From a therapeutic standpoint, manipulating the response of the cell to energetic status through clock genes and sleep-related waveforms may provide novel therapeutic inroads in stroke and other conditions impacted by abnormalities in the processing of glycolytic fuels.

## REFERENCES

1.  Achermann P, Borbely AA (1997) Low-frequency (<1 Hz) oscillations in the human sleep electroencephalogram. Neuroscience 81:213–222

2.  Ahnaou A, Drinkenburg WH (2010) Disruption of glycogen synthase kinase-3-beta activity leads to abnormalities in physiological measures in mice. Behav Brain Res 221:246–252

3.  Alcain FJ, Villalba JM (2009) Sirtuin inhibitors. Expert Opin Ther Pat 19:283–294

4.  Alle H, Roth A, Geiger JR (2009) Energy-efficient action potentials in hippocampal mossy fibers. Science 325:1405–1408

5.  Asher G, Schibler U (2011) Crosstalk between components of circadian and metabolic cycles in mammals. Cell Metab 13:125–137

6.  Asher G, Gatfield D, Stratmann M, Reinke H, Dibner C, Kreppel F, Mostoslavsky R, Alt FW, Schibler U (2008) SIRT1 regulates circadian clock gene expression through PER2 deacetylation. Cell 134:317–328

7.  Asher G, Reinke H, Altmeyer M, Gutierrez-Arcelus M, Hottiger MO, Schibler U (2010) Poly(ADP-ribose) polymerase 1 participates in the phase entrainment of circadian clocks to feeding. Cell 142:943–953

8.  Attwell D, Laughlin SB (2001) An energy budget for signaling in the grey matter of the brain. J Cereb Blood Flow Metab 21:1133–1145

9.  Bechtold DA (2008) Energy-responsive timekeeping. J Genet 87:447–458

10. Benington JH, Heller HC (1995) Restoration of brain energy metabolism as the function of sleep. Prog Neurobiol 45:347–360

11. Boger DL, Henriksen SJ, Cravatt BF (1998) Oleamide: an endogenous sleep-inducing lipid and prototypical member of a new class of biological signaling molecules. Curr Pharm Des 4:303–314

12. Borbely AA, Achermann P (2004) Sleep homeostasis and models of sleep regulation. In: Kryger MH, Roth T, Dement WC (eds) Principles and practice of sleep medicine. Saunders, Philadelphia, pp 377–390

13. Bouaboula M, Hilairet S, Marchand J, Fajas L, Le Fur G, Casellas P (2005) Anandamide induced PPARgamma transcriptional activation and 3T3-L1 preadipocyte differentiation. Eur J Pharmacol 517:174–181

14. Buchsbaum MS, Gillin JC, Wu J, Hazlett E, Sicotte N, Dupont RM, Bunney WE Jr (1989) Regional cerebral glucose metabolic rate in human sleep assessed by positron emission tomography. Life Sci 45:1349–1356

15. Buzsaki G, Kaila K, Raichle M (2007) Inhibition and brain work. Neuron 56:771–783

16. Canaple L, Rambaud J, Dkhissi-Benyahya O, Rayet B, Tan NS, Michalik L, Delaunay F, Wahli W, Laudet V (2006) Reciprocal regulation of brain and muscle Arnt-like protein 1 and peroxisome proliferator-activated receptor alpha defines a novel positive feedback loop in the rodent liver circadian clock. Mol Endocrinol 20:1715–1727

17. Chikahisa S, Tominaga K, Kawai T, Kitaoka K, Oishi K, Ishida N, Rokutan K, Sei H (2008) Bezafibrate, a PPARs agonist, decreases body temperature and enhances EEG delta oscillation during sleep in mice. Endocrinology 149:5262–5271

18. Chikahisa S, Fujiki N, Kitaoka K, Shimizu N, Sei H (2009) Central AMPK contributes to sleep homeostasis in mice. Neuropharmacology 57:369–374

19. Cirelli C (2006) Cellular consequences of sleep deprivation in the brain. Sleep Med Rev 10:307–321

20. Cirelli C, Tononi G (1998) Differences in gene expression between sleep and waking as revealed by mRNA differential display. Brain Res Mol Brain Res 56:293–305

21. Cravatt BF, Prospero-Garcia O, Siuzdak G, Gilula NB, Henriksen SJ, Boger DL, Lerner RA (1995) Chemical characterization of a family of brain lipids that induce sleep. Science 268:1506–1509

22. Dauvilliers Y, Tafti M (2008) The genetic basis of sleep disorders. Curr Pharm Des 14:3386–3395

23. DeBruyne JP, Noton E, Lambert CM, Maywood ES, Weaver DR, Reppert SM (2006) A clock shock: mouse CLOCK is not required for circadian oscillator function. Neuron 50:465

24. Destexhe A, Contreras D, Steriade M (1999) Spatiotemporal analysis of local field potentials and unit discharges in cat cerebral cortex during natural wake and sleep states. J Neurosci 19:4595–4608

25. Dworak M, McCarley RW, Kim T, Kalinchuk AV, Basheer R (2010) Sleep and brain energy levels: ATP changes during sleep. J Neurosci 30:9007–9016

26. Etchegaray JP, Machida KK, Noton E, Constance CM, Dallmann R, Di Napoli MN, DeBruyne JP, Lambert CM, Yu EA, Reppert SM, Weaver DR (2009) Casein kinase 1 delta regulates the pace of the mammalian circadian clock. Mol Cell Biol 29:3853–3866

27. Franken P, Dijk DJ (2009) Circadian clock genes and sleep homeostasis. Eur J Neurosci 29:1820–1829

28. Franken P, Thomason R, Heller HC, O'Hara BF (2007) A non-circadian role for clock-genes in sleep homeostasis: a strain comparison. BMC Neurosci 8:87

29. Fu J, Gaetani S, Oveisi F, Lo Verme J, Serrano A, Rodriguez De Fonseca F, Rosengarth A, Luecke H, Di Giacomo B, Tarzia G, Piomelli D (2003) Oleylethanolamide regulates feeding and body weight through activation of the nuclear receptor PPAR-alpha. Nature 425:90–93

30. Gamble KL, Allen GC, Zhou T, McMahon DG (2007) Gastrin-releasing peptide mediates light-like resetting of the suprachiasmatic nucleus circadian pacemaker through cAMP response element-binding protein and Per1 activation. J Neurosci 27:12078–12087

31. Haque R, Ali FG, Biscoglia R, Abey J, Weller J, Klein D, Iuvone PM (2011) CLOCK and NPAS2 have overlapping roles in the circadian oscillation of arylalkylamine N-acetyltransferase mRNA in chicken cone photoreceptors. J Neurochem 113:1296–1306

32. Hardie DG (2007) AMP-activated/SNF1 protein kinases: conserved guardians of cellular energy. Nat Rev Mol Cell Biol 8:774–785

33. Hassa PO, Haenni SS, Elser M, Hottiger MO (2006) Nuclear ADP-ribosylation reactions in mammalian cells: where are we today and where are we going? Microbiol Mol Biol Rev 70:789–829

34. He Y, Jones CR, Fujiki N, Xu Y, Guo B, Holder JL Jr, Rossner MJ, Nishino S, Fu YH (2009) The transcriptional repressor DEC2 regulates sleep length in mammals. Science 325:866–870

35. Heiss WD, Pawlik G, Herholz K, Wagner R, Wienhard K (1985) Regional cerebral glucose metabolism in man during wakefulness, sleep, and dreaming. Brain Res 327:362–366

36. Hirayama J, Sahar S, Grimaldi B, Tamaru T, Takamatsu K, Nakahata Y, Sassone-Corsi P (2007) CLOCK-mediated acetylation of BMAL1 controls circadian function. Nature 450:1086–1090

37. Hong HK, Chong JL, Song W, Song EJ, Jyawook AA, Schook AC, Ko CH, Taka-hashi JS (2007) Inducible and reversible Clock gene expression in brain using the tTA system for the study of circadian behavior. PLoS Genet 3:e33

38. Hottiger MO, Boothby M, Koch-Nolte F, Luscher B, Martin NM, Plummer R, Wang ZQ, Ziegler M (2011) Progress in the function and regulation of ADP-ribosylation. Sci Signal 4:mr5

39. Huang W, Ramsey KM, Marcheva B, Bass J (2011) Circadian rhythms, sleep, and metabolism. J Clin Invest 121:2133–2141

40. Iitaka C, Miyazaki K, Akaike T, Ishida N (2005) A role for glycogen synthase ki-nase-3beta in the mammalian circadian clock. J Biol Chem 280:29397–29402

41. Johnson LA, Euston DR, Tatsuno M, McNaughton BL (2008) Stored-trace reactiva-tion in rat prefrontal cortex is correlated with down-to-up state fluctuation density. J Neurosci 30:2650–2661

42. Jones BE (2004) Activity, modulation and role of basal forebrain cholinergic neu-rons innervating the cerebral cortex. Prog Brain Res 145:157–169

43. Karnovsky ML, Reich P, Anchors JM, Burrows BL (1983) Changes in brain glyco-gen during slow-wave sleep in the rat. J Neurochem 41:1498–1501

44. Kennedy C, Gillin JC, Mendelson W, Suda S, Miyaoka M, Ito M, Nakamura RK, Storch FI, Pettigrew K, Mishkin M, Sokoloff L (1982) Local cerebral glucose utili-zation in non-rapid eye movement sleep. Nature 297:325–327

45. Koethe D, Schreiber D, Giuffrida A, Mauss C, Faulhaber J, Heydenreich B, Hellmich M, Graf R, Klosterkotter J, Piomelli D, Leweke FM (2009) Sleep depriva-tion increases oleoylethanolamide in human cerebrospinal fluid. J Neural Transm 116:301–305

46. Krishnakumar R, Kraus WL The PARP side of the nucleus: molecular actions, physi-ological outcomes, and clinical targets. Mol Cell 39:8–24

47. Krueger JM, Rector DM, Roy S, Van Dongen HP, Belenky G, Panksepp J (2008) Sleep as a fundamental property of neuronal assemblies. Nat Rev Neurosci 9:910–919

48. Lamia KA, Sachdeva UM, DiTacchio L, Williams EC, Alvarez JG, Egan DF, Vasquez DS, Juguilon H, Panda S, Shaw RJ, Thompson CB, Evans RM (2009) AMPK regulates the circadian clock by cryptochrome phosphorylation and degra-dation. Science 326:437–440

49. Landgraf D, Shostak A, Oster H (2011) Clock genes and sleep. Pfluger's Archives Euro J Physiol, in press.

50. Mackiewicz M, Shockley KR, Romer MA, Galante RJ, Zimmerman JE, Naidoo N, Baldwin DA, Jensen ST, Churchill GA, Pack AI (2007) Macromolecule biosynthe-sis: a key function of sleep. Physiol Genomics 31:441–457

51. Maquet P (1995) Sleep function(s) and cerebral metabolism. Behav Brain Res 69:75–83

52. Maquet P, Dive D, Salmon E, Sadzot B, Franco G, Poirrier R, von Frenckell R, Franck G (1990) Cerebral glucose utilization during sleep–wake cycle in man de-termined by positron emission tomography and [18F]2-fluoro-2-deoxy-d-glucose method. Brain Res 513:136–143

53. Martinek S, Inonog S, Manoukian AS, Young MW (2001) A role for the segment polarity gene shaggy/GSK-3 in the Drosophila circadian clock. Cell 105:769–779

54. McMurry J, Castellion ME (1976) The generation of biochemical energy, organic and biological chemistry. Prentice-Hall, Upper Saddle River, NJ, pp 590–619

55. Morgenthaler FD, Lanz BR, Petit JM, Frenkel H, Magistretti PJ, Gruetter R (2009) Alteration of brain glycogen turnover in the conscious rat after 5 h of prolonged wakefulness. Neurochem Int 55:45–51

56. Mukovski M, Chauvette S, Timofeev I, Volgushev M (2007) Detection of active and silent states in neocortical neurons from the field potential signal during slow-wave sleep. Cereb Cortex 17:400–414

57. Naylor E, Aillon DV, Gabbert S, Harmon H, Johnson DA, Wilson GS, Petillo PA (2011) Real-time measurement of EEG/EMG and l-glutamate in mice: a biosensor study of neuronal activity during sleep. J Electroanal Chem 656:106–113

58. Nelson DL, Cox MM (2008) Bioenergetics and biochemical reaction types. Lehninger principles of biochemistry. Freeman, New York, pp 485–519

59. Nelson DL, Cox MM (2008) The citric acid cycle. Lehninger principles of biochemistry. Freeman, New York, pp 615–646

60. Nelson DL, Cox MM (2008) Principles of metabolic regulation. Lehninger principles of biochemistry. Freeman, New York, pp 569–614

61. Nir Y, Staba RJ, Andrillon T, Vyazovskiy VV, Cirelli C, Fried I, Tononi G (2011) Regional slow waves and spindles in human sleep. Neuron 70:153–169

62. Nonaka K, Nakazawa Y, Kotorii T (1983) Effects of antibiotics, minocycline and ampicillin, on human sleep. Brain Res 288:253–259

63. Oishi K, Miyazaki K, Kadota K, Kikuno R, Nagase T, Atsumi G, Ohkura N, Azama T, Mesaki M, Yukimasa S, Kobayashi H, Iitaka C, Umehara T, Horikoshi M, Kudo T, Shimizu Y, Yano M, Monden M, Machida K, Matsuda J, Horie S, Todo T, Ishida N (2003) Genome-wide expression analysis of mouse liver reveals CLOCK-regulated circadian output genes. J Biol Chem 278:41519–41527

64. Panda S, Antoch MP, Miller BH, Su AI, Schook AB, Straume M, Schultz PG, Kay SA, Takahashi JS, Hogenesch JB (2002) Coordinated transcription of key pathways in the mouse by the circadian clock. Cell 109:307–320

65. Panossian L, Fenik P, Zhu Y, Zhan G, McBurney MW, Veasey S (2010) SIRT1 regulation of wakefulness and senescence-like phenotype in wake neurons. J Neurosci 31:4025–4036

66. Petit JM, Tobler I, Kopp C, Morgenthaler F, Borbely AA, Magistretti PJ (2010) Metabolic response of the cerebral cortex following gentle sleep deprivation and modafinil administration. Sleep 33:901–908

67. Raizen DM, Wu MN (2010) Genome-wide association studies of sleep disorders. Chest 139:446–452

68. Ramanathan L, Hu S, Frautschy SA, Siegel JM (2010) Short-term total sleep deprivation in the rat increases antioxidant responses in multiple brain regions without impairing spontaneous alternation behavior. Behav Brain Res 207:305–309

69. Rector DM (2010) Local functional state differences between rat cortical columns. Curr Topics Med Chem, in press

70. Rutter J, Reick M, Wu LC, McKnight SL (2001) Regulation of clock and NPAS2 DNA binding by the redox state of NAD cofactors. Science 293:510–514
71. Scharf MT, Naidoo N, Zimmerman JE, Pack AI (2008) The energy hypothesis of sleep revisited. Prog Neurobiol 86:264–280
72. Siegel JM (2011) REM sleep: a biological and psychological paradox. Sleep Med 15:139–142
73. Silva RH, Abilio VC, Takatsu AL, Kameda SR, Grassl C, Chehin AB, Medrano WA, Calzavara MB, Registro S, Andersen ML, Machado RB, Carvalho RC, Ribeiro Rde A, Tufik S, Frussa-Filho R (2004) Role of hippocampal oxidative stress in memory deficits induced by sleep deprivation in mice. Neuropharmacology 46:895–903
74. Smith SA (2002) Peroxisome proliferator-activated receptors and the regulation of mammalian lipid metabolism. Biochem Soc Trans 30:1086–1090
75. Szymusiak R (2010) Hypothalamic versus neocortical control of sleep. Curr Opin Pulm Med 16:530–535
76. Thakkar M, Mallick BN (1993) Rapid eye movement sleep-deprivation-induced changes in glucose metabolic enzymes in rat brain. Sleep 16:691–694
77. Tu BP, McKnight SL (2006) Metabolic cycles as an underlying basis of biological oscillations. Nat Rev Mol Cell Biol 7:696–701
78. Van den Noort S, Brine K (1970) Effect of sleep on brain labile phosphates and metabolic rate. Am J Physiol 218:1434–1439
79. Vaziri H, Dessain SK, Ng Eaton E, Imai SI, Frye RA, Pandita TK, Guarente L, Weinberg RA (2001) hSIR2(SIRT1) functions as an NAD-dependent p53 deacetylase. Cell 107:149–159
80. Vyazovskiy VV, Cirelli C, Pfister-Genskow M, Faraguna U, Tononi G (2008) Molecular and electrophysiological evidence for net synaptic potentiation in wake and depression in sleep. Nat Neurosci 11:200–208
81. Vyazovskiy VV, Olcese U, Lazimy YM, Faraguna U, Esser SK, Williams JC, Cirelli C, Tononi G (2009) Cortical firing and sleep homeostasis. Neuron 63:865–878
82. Walker JW, Jijon HB, Madsen KL (2006) AMP-activated protein kinase is a positive regulator of poly(ADP-ribose) polymerase. Biochem Biophys Res Commun 342:336–341
83. Wang N, Yang G, Jia Z, Zhang H, Aoyagi T, Soodvilai S, Symons JD, Schnermann JB, Gonzalez FJ, Litwin SE, Yang T (2008) Vascular PPARgamma controls circadian variation in blood pressure and heart rate through Bmal1. Cell Metab 8:482–491
84. Wigren HK, Rytkonen KM, Porkka-Heiskanen T (2009) Basal forebrain lactate release and promotion of cortical arousal during prolonged waking is attenuated in aging. J Neurosci 29:11698–11707
85. Wisor JP, Clegern WC (2011) Quantification of short-term slow wave sleep homeostasis and its disruption by minocycline in the laboratory mouse. Neurosci Lett 490:165–169
86. Wisor JP, Kilduff TS (2005) Molecular genetic advances in sleep research and their relevance to sleep medicine. Sleep 28:357–367
87. Wisor JP, O'Hara BF, Terao A, Selby CP, Kilduff TS, Sancar A, Edgar DM, Franken P (2002) A role for cryptochromes in sleep regulation. BMC Neurosci 3:20

88. Wisor JP, Pasumarthi RK, Gerashchenko D, Thompson CL, Pathak S, Sancar A, Franken P, Lein ES, Kilduff TS (2008) Sleep deprivation effects on circadian clock gene expression in the cerebral cortex parallel electroencephalographic differences among mouse strains. J Neurosci 28:7193–7201

89. Wisor JP, Schmidt MA, Clegern WC (2011) Evidence for neuroinflammatory and microglial changes in the cerebral response to sleep loss. Sleep 34:261–272

# PART III

# EFFECTS OF ARTIFICIAL LIGHT
# AND SLEEP DISRUPTION
# ON METABOLISM

# CHAPTER 10

# PATHOPHYSIOLOGY AND PATHOGENESIS OF CIRCADIAN RHYTHM SLEEP DISORDERS

AKIKO HIDA, SHINGO KITAMURA, AND KAZUO MISHIMA

## 10.1 MAMMALIAN CIRCADIAN CLOCK SYSTEM

The circadian clock system regulates daily rhythms of physiology and behavior, such as the sleep-wake cycle and hormonal secretion, body temperature and mood [1]. These rhythms are entrained by environmental cues, light-dark (LD) cycles and food intake. In mammals, the master clock in the suprachiasmatic nuclei (SCN) of the hypothalamus incorporates environmental information and coordinates the phase of oscillators in peripheral cells, tissues and organs [2,3]. Light is one of the most potent environmental cues that enable the organisms to adapt to the 24-hour environmental LD cycle. Photic signals are delivered from the eye to the SCN via the retinohypothalamic tract, thereby mediating the entrainment of the circadian clock system [4]. The circadian clock system involves transcription-translation negative feedback loops of multiple clock genes and posttranscriptional modification and degradation of clock proteins [4-6] (Figure 1). The basic helix-loop-helix and Per-Arnt-Sim transcription fac-

*This chapter was originally published under the Creative Commons Attribution License. Hida A, Kitamura S, and Mishima K. Pathophysiology and Pathogenesis of Circadian Rhythm Sleep Disorders.* Journal of Physiological Anthropology *31,7 (2012). doi:10.1186/1880-6805-31-7.*

tors CLOCK and BMAL1 form heterodimers and activate transcription of *Period 1 (Per1), Per2, Per3, Cryptochrome 1 (Cry1), Cry2* and *retinoid-related orphan receptor α (Rorα), Rorβ, Rorγ, Rev-Erbα* and *Rev-Erbβ* by binding to E-box motifs on their promoter regions. PER and CRY proteins gradually accumulate in the cytoplasm and phosphorylation of PER and CRY occurs with casein kinase Iδ (CKIδ) and CKIε. PER, CRY and CKI proteins form complexes that translocate to the nucleus and interact with CLOCK-BMAL1 heterodimers, thereby inhibiting transcription of the *Per, Cry, Ror* and *Rev-Erb* genes. Meanwhile, *Bmal1* transcription is regulated positively by retinoid-related orphan receptor (ROR) and negatively by REV-ERB via the ROR element (RORE) motif on the *Bmal1* promoter.

## 10.2 CIRCADIAN RHYTHM SLEEP DISORDERS

A two-process model is a major model of sleep regulation. Two components, homeostatic drive and circadian drive, interact with each other and regulate the sleep-wake cycle [7]. The sleep-wake cycle is controlled by sleep homeostasis. The desire to sleep increases gradually with extended wakefulness and decreases during sleep. Additionally, sleep and wakefulness occur in turn, and the timing of their occurrence is controlled by the circadian clock system. Circadian rhythm sleep disorders (CRSDs) are defined by a persistently or recurrently disturbed sleep pattern. CRSD is attributed etiologically to alterations of the circadian timekeeping system and/or a misalignment between endogenous circadian rhythm and exogenous factors that affect sleep timing [8]. The intrinsic circadian period (τ, the free-running period of circadian rhythms in the absence of external cues) is considered to be a critical factor in the pathophysiology of CRSD [9,10].

### 10.2.1 FAMILIAL ADVANCED SLEEP PHASE TYPE

Familial advanced sleep phase type (FASPT) is an autosomal dominant genetic disease characterized by extremely early involuntary sleep timing. A missense mutation in the *PER2* gene has been identified in a large pedi-

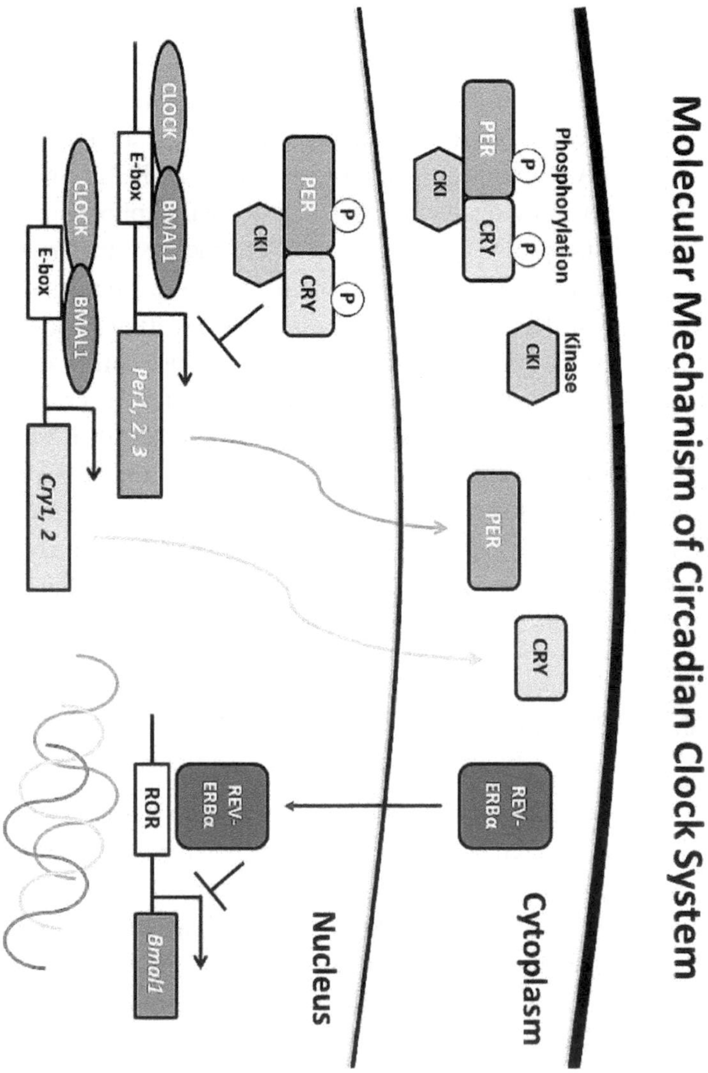

**FIGURE 1:** Molecular mechanism of circadian clock system.

gree with FASPT. This mutation caused a change from serine to glycine at amino acid 662 (S662G) located in the CKIε binding domain of the PER2 protein and resulted in decreased PER2 phosphorylation [11]. Transgenic mice carrying the mutant S662G *PER2* gene showed a shorter free-running period, $\tau$ [12]. In addition, a missense mutation in the CKIδ gene was found in another FASPT pedigree. The substitution of threonine with alanine at amino acid 44 of CKIδ reduced enzymatic activity of CKIδ, leading to decreased phosphorylation level of PER2, a target of CKI [13]. The CKIδ T44A mutation shortened $\tau$, as well as the PER2 S662G mutation, in mice. It was previously proposed that decreased phosphorylation of PER2 stabilizes the PER2 protein, thereby enhancing nuclear accumulation of PER2 and leading to a shorter circadian period. Recent studies, however, have shown that decreased PER2 phosphorylation enhances destabilization of PER2 by increasing turnover and degradation of PER2 [14,15]. These findings suggest that the shortening of $\tau$ observed in the FASPT models results from enhanced turnover of nuclear PER2 caused either by increased degradation or by reduced nuclear retention. FASPT patients have been reported to have a shorter period of physiological rhythms [16]. Several studies have indicated that the phosphorylation status of circadian clock proteins plays a critical role in regulating circadian periods [17,18]. Altered $\tau$ seems to contribute to the pathogenesis of CRSD.

### 10.2.2 DELAYED SLEEP PHASE TYPE

Delayed sleep phase type (DSPT) is characterized by the inability to fall asleep and awaken at a desired time, leading to significantly later sleep onset and wake times. The pathophysiology of DSPT is attributed to longer $\tau$, misaligned phase relationship between endogenous clock and sleep-wake cycles, reduced photic entrainment and/or altered sleep homeostasis. The human *PER3* gene has multiple missense polymorphisms that cause amino acid substitution and a variable number tandem repeat (VNTR) polymorphism that encodes either four or five copies of eighteen amino acids [19]. Association studies have shown that the longer allele (five copies) in *PER3* VNTR polymorphism (*PER3⁵*) is associated with extreme morning preference and that the shorter allele (four copies) is associated with extreme evening preference and DSPT [20]. *PER3⁵* homozygotes have been reported to show increased slow-wave sleep in non-rapid eye movement sleep and θ/α activity during wakefulness compared to homozygotes for *PER3⁴* [21]. These results suggest that the *PER3* polymorphism may be linked to homeostatic regulation of human sleep. The mouse *Per3* gene was thought to be dispensable for circadian rhythm, as PER3-deficient mice did not show altered expression patterns of circadian clock genes in the SCN or altered behavioral rhythm [22]. However, PER3-deficient mice have recently been reported to have a shorter τ and advanced phase of *Per1* rhythm in peripheral tissues compared to wild-type mice. The results suggest that *Per3* may play a role in regulating circadian rhythms in the periphery [23]. Another group has found that PER3-deficient mice had a lower light sensitivity and suggested that *Per3* may be involved in the light input pathway [24]. These findings imply that the function of the *PER3* gene may contribute to the interaction between the circadian system and sleep homeostasis.

## 10.2.3 NONENTRAINED TYPE (FREE-RUNNING TYPE)

Nonentrained type is characterized by sleep timing that occurs with a 30-minute to 1-hour delay each day. Nonentrained sleep-wake patterns are usually observed in totally blind people [25-27], whereas the nonentrained patterns are rarely observed in sighted people. It is likely that blind individuals have free-running rhythms due to the loss of photic reception (photic entrainment). Because the τ in humans is not extensively longer than 24 hours (average τ = 24.18 hours) [28] and sighted people are capable of perceiving photic signals, impaired photic entrainment as well as prolonged τ may underlie the pathophysiology of sighted patients with the nonentrained type.

## 10.3 EVALUATION OF INDIVIDUAL CIRCADIAN PHENOTYPES

FASPT, DSPT and nonentrained type of CRSDs are thought to result from malfunction and/or maladaptation of the circadian system. Evaluation of

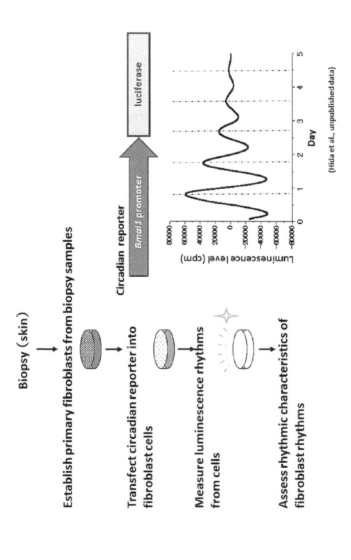

**FIGURE 2:** Surrogate measurements for circadian phenotypes.

an individual's circadian phenotype is indispensable to understanding the pathophysiology of CRSD. Individual subjects are required to stay in a laboratory environment free from external cues during a couple of weeks' time to assess circadian rhythms precisely [28-30]. First, rhythmic characteristics of physiological functions (core body temperature, plasma melatonin and plasma cortisol levels) are measured to estimate individual circadian phases. Blood samples are collected over a 40-hour period under constant routine (CR) conditions where masking effects (for example, physical movement, food intake, ambient temperature and light intensity) are minimized (first CR). Next, patients undergo a 28-hour forced desynchrony (FD) protocol (9.33-hour sleep and 18.67-hour wake cycle) followed by a 40-hour CR (second CR). Individual circadian phases are assessed again during the second CR. The intrinsic circadian period, $\tau$, is determined by the difference in circadian phase between the first and second CRs. As described herein, the CR and FD protocols are laborious and costly to perform in a clinical setting. More convenient measurements of circadian phenotypes are required to reduce the patients' burden.

## 10.4 SURROGATE MEASUREMENTS FOR ASSESSING CIRCADIAN PHENOTYPES

Most cells in peripheral tissues as well as cells in the SCN are equipped with circadian clock components. Brown et al. developed a lentiviral luminescence assay system using biopsy samples to measure individual circadian rhythms in fibroblasts [31]. Primary cells derived from skin biopsy samples were introduced with a circadian reporter: the Bmal1 promoter-driven luciferase gene (Bmal1-luc). The luciferase activity under the control of the Bmal1 promoter showed robust daily rhythms in individual primary fibroblast cells. Bmal1-luc rhythms were monitored for several days, and rhythmic characteristics of the luminescence rhythms were evaluated. Independently, we measured clock gene expression in primary fibroblast cells established from individual skin biopsies and observed robust Bmal1-luc rhythms (Figure 2). Brown et al. found that extreme morning types had shorter periods of fibroblast rhythms compared to extreme evening types [32]. Furthermore, they compared the period length of fibroblast rhythms with that of physiological rhythms in the same subjects and observed a significant correlation between the two rhythms. However, they did not observe long fibroblast periods in blind subjects, who had significantly longer physiological rhythms than sighted subjects [33]. The prolonged physiological period observed in the blind subjects may be caused by their previous sleep-wake cycles under constant darkness. The unaltered fibroblast period may be attributed to experimental conditions. Although the reason for this discrepancy is not yet fully understood and further studies are required, surrogate measurements using fibroblast cells should be a powerful tool for assessing individual circadian properties.

## 10.5 CONCLUSIONS

Evaluation of circadian phenotypes is indispensable to understanding the pathophysiology and pathogenesis of CRSD. Because conventional protocols for examining individual circadian characteristics are laborious and costly, more convenient measurement methods are required in the clinical setting. The circadian reporter Bmal1-luc showed robust daily rhythms in primary fibroblast cells derived from individual skin biopsies. The fibroblast rhythms are associated with chronotypes (morningness vs eveningness preference) and physiological rhythms. Surrogate measurements using fibroblast cells would be a powerful tool for the assessment of individual circadian properties and could lead to providing personalized medicine for CRSD.

## REFERENCES

1. Pittendrigh CS: Temporal organization: reflections of a Darwinian clock-watcher. Annu Rev Physiol 1993, 55:16-54.
2. Yamazaki S, Numano R, Abe M, Hida A, Takahashi R, Ueda M, Block GD, Sakaki Y, Menaker M, Tei H: Resetting central and peripheral circadian oscillators in transgenic rats. Science 2000, 288:682-585.
3. Yoo SH, Yamazaki S, Lowrey PL, Shimomura K, Ko CH, Buhr ED, Siepka SM, Hong HK, Oh WJ, Yoo OJ, Menaker M, Takahashi JS: PERIOD2::LUCIFERASE real-time reporting of circadian dynamics reveals persistent circadian oscillations in mouse peripheral tissues. Proc Natl Acad Sci USA 2004, 101:5339-5346.

4.  Lowrey PL, Takahashi JS: Mammalian circadian biology: elucidating genome-wide levels of temporal organization. Annu Rev Genomics Hum Genet 2004, 5:407-441.

5.  Reppert SM, Weaver DR: Coordination of circadian timing in mammals. Nature 2002, 418:935-941.

6.  Takahashi JS, Hong HK, Ko CH, McDearmon EL: The genetics of mammalian circadian order and disorder: implications for physiology and disease. Nat Rev Genet 2008, 9:764-775.

7.  Daan S, Beersma DG, Borbely AA: Timing of human sleep: recovery process gated by a circadian pacemaker. Am J Physiol 1984, 246:R161-R183.

8.  International Classification of Sleep Disorders: Diagnostic and Coding Manual. 2nd edition (ICSD-II). Darien, IL: American Academy of Sleep Medicine; 2005.

9.  Barion A, Zee PC: A clinical approach to circadian rhythm sleep disorders. Sleep Med 2007, 8:566-577.

10. Okawa M, Uchiyama M: Circadian rhythm sleep disorders: characteristics and entrainment pathology in delayed sleep phase and non-24-h sleep-wake syndrome. Sleep Med Rev 2007, 11:485-496.

11. Toh KL, Jones CR, He Y, Eide EJ, Hinz WA, Virshup DM, Ptácek LJ, Fu YH: An hPer2 phosphorylation site mutation in familial advanced sleep phase syndrome. Science 2001, 291:1040-1043.

12. Xu Y, Toh KL, Jones CR, Shin JY, Fu YH, Ptácek LJ: Modeling of a human circadian mutation yields insights into clock regulation by PER2. Cell 2007, 128:59-70.

13. Xu Y, Padiath QS, Shapiro RE, Jones CR, Wu SC, Saigoh N, Saigoh K, Ptácek LJ, Fu YH: Functional consequences of a CKIδ mutation causing familial advanced sleep phase syndrome. Nature 2005, 434:640-644.

14. Gallego M, Eide EJ, Woolf MF, Virshup DM, Forger DB: An opposite role for tau in circadian rhythms revealed by mathematical modeling. Proc Natl Acad Sci USA 2006, 103:10618-10623.

15. Vanselow K, Vanselow JT, Westermark PO, Reischl S, Maier B, Korte T, Herrmann A, Herzel H, Schlosser A, Kramer A: Differential effects of PER2 phosphorylation: molecular basis for the human familial advanced sleep phase syndrome (FASPS). Genes Dev 2006, 20:2660-2672.

16. Jones CR, Campbell SS, Zone SE, Cooper F, DeSano A, Murphy PJ, Jones B, Czajkowski L, Ptácek LJ: Familial advanced sleep-phase syndrome: a short-period circadian rhythm variant in humans. Nat Med 1999, 5:1062-1065.

17. Hirota T, Lewis WG, Liu AC, Lee JW, Schultz PG, Kay SA: A chemical biology approach reveals period shortening of the mammalian circadian clock by specific inhibition of GSK-3β. Proc Natl Acad Sci USA 2008, 105:20746-20751.

18. Isojima Y, Nakajima M, Ukai H, Fujishima H, Yamada RG, Masumoto KH, Kiuchi R, Ishida M, Ukai-Tadenuma M, Minami Y, Kito R, Nakao K, Kishimoto W, Yoo SH, Shimomura K, Takao T, Takano A, Kojima T, Nagai K, Sakaki Y, Takahashi JS, Ueda HR: CKIε/δ-dependent phosphorylation is a temperature-insensitive, period-determining process in the mammalian circadian clock. Proc Natl Acad Sci USA 2009, 106:15744-15749.

19. Ebisawa T, Uchiyama M, Kajimura N, Mishima K, Kamei Y, Katoh M, Watanabe T, Sekimoto M, Shibui K, Kim K, Kudo Y, Ozeki Y, Sugishita M, Toyoshima R, Inoue Y, Yamada N, Nagase T, Ozaki N, Ohara O, Ishida N, Okawa M, Takahashi K, Ya-

mauchi T: Association of structural polymorphisms in the human period3 gene with delayed sleep phase syndrome. EMBO Rep 2001, 2:342-346.

20. Dijk DJ, Archer SN: PERIOD3, circadian phenotypes, and sleep homeostasis. Sleep Med Rev 2009, 14:151-160.

21. Viola AU, Archer SN, James LM, Groeger JA, Lo JC, Skene DJ, von Schantz M, Dijk DJ: PER3 polymorphism predicts sleep structure and waking performance. Curr Biol 2007, 17:613-618.

22. Shearman LP, Jin X, Lee C, Reppert SM, Weaver DR: Targeted disruption of the mPer3 gene: subtle effects on circadian clock function. Mol Cell Biol 2000, 20:6269-6275.

23. Pendergast JS, Friday RC, Yamazaki S: Distinct functions of Period2 and Period3 in the mouse circadian system revealed by in vitro analysis. PLoS One 2010, 5:e8552.

24. van der Veen DR, Archer SN: Light-dependent behavioral phenotypes in PER3-deficient mice. J Biol Rhythms 2010, 25:3-8. A published erratum appears in J Biol Rhythms 2010, 25:150

25. Sack RL, Lewy AJ, Blood ML, Keith LD, Nakagawa H: Circadian rhythm abnormalities in totally blind people: incidence and clinical significance. J Clin Endocrinol Metab 1992, 75:127-134.

26. Lockley SW, Skene DJ, Arendt J, Tabandeh H, Bird AC, Defrance R: Relationship between melatonin rhythms and visual loss in the blind. J Clin Endocrinol Metab 1997, 82:3763-3770.

27. Lockley SW, Skene DJ, Tabandeh H, Bird AC, Defrance R, Arendt J: Relationship between napping and melatonin in the blind. J Biol Rhythms 1997, 12:16-25.

28. Czeisler CA, Duffy JF, Shanahan TL, Brown EN, Mitchell JF, Rimmer DW, Ronda JM, Silva EJ, Allan JS, Emens JS, Dijk DJ, Kronauer RE: Stability, precision, and near-24-hour period of the human circadian pacemaker. Science 1999, 284:2177-2181.

29. Wright KP Jr, Hughes RJ, Kronauer RE, Dijk DJ, Czeisler CA: Intrinsic near-24-h pacemaker period determines limits of circadian entrainment to a weak synchronizer in humans. Proc Natl Acad Sci USA 2001, 98:14027-14032.

30. Gronfier C, Wright KP Jr, Kronauer RE, Czeisler CA: Entrainment of the human circadian pacemaker to longer-than-24-h days. Proc Natl Acad Sci USA 2007, 104:9081-9086.

31. Brown SA, Fleury-Olela F, Nagoshi E, Hauser C, Juge C, Meier CA, Chicheportiche R, Dayer JM, Albrecht U, Schibler U: The period length of fibroblast circadian gene expression varies widely among human individuals. PLoS Biol 2005, 3:e338.

32. Brown SA, Kunz D, Dumas A, Westermark PO, Vanselow K, Tilmann-Wahnschaffe A, Herzel H, Kramer A: Molecular insights into human daily behavior. Proc Natl Acad Sci USA 2008, 105:1602-1607.

33. Pagani L, Semenova EA, Moriggi E, Revell VL, Hack LM, Lockley SW, Arendt J, Skene DJ, Meier F, Izakovic J, Wirz-Justice A, Cajochen C, Sergeeva OJ, Cheresiz SV, Danilenko KV, Eckert A, Brown SA: The physiological period length of the human circadian clock in vivo is directly proportional to period in human fibroblasts. PLoS One 2010, 5:e13376.

# CHAPTER 11

# SHIFT WORK, JET LAG, AND FEMALE REPRODUCTION

MEGAN M. MAHONEY

## 11.1 INTRODUCTION

In mammals, the 24-hour clock mechanism, or circadian oscillator, is critical for the function and coordination of a broad range of biological processes, from hormone secretion to locomotor activity. This biological timing system is vital for successful reproduction. Animals are more likely to gain mating opportunities if they coordinate their sexual behavior with that of their potential partners. Females benefit from synchronizing the timing of pregnancy to seasons with favorable food and weather conditions, and it is advantageous for an animal to give birth at a time of day when it is most likely to be in a safe place such as a burrow rather than out foraging. A mounting body of evidence indicates that disruptions in normally synchronized, or entrained, biological rhythms are associated with a broad range of pathologies including reproductive dysfunction in females.

This review will describe how the endogenous timing system interacts with the hypothalamic-pituitary-gonadal axis to regulate female reproductive cyclicity. I will address how disruptions in the alignment of

*This chapter was originally published under the Creative Commons Attribution License. Mahoney MM. Shift Work, Jet Lag, and Female Reproduction.* International Journal of Endocrinology **2010** (2010). http://dx.doi.org/10.1155/2010/813764.

these rhythms, as occurs in shift work or jet lag, are strongly associated with reproductive dysfunction in women. Animal models will highlight the relationship between circadian desynchrony and prevalence of disease states. I will lastly address how "clock genes," the genetic components underlying the circadian mechanism, relate to reproductive function, and how hormone secretion in turn can alter clock gene rhythmicity.

## 11.2 SHIFT WORK AND JET LAG

The Bureau of Labor Statistics reported that in 2004 over 27 million Americans had flexible or shift work schedules. Shift work is defined as any employment after 7 pm and before 9 am. Women working non-daytime shifts equaled 12.4% or over 3 million women. Shift work is found in services such as healthcare, military, and protection (police, firefighters). Shift-workers tend to have activity, body temperature, and hormonal rhythms that are out of phase with environmental cues and often the behavioral rhythms of their family and friends. Some workers are able to adapt or synchronize their rhythms (sleep schedules, melatonin secretion patterns) to an alternative work schedule [1]. Even so, adapting to a shift work schedule can be hindered when workers have weekends off and encounter a world operating on a standard schedule [2]. A number of individuals are never able to adjust to shift work.

Jet lag is caused by shifts in the environmental light:dark cycle, or photic phase, that result in an organism's internal rhythms becoming transiently out of phase with the environment and each other [3]. Similar to shift work, jet lag also causes a myriad of physical, emotional, and psychiatric problems in humans [4–7]. It is likely that these disruptions in circadian rhythms are even more extreme for transmeridian travelers than those of shift workers. These individuals do not have a regular schedule to enable entrainment, they travel through different time zones which provide constantly changing light:dark schedules, and they experience light exposure at times when their internal clock mechanism indicates it should be night. All of these signals can continuously reset and disrupt internal circadian rhythms (e.g., sleep patterns).

Shift work, jet lag, and other forms of circadian disruption including sleep deprivation increase the risk of individuals acquiring a disease or exacerbate the symptoms of a preexisting condition. Shift-work, jet lag, and sleep deprivation have been associated with an increased risk of mood disorders, depression, cardiovascular disease, endometriosis, dysmenorrhea, as well as an increased incidence and risk of breast cancer [8–11]. Shift workers and transmeridian travelers report increased fatigue and sleep disturbances relative to individuals working daytime shifts [2]. Women with chronic sleep deprivation or insomnia are more likely to have circadian rhythm disruptions and clinical depression [11]. Sleep disturbance in late pregnancy is associated with increased labor duration and increased likelihood of requiring medical intervention such as cesarean section [12].

These relationships between work schedules and health have gained considerable attention from society and the scientific community. The American Academy of Sleep Medicine recognizes jet lag as a sleep disorder typified by excessive daytime sleepiness and associated physiological impairments [13]. In 2007, night shift work was reclassified from a possible to a probable human carcinogen (class 2A) by the International Agency for Research on Cancer. In fact, this ruling formed the basis for a recent decision by a Danish industrial injuries board to award compensation to women shift workers. These women had worked more than 20 years as a shift worker and developed cancer [14].

## 11.3 THE HYPOTHALAMUS-PITUITARY-GONADAL AXIS AND THE CIRCADIAN SYSTEM REGULATE REPRODUCTIVE CYCLES

Female mammals have a cyclical change in hormone secretion and ovulation. The most-studied animal models of female reproductive cyclicity are laboratory muroid rodents (i.e., rat, hamster, mouse), which have an estrous cycle characterized by a short total duration (4-5 days), spontaneous follicular development and spontaneous ovulation. The menstrual cycles of women and the estrous cycles of these rodents have several features in common including a series of tightly orchestrated events that result in increased activity in gonadotropin releasing hormone (GnRH) neurons, a hormone surge, and ovulation (Figure 1). During the follicular phase of the cycle, maturing follicles in the ovary release increasing levels of estradiol. When estradiol concentrations reach a threshold, a surge of GnRH is released from cells in the hypothalamus into the hypophyseal portal blood system. This surge of GnRH triggers a surge of luteinizing hormone (LH) from the anterior pituitary, and this hormone acts on the ovary to induce ovulation. Following ovulation the follicles rupture then are luteinized. During this cycle stage progesterone is the dominant hormone (secreted by the corpora lutea). This luteal phase lasts for 10–16 days in women. Rats and mice have corpora lutea that function for 1–3 days but do not have a true extended luteal phase without coitus or vaginal stimulation [15].

In rodents these reproductive events occur in a cyclical and circadian manner. In rats GnRH neurons become active just before lights-off as indicated by the presence of the immediate early gene Fos within the nucleus [16]. This rhythm is endogenous, as ovariectomized rats given steroid hormones only have a rise in GnRH cell activation at one time of day, and this rhythm persists in animals housed in constant darkness [17]. The LH surge is concurrent with the GnRH cell activation and occurs just before lights-off [18]. Ovulation occurs 6–15 hours later [19]. These latter two events occur at precise circadian intervals. For example, in hamsters housed in a light:dark cycle, the estrous cycle occurs every 96 hours (4 periods of 24 hours). When animals are housed in constant conditions this rhythm continues (range 95.35–97.54 h), indicating that an endogenous circadian mechanism (rather than the environmental light:dark cycle) is regulating the estrous cycle [20]. Rodents also exhibit a daily rhythm in the timing of mating behavior; typically this occurs around the onset of their active period [21, 22].

In laboratory rodents the precise timing of this cascade of estrous cycle events is regulated by a small number of cells located in a brain region called the suprachiasmatic nucleus (SCN). The SCN contains the primary circadian mechanism and regulates the timing of central and peripheral oscillators [23]. Rats and hamsters with bilateral SCN lesions lack a rhythm in sexual behavior, the preovulatory LH surge, corticosteroid rhythms, and a consistently functional estrous cycle [24–28]. Transplants of fetal SCN tissue restore some behavioral rhythms but do not restore estrous rhythms, indicating that synaptic inputs from the circadian clock are critical for mediating these systems [28].

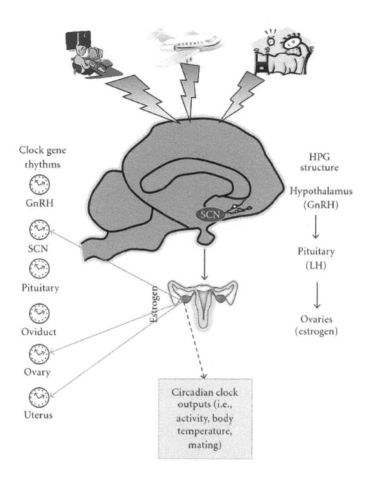

**FIGURE 1:** The hypothalamus-pituitary-gonadal axis regulates reproductive cycles in female mammals. Increasing levels of estrogens released from the ovaries feedback onto the hypothalamus. When estrogen stimulation reaches a threshold, gonadotropin releasing hormone (GnRH) neurons release their product into the blood stream. GnRH acts on the pituitary to trigger a surge of luteinizing hormone (LH) which then induces ovulation. In rodents, the suprachiasmatic nucleus (SCN) of the hypothalamus provides an additional signal which regulates the timing of reproductive events. Shift work schedules, jet lag, and sleep deprivation can perturb the daily (circadian) rhythms in reproduction and "clock gene" expression. Clock gene expression has been detected in the SCN, GnRH neurons and female reproductive tissues. Estrogen can influence the pattern of expression of gene expression in some of these tissues (solid arrows). Estrogen also influences the rhythmic expression of clock-controlled outputs such as activity and body temperature (dashed arrow).

Women also exhibit daily rhythms in the timing of reproductive cycle events and hormone secretion patterns. The preovulatory LH surge acrophase typically occurs between midnight and 8 am [29]. A second study examining the timing of the LH surge in 155 cycles (from 35 women) found that 48% of the surges occurred between 4 and 8 am and 37% of the surges occurred between midnight and 4 am [30]. In women, the precise timing of ovulation has not been determined but is estimated to occur 24–40 h later [19, 30, 31]. In humans, the LH surge occurs before the active period (daytime) as is the case for other day-active or diurnal species [32]. In nocturnal rodents, these events also occur just before their active period at the time of lights-off [21].

Women express other daily rhythms related to reproduction. There is diurnal variation in the pattern of pulsatile LH secretion; this rhythm of peaks and troughs remains evident even in the reduction or absence of ovarian hormones, as is seen in hypogonadal women [33]. The timing of the onset of labor and the timing of birth also exhibit strong diurnal rhythmicity with respect to time of day. The rupture of membranes is reported to occur between midnight and 4 am [34]. A study of over 17,000 term singleton deliveries found the majority of women going into labor between midnight and 8 am with 01:45 AM as the peak time of labor onset [35]. In a second study of over 15,000 women, the onset of labor had a 24-hour rhythm, with a nadir in the middle of the day and peaks around dawn and dusk [36]. The timing of birth typically occurs in the middle of the afternoon. In two retrospective studies (6608 and 15,000 women, resp.), the majority of births following a spontaneous onset of labor occurred between 1 and 2 pm [36, 37]. Interestingly, multiparous women were more likely to deliver babies earlier in the morning, between 8 and 11 am when compared to nulliparous mothers, the authors speculated this difference may be related to the timing of fetal and maternal hormone secretions [37]. A clinical study was conducted to determine if this diurnal rhythm in the onset of labor was also important to women in whom labor was induced. Women which had labor induced in the morning required less uterine stimulation (i.e., oxytocin), had a shorter interval from induction to birth, and were less likely to require operative assistance with the delivery when compared to women that had their labor induced in the evening hours [38].

These reproductive events in women occur with a diurnal rhythmicity; however, it remains possible that the circadian system does not control the timing of reproductive events in humans as tightly as it does in rodents. For example, humans and primates are able to copulate throughout the ovarian cycle and are not limited to a particular time of day or specific duration of exposure to steroid hormones [39]. In primates a surge in LH can be induced at any time of day with the proper strength and interval of steroid hormone treatment [40]. This does not eliminate the possibility that appropriate and successful reproduction in women is regulated by the light:dark cycle and/or a circadian timing mechanism. Nearly all of the available data indicate that alteration of the phase relationship between an animal, human or otherwise, and the light:dark cycle has adverse effects on the physiology of the affected organism. In support of this hypothesis, alterations or disruptions in the daily (and potentially circadian) rhythms of women are linked to significant disruptions in reproductive function.

## 11.4 DISRUPTION OF DIURNAL RHYTHMS IS ASSOCIATED WITH REPRODUCTIVE DYSFUNCTION

Women working an evening shift, night shift, or have irregularly scheduled shifts (such as days-off or flexible schedules) report altered menstrual cycle length (both increases and decreases), increased menstrual pain, and changes in the duration and amount of menstrual bleeding [41, 42]. These symptoms are accompanied by changes in patterns of ovarian and pituitary hormone secretion, such as an increase in follicular stage length and changes in follicular stimulating hormone (FSH) concentrations [8, 10, 42, 43]. These effects are apparent even when the studies controlled for health, lifestyle, or job environment (i.e., stress) [43].

Pregnancy outcomes are also affected by the working environment. Female shift workers have a higher risk of producing premature and/or low birth weight babies, spontaneous abortion and subfecundity [10, 44]. Flight attendants who worked while they were pregnant were twice as likely to have a spontaneous abortion when compared to flight attendants who did not work during their pregnancy [45]. Some studies on pregnancy outcomes in flight attendants indicate that this risk of miscarriage is moderate compared to the general population of women [45, 46]. In a mouse model of shift work, there was a significant reduction in the percent of animals that mated when they were housed in a 22 hours (11 h light : 11 h dark) or 26 hours (13 h light : 13 h dark) light-dark cycles for 2 or more weeks prior to mating [47]. Interestingly, if pregnant animals were taken from a 24 hours light:dark cycle and moved to a 22 or 26 hours light:dark cycle there was very little effect on the pregnancy outcomes. Entrainment to the light:dark cycle in women and rodents may be essential for successful copulation and conception, however, once pregnancy is achieved, female hormonal secretion patterns may be less sensitive to environmental changes [47].

Shift work and jet lag may exert their effects on health and physiology by reducing the total amount of sleep for an individual. Women working the night shift or experiencing transmeridian travel report a decrease in the amount of sleep and an increase in fatigue and insomnia [13, 41]. This reduction in sleep duration is not trivial as it has an effect on hormone secretion patterns. For example women with less than 8 hours of sleep secrete 20% less FSH compared to women with longer sleep durations [48]. Total or partial sleep deprivation increases LH amplitude, estradiol and FSH concentrations in normal cycling women [49]. Increased estrogen is associated with an increased risk of breast cancer (discussed below). It is possible that the altered menstrual cycle physiology associated with circadian misalignment is due to a direct effect of sleep state on ovarian and pituitary hormone secretion. It remains to be eluciated if circadian disruption, while significant to emotional well being and other physiological aspects, is a critical mechanism underlying the reproductive dysfunctions [41].

## 11.5 BREAST CANCER AND BIOLOGICAL RHYTHMS

In the last decade there has been a strong link between shift work and incidence of breast cancer. As a number of recent reviews discuss this issue in depth, this topic will only be highlighted here [50, 51]. There is a substantial literature which links light exposure at night, shift work or transmeridian travel, and an increased risk of breast cancer [9, 51–54].

One report examining over 85,000 women enrolled in the Nurses' Health Study found that a woman's relative risk of getting breast cancer was amplified if she worked the night shift or had rotating shifts [52, 55]. Similar risk levels have been determined for female flight attendants [53]. Animal cancer models indicate that altered circadian function exacerbates cancer symptomology. In a series of elegant studies, Filipski et al. disrupted circadian rhythms in mice either through SCN ablation or jet-lag schedules (repeated advances of the light:dark cycle). Mice experiencing this desynchrony had significantly accelerated growth of inoculated tumor cells [56–58].

One hypothesis which addresses the mechanism underlying this risk of breast cancer in shift workers is the "light at night theory" [51]. This postulates that the increased exposure to light during evening working hours decreases melatonin secretion. Melatonin is a pineal hormone that is secreted during the dark phase of the light:dark cycle and is suppressed when an individual is exposed to light including artificial light. Melatonin concentration, diurnal pattern of melatonin secretion, and the relationship of this pineal hormone rhythm to other physiological rhythms are altered in shift workers compared to daytime employees [13]. When compared to day-shift workers, women working the second or third shift have altered melatonin rhythms as measured by the urinary melatonin breakdown product 6-hydroxymelatonin sulfate [2]. This hormone has a protective effect against cancer, and can inhibit the growth of metastatic cells. In in vitro studies melatonin can suppress the growth of malignant breast cancer cells (reviewed in [59]).

Melatonin-rich blood (collected at night from healthy women) suppresses tumor growth in immunodeficient rats carrying a human breast cancer xenograft. When these animals were given the melatonin rich blood and a melatonin receptor inhibitor, or blood collected during the day, the tumor suppressive effects were eliminated [50].

There is a strong link between light at night, melatonin, and breast cancer risk However, shift work or sleep deprivation may not be the direct cause of cancer. Rather the exposure to light at night suppresses the oncostatic hormone melatonin and accelerates the development of cancer symptoms. Additionally, as mentioned above, sleep deprivation can alter gonadal and pituitary hormone secretion patterns which may influence tumor cell growth. It is clear that shift work, jet lag, and sleep disturbances put a woman at increased risk for acquiring this pathology and this will require additional research to determine the causal relationships.

## 11.6 CLOCK GENES AND REPRODUCTION

The link between circadian rhythms and reproductive function also functions at the molecular level. In the last decade a family of "clock" gene and protein transcription and translation feedback loops have been identified. These clock genes play a role in an individual's rhythmicity, entrainment and responsiveness to light [60–62]. In mammals, the proteins CLOCK and BMAL1 form heterodimers. This complex then activates the transcription of thee *Period* genes known as *Per1, Per2*, and *Per3*. This CLOCK/BMAL1 heterodimer also turns on the transcription of two *cryptochome* genes known as *Cry1* and *Cry2*. The protein products of the *Per* and *Cry* genes heterodimerize, then act as repressors and turn off the transcription of *Clock* and *Bmal1*. A second protein, NPAS2 also forms heterodimers with BMAL and this protein complex also initiates *Per* and *Cry* transcription [63].

The initial identification of rhythmic expression of clock gene transcription and translation was within individual cells of the SCN. These molecular rhythms have also been found in peripheral organs including female reproductive tissues such as the ovary [64, 65], uterus [66–68], and oviducts [69] (Figure 1).

Daily rhythms in clock gene expression have been found in an additional component of the HPG system; the GnRH neurons themselves. In cell cultures of GnRH GT1-7 cells, mRNA of *Clock, Bmal1, Per1* and *Per2*, and the protein BMAL1 have a diurnal pattern of expression [70, 71]. Transfecting these cells with an altered CLOCK protein (Clock$^{\Delta19}$) or the addition of the CRY protein to the culture alters the amplitude and frequency of GnRH pulsatility [70]. The exact role of the molecular clock within these neuroendocrine cells has not been determined. It is possible that this is a mechanism which alters cellular activity of GnRH neurons, or modifies their sensitivity to estradiol [72].

Further evidence that clock gene rhythmicity is critical for reproductive function is seen in knock out or transgenic animal models. Disruptions in known circadian clock genes disrupts reproductive processes in female rodents; several detailed reviews have been published recently [19, 73]. In knock-out mice missing either the *Per1* or *Per2* gene, estrous cycles are irregular or absent, and animals have decreased fertility. This reduced fertility is more pronounced in "middle aged" mice compared to young mice, suggesting that mutations in this gene accelerate ageing at least with respect to reproductive function [74]. *Bmal1* knock-out female mice are able to mate but are not able to produce young [75]. Mice expressing a homozygous genotype of a mutated CLOCK protein (Clock$^{\Delta19/\Delta19}$) have a dampened LH surge, disrupted and irregular estrous cycles and difficulties with pregnancy [76]. Not all clock genes have an equal effect on reproduction as mice lacking, *Per3, Cry1,* or *Cry2* (or combinations of these genes) are able to breed and reproduce [19].

Fertility and reproductive cyclicity may depend upon the precise phase relationship between the "master" clock contained in the SCN and the clocks contained within reproductive tissues and GnRH neurons. Clock gene rhythms within the SCN and peripheral tissues have a phase relationship. The peak expression of *Bmal1* in the rat ovary is about 4 hours delayed relative to the acrophase of *Bmal1* mRNA in the SCN. Similarly, the *Per2* rhythm in the ovary peaks 4 hours after lights off, whereas it peaks 6 hours earlier in the SCN [65]. If a female experiences a shift in the light:dark cycle, it is unknown how long it takes the circadian clock genes in the SCN, ovary and uterus to resynchronize to one another. It is known that in mice experiencing a phase advance, *Per1* mRNA rhythms in the SCN rapidly readjust to the new light:dark cycle but the peripheral organs (liver, lung, muscle) take nearly 6 times as long as the SCN to recover [77]. Rhythms in clock gene expression thus adjust to jet lag at different rates relative to one another, and relative to the peripheral organs. It is this mismatch of rhythms within the body that may underlie the reproductive deficits experienced by women experiencing disrupted biological rhythms [77, 78].

The relationship between clock genes and female health has not yet been examined closely in women; however, several studies have correlated circadian clock gene polymorphisms with reproductive disorders. The expression of three different polymorphisms of the NPAS2 gene was examined in control (n = 476) and breast cancer cases (n= 431). This gene is part of the transcription-translation loop of clock genes. A significant association was found between breast cancer risk and one of the heterozygous gene polymorphisms (compared to homozygous genotype) [63]. This same research group also found a 1.7 fold increased risk of breast cancer in women with a heterozygous genotype for a *Per3* length polymorphism compared to women with a homozygous genotype [79]. In contrast no link was found between endometriosis, shift work, and the expression of a polymorphism of the *Clock* gene (hT3111C) in humans. This gene is correlated with mood disorders and in *Clock* mutant mice estrous cyclicity is impaired [76, 80]. Despite these data, the authors did find that women working the night shift had a nearly doubled increase in risk of endometriosis and this was further increased if women had altered sleep rhythms on their days off. Circadian gene markers may provide a valuable tool for identifying individuals in shift work environments that may be particularly susceptible to developing diseases. These markers may also help identify those individuals that may be better able to adapt to or accommodate a changing work schedule.

## 11.7 INTERACTION BETWEEN CIRCADIAN TIMING MECHANISMS AND OVARIAN HORMONES

A reciprocal interaction exists between the circadian timing mechanisms and gonadal hormones. As described above, the timing of estrus-related events including hormone secretion is regulated in part by the SCN and circadian system. Ovarian hormones in turn influence the behavioral and molecular circadian rhythms [81, 82]. On the day of sexual receptivity (estrus), female rats, hamsters, and degus (*Octodon degus*, an hystricomorph rodent) advance the onset of their daily activity rhythms [83–85]. Ovariectomized female hamsters and rats have given a capsule containing estrogen similarly advance the onset of their activity rhythms and have a shorter free running period when compared to control animals [86, 87].

Ovarian hormones appear to have a similar effect in women as diurnal and circadian rhythms including sleep-wake cycles and endocrine rhythms (cortisol, melatonin) change between the follicular and luteal phases of the reproductive cycle [88–90]. There are relatively few studies that have examined these rhythms in a controlled environment but one generalization is that ovarian hormones modify the amplitude but not the phase of various physiological rhythms. For example, humans have a daily rhythm in the fluctuation of body temperature, the nadir occurs after lights-off, and the temperature remains relatively low until the time of lights-on. In females, this general pattern remains consistent across the menstrual cycle but the amplitude of the rhythm is reduced during the luteal compared to follicular phase [91]. Similarly, when women were studied in an ultrashort sleep-wake protocol (which separates the endogenous rhythms from the influence of the environmental cues) the daily rhythm in cortisol was blunted during the luteal compared to follicular phase [90].

Ovarian hormones also influence the expression of circadian clock genes both within and outside of the SCN. Importantly, the effects of estrogen on the rhythm of clock gene expression are both tissue and gene specific. In ovariectomized female rats, chronic estrogen treatment significantly phase advances the acrophase of $Per2$ mRNA expression, but not that of $Per1$, in the SCN [67]. An injection with estrogen significantly decreases the amount of $Cry2$ mRNA within the SCN, but does not change the amount of $Cry1$ mRNA [92]. In the uterus, estradiol treatment results in bimodal $Per1$ and $Per2$ expression whereas control animals had a single peak and estrogen shortens the period of $Per2$ expression [67, 93]. On the day of proestrus (high estradiol), $Bmal1$ mRNA levels are increased relative to diestrus [65]. Data on clock gene expression in reproductive tissue of women is limited; breast and endometrial cancer lines and tissue from breast cancer patients express clock genes and their protein products [94, 95]. Additionally, $Per2$ expression inhibits the expression of estrogen receptors in breast cancer cell lines [94]. Lastly, it is possible for estrogen to have a direct effect on the circadian timing system as estrogen receptors have been detected in the human SCN [96].

In rodent studies, changing concentrations of estradiol, either though the endogenous estrous cycle, or though disrupted ovarian function can phase shift or desynchronize circadian genes in both a tissue specific and clock gene specific manner [67]. This perturbation in the steroid hormone signal can lead to a change in the expression of circadian clock genes both within the SCN and in peripheral tissues including female reproductive organs. It will be important to determine if these factors also play a role in human reproductive health and disease.

## 11.8 CONCLUSIONS

The general mechanisms by which the SCN and circadian system regulate the physiological rhythms are still being elucidated. The investigation of specific central (SCN) or peripheral oscillators that regulate rhythms in the well-described hypothalamic-pituitary-gonadal system will provide a more general understanding of how the circadian clock mechanism regulates rhythmic outputs. Future work will also clarify the relationship between the circadian timing system and the contribution of other factors that impact women's reproductive health. Life or work stressors, sleep deprivation and fatigue, smoking habits, age, weight, and environmental conditions such as exposure to solvents all impact female reproductive function [97].

The circadian timing system and SCN regulate the onset of the pre-ovulatory LH surge, ovulation, and mating behavior in rodents. Rhythmic clock gene expression within the SCN and peripheral reproductive tissues in females, and the relationship of these rhythms to one another, may be critical for successful reproduction. I hypothesize those disruptions in the endogenous circadian timing mechanism underlie reproductive deficits. In animal models, disruptions in these rhythms, as seen in transgenic and knockout mice, SCN lesioned animals, or individuals experiencing changes in the light:dark cycle, lead to changes in estrous cyclicity and altered patterns of hormonal secretion. The desynchrony of gene expression within a tissue and between central and peripheral tissues may also impact upon an individual's ability to establish phase relationships to environmental cues. In women, perturbations in daily rhythms, as occurs in shift work, jet lag, and sleep deprivation is associated with an increased menstrual cycle irregularity, increased risk of miscarriage, difficulty in conceiving, and a higher risk of breast cancer. Females' health and physiology may be particularly vulnerable to circadian disruption as the resulting changes in steroid hormones secretion patterns can further alter clock gene rhythms. Further investigations are needed to examine how reproductive cycles are regulated in women, the impact of disturbed biological rhythms on reproductive physiology, and how to reduce the health risks associated with altered rhythms.

## REFERENCES

1. T. S. Horowitz, B. E. Cade, J. M. Wolfe, and C. A. Czeisler, "Efficacy of bright light and sleep/darkness scheduling in alleviating circadian maladaptation to night work," American Journal of Physiology, vol. 281, no. 2, pp. E384–E391, 2001.

2. J. B. Burch, M. G. Yost, W. Johnson, and E. Allen, "Melatonin, sleep, and shift work adaptation," Journal of Occupational and Environmental Medicine, vol. 47, no. 9, pp. 893–901, 2005.

3. W. N. Tapp and B. H. Natelson, "Circadian rhythms and patterns of performance before and after simulated jet lag," American Journal of Physiology, vol. 257, no. 4, pp. R796–R803, 1989.

4. C. M. Winget, C. W. Deroshia, C. L. Markley, and D. C. Holley, "A review of human physiological and performance changes associated with desynchronosis of biological rhythms," Aviation Space and Environmental Medicine, vol. 55, no. 12, pp. 1085–1096, 1984.

5. K. Cho, A. Ennaceur, J. C. Cole, and C. K. Suh, "Chronic jet lag produces cognitive deficits," The Journal of Neuroscience, vol. 20, no. 6, p. RC66, 2000.

6. K. Cho, "Chronic 'jet lag' produces temporal lobe atrophy and spatial cognitive deficits," Nature Neuroscience, vol. 4, no. 6, pp. 567–568, 2001.

7. G. Katz, R. Durst, Y. Zislin, Y. Barel, and H. Y. Knobler, "Psychiatric aspects of jet lag: review and hypothesis," Medical Hypotheses, vol. 56, no. 1, pp. 20–23, 2001.

8. A. J. Scott, "Shift work and health," Primary Care, vol. 27, no. 4, pp. 1057–1078, 2000.

9. S. Davis, D. K. Mirick, and R. G. Stevens, "Night shift work, light at night, and risk of breast cancer," Journal of the National Cancer Institute, vol. 93, no. 20, pp. 1557–1562, 2001.

10. A. Knutsson, "Health disorders of shift workers," Occupational Medicine, vol. 53, no. 2, pp. 103–108, 2003.

11. F. W. Turek, "From circadian rhythms to clock genes in depression," International Clinical Psychopharmacology, vol. 22, supplement 2, pp. S1–S8, 2007.

12. K. A. Lee and C. L. Gay, "Sleep in late pregnancy predicts length of labor and type of delivery," American Journal of Obstetrics and Gynecology, vol. 191, no. 6, pp. 2041–2046, 2004.

13. R. L. Sack, "The pathophysiology of jet lag," Travel Medicine and Infectious Disease, vol. 7, no. 2, pp. 102–110, 2009.

14. J. Wise, "Danish night shift workers with breast cancer awarded compensation," British Medical Journal, vol. 338, article b1152, 2009.

15. F. W. Turek and E. Van Cauter, "Rhythms in reproduction," in The Physiology of Reproduction, E. Knobil and J. D. Neill, Eds., pp. 487–540, Raven Press, New York, NY, USA, 1994.

16. G. E. Hoffman, W.-S. Lee, B. Attardi, V. Yann, and M. D. Fitzsimmons, "Luteinizing hormone-releasing hormone neurons express c-fos antigen after steroid activation," Endocrinology, vol. 126, no. 3, pp. 1736–1741, 1990.

17. M. M. Mahoney, C. Sisk, H. E. Ross, and L. Smale, "Circadian regulation of gonadotropin-releasing hormone neurons and the preovulatory surge in luteinizing hormone in the diurnal rodent, Arvicanthis niloticus, and in a nocturnal rodent, Rattus norvegicus," Biology of Reproduction, vol. 70, no. 4, pp. 1049–1054, 2004.

18. W.-S. Lee, M. S. Smith, and G. E. Hoffman, "Luteinizing hormone-releasing hormone neurons express Fos protein during the proestrous surge of luteinizing hormone," Proceedings of the National Academy of Sciences of the United States of America, vol. 87, no. 13, pp. 5163–5167, 1990.

19. M. J. Boden and D. J. Kennaway, "Circadian rhythms and reproduction," Reproduction, vol. 132, no. 3, pp. 379–392, 2006.

20. J. J. Alleva, M. V. Waleski, and F. R. Alleva, "A biological clock controlling the estrous cycle of the hamster," Endocrinology, vol. 88, no. 6, pp. 1368–1379, 1971.

21. P. Sodersten, "Hormonal and behavioral rhythms related to reproduction," in Advances in Comparative and Environmental Physiology, J. Balthazart, Ed., vol. 3 of Molecular and Cellular Basis of Social Behavior in Vertebrates, pp. 1–29, Springer, New York, NY, USA, 1989.

22. T. L. McElhinny, L. Smale, and K. E. Holekamp, "Patterns of body temperature, activity, and reproductive behavior in a tropical murid rodent, Arvicanthis niloticus," Physiology and Behavior, vol. 62, no. 1, pp. 91–96, 1997.

23. D. C. Klein, R. Y. Moore, et al., Eds., Suprachiasmatic Nucleus: The Mind's Clock, Oxford University Press, New York, , NY, USA, 1991.

24. G. D. Gray, P. Soderstein, D. Tallentire, and J. M. Davidson, "Effects of lesions in various structures of the suprachiasmatic preoptic region on LH regulation and sexual behavior in female rats," Neuroendocrinology, vol. 25, no. 3, pp. 174–191, 1978.

25. M. Kawakami, J. Arita, and E. Yoshioka, "Loss of estrogen-induced daily surges of prolactin and gonadotropins by suprachiasmatic nucleus lesions in ovariectomized rats," Endocrinology, vol. 106, no. 4, pp. 1087–1092, 1980.

26. S. J. Wiegand and E. Terasawa, "Discrete lesions reveal functional heterogeneity of suprachiasmatic structures in regulation of gonadotropin secretion in the female rat," Neuroendocrinology, vol. 34, no. 6, pp. 395–404, 1982.

27. R. M. Buijs, A. Kalsbeek, T. P. Van der Woude, J. J. Van Heerikhuize, and S. Shinn, "Suprachiasmatic nucleus lesion increases corticosterone secretion," American Journal of Physiology, vol. 264, no. 6, pp. R1186–R1192, 1993.

28. E. L. Meyer-Bernstein, A. E. Jetton, S.-I. Matsumoto, J. F. Markuns, M. N. Lehman, and E. L. Bittman, "Effects of suprachiasmatic transplants on circadian rhythms of

neuroendocrine function in golden hamsters," Endocrinology, vol. 140, no. 1, pp. 207–218, 1999.

29. B. Kerdelhue, S. Brown, V. Lenoir, et al., "Timing of initiation of the preovulatory luteinizing hormone surge and its relationship with the circadian cortisol rhythm in the human," Neuroendocrinology, vol. 75, no. 3, pp. 158–163, 2002.

30. D. J. Cahill, P. G. Wardle, C. R. Harlow, and M. G. R. Hull, "Onset of the preovulatory luteinizing hormone surge: diurnal timing and critical follicular prerequisites," Fertility and Sterility, vol. 70, no. 1, pp. 56–59, 1998.

31. A. F. Khattab, F. A. Mustafa, and P. J. Taylor, "The use of urine LH detection kits to time intrauterine insemination with donor sperm," Human Reproduction, vol. 20, no. 9, pp. 2542–2545, 2005.

32. T. L. McElhinny, C. L. Sisk, K. E. Holekamp, and L. Smale, "A morning surge in plasma luteinizing hormone coincides with elevated fos expression in gonadotropin-releasing hormone-immunoreactive neurons in the diurnal rodent, Arvicanthis niloticus," Biology of Reproduction, vol. 61, no. 4, pp. 1115–1122, 1999.

33. W. G. Rossmanith, "Ultradian and circadian patterns in luteinizing hormone secretion during reproductive life in women," Human Reproduction, vol. 8, supplement 2, pp. 77–83, 1993.

34. S. Ngwenya and S. W. Lindow, "24 Hour rhythm in the timing of pre-labour spontaneous rupture of membranes at term," European Journal of Obstetrics Gynecology and Reproductive Biology, vol. 112, no. 2, pp. 151–153, 2004.

35. M. Cooperstock, J. E. England, and R. A. Wolfe, "Circadian incidence of labor onset hour in preterm birth and chorioamnionitis," Obstetrics and Gynecology, vol. 70, no. 6, pp. 852–855, 1987.

36. A. Cagnacci, R. Soldani, G. B. Melis, and A. Volpe, "Diurnal rhythms of labor and delivery in women: modulation by parity and seasons," American Journal of Obstetrics and Gynecology, vol. 178, no. 1 I, pp. 140–145, 1998.

37. P. J. Mancuso, J. M. Alexander, D. D. McIntire, E. Davis, G. Burke, and K. J. Leveno, "Timing of birth after spontaneous onset of labor," Obstetrics and Gynecology, vol. 103, no. 4, pp. 653–656, 2004.

38. J. M. Dodd, C. A. Crowther, and J. S. Robinson, "Morning compared with evening induction of labor: a nested randomized controlled trial," Obstetrics and Gynecology, vol. 108, no. 2, pp. 350–360, 2006.

39. K. Wallen, "Desire and ability: hormones and the regulation of female sexual behavior," Neuroscience and Biobehavioral Reviews, vol. 14, no. 2, pp. 233–241, 1990.

40. F. J. Karsch, R. F. Weick, and W. R. Butler, "Induced LH surges in the rhesus monkey: strength duration characteristics of the estrogen stimulus," Endocrinology, vol. 92, no. 6, pp. 1740–1747, 1973.

41. S. Labyak, S. Lava, F. Turek, and P. Zee, "Effects of shiftwork on sleep and menstrual function in nurses," Health Care for Women International, vol. 23, no. 6-7, pp. 703–714, 2002.

42. F.-F. Chung, C.-C. C. Yao, and G.-H. Wan, "The associations between menstrual function and life style/working conditions among nurses in Taiwan," Journal of Occupational Health, vol. 47, no. 2, pp. 149–156, 2005.

43. P. N. Lohstroh, J. Chen, J. Ba, et al., "Bone resorption is affected by follicular phase length in female rotating shift workers," Environmental Health Perspectives, vol. 111, no. 4, pp. 618–622, 2003.

44. L. Bisanti, J. Olsen, O. Basso, P. Thonneau, and W. Karmaus, "Shift work and subfecundity: a European multicenter study," Journal of Occupational and Environmental Medicine, vol. 38, no. 4, pp. 352–358, 1996.

45. J. E. Cone, L. M. Vaughan, A. Huete, and S. J. Samuels, "Reproductive health outcomes among female flight attendants: an exploratory study," Journal of Occupational and Environmental Medicine, vol. 40, no. 3, pp. 210–216, 1998.

46. R. Aspholm, M.-L. Lindbohm, H. Paakkulainen, H. Taskinen, T. Nurminen, and A. Tiitinen, "Spontaneous abortions among Finnish flight attendants," Journal of Occupational and Environmental Medicine, vol. 41, no. 6, pp. 486–491, 1999.

47. A. Endo and T. Watanabe, "Effects of non-24-hour days on reproductive efficacy and embryonic development in mice," Gamete Research, vol. 22, no. 4, pp. 435–441, 1989.

48. S. Touzet, M. Rabilloud, H. Boehringer, E. Barranco, and R. Ecochard, "Relationship between sleep and secretion of gonadotropin and ovarian hormones in women with normal cycles," Fertility and Sterility, vol. 77, no. 4, pp. 738–744, 2002.

49. A. Baumgartner, M. Dietzel, B. Saletu, et al., "Influence of partial sleep deprivation on the secretion of thyrotropin, thyroid hormones, growth hormone, prolactin, luteinizing hormone, follicle stimulating hormone, and estradiol in healthy young women," Psychiatry Research, vol. 48, no. 2, pp. 153–178, 1993.

50. D. E. Blask, "Melatonin, sleep disturbance and cancer risk," Sleep Medicine Reviews, vol. 13, no. 4, pp. 257–264, 2009.

51. R. G. Stevens, "Working against our endogenous circadian clock: breast cancer and electric lighting in the modern world," Mutation Research, vol. 679, no. 1-2, pp. 6–8, 2009.

52. E. S. Schernhammer, F. Laden, F. E. Speizer, et al., "Rotating night shifts and risk of breast cancer in women participating in the nurses' health study," Journal of the National Cancer Institute, vol. 93, no. 20, pp. 1563–1568, 2001.

53. S. P. Megdal, C. H. Kroenke, F. Laden, E. Pukkala, and E. S. Schernhammer, "Night work and breast cancer risk: a systematic review and meta-analysis," European Journal of Cancer, vol. 41, no. 13, pp. 2023–2032, 2005.

54. M. Moser, K. Schaumberger, E. Schernhammer, and R. G. Stevens, "Cancer and rhythm," Cancer Causes and Control, vol. 17, no. 4, pp. 483–487, 2006.

55. E. S. Schernhammer, C. H. Kroenke, F. Laden, and S. E. Hankinson, "Night work and risk of breast cancer," Epidemiology, vol. 17, no. 1, pp. 108–111, 2006.

56. E. Filipski, V. M. King, X. M. Li, et al., "Disruption of circadian coordination accelerates malignant growth in mice," Pathologie Biologie, vol. 51, no. 4, pp. 216–219, 2003.

57. E. Filipski, F. Delaunay, V. M. King, et al., "Effects of chronic jet lag on tumor progression in mice," Cancer Research, vol. 64, no. 21, pp. 7879–7885, 2004.

58. E. Filipski, X. M. Li, and F. Lévi, "Disruption of circadian coordination and malignant growth," Cancer Causes and Control, vol. 17, no. 4, pp. 509–514, 2006.

59. S. Davis and D. K. Mirick, "Circadian disruption, shift work and the risk of cancer: a summary of the evidence and studies in Seattle," Cancer Causes and Control, vol. 17, no. 4, pp. 539–545, 2006.

60. L. P. Shearman, M. J. Zylka, D. R. Weaver, L. F. Kolakowski Jr., and S. M. Reppert, "Two period homologs: circadian expression and photic regulation in the suprachiasmatic nuclei," Neuron, vol. 19, no. 6, pp. 1261–1269, 1997.

61. Y. Shigeyoshi, K. Taguchi, S. Yamamoto, et al., "Light-induced resetting of a mammalian circadian clock is associated with rapid induction of the mPer1 transcript," Cell, vol. 91, no. 7, pp. 1043–1053, 1997.

62. M. J. Zylka, L. P. Shearman, D. R. Weaver, and S. M. Reppert, "Three period homologs in mammals: differential light responses in the suprachiasmatic circadian clock and oscillating transcripts outside of brain," Neuron, vol. 20, no. 6, pp. 1103–1110, 1998.

63. Y. Zhu, R. G. Stevens, D. Leaderer, et al., "Non-synonymous polymorphisms in the circadian gene NPAS2 and breast cancer risk," Breast Cancer Research and Treatment, vol. 107, no. 3, pp. 421–425, 2008.

64. J. Fahrenkrug, B. Georg, J. Hannibal, P. Hindersson, and S. Graäs, "Diurnal rhythmicity of the clock genes Per1 and Per2 in the rat ovary," Endocrinology, vol. 147, no. 8, pp. 3769–3776, 2006.

65. B. N. Karman and S. A. Tischkau, "Circadian clock gene expression in the ovary: effects of luteinizing hormone," Biology of Reproduction, vol. 75, no. 4, pp. 624–632, 2006.

66. B. Horard, B. Rayet, G. Triqueneaux, V. Laudet, F. Delaunay, and J.-M. Vanacker, "Expression of the orphan nuclear receptor ERRα is under circadian regulation in estrogen-responsive tissues," Journal of Molecular Endocrinology, vol. 33, no. 1, pp. 87–97, 2004.

67. T. J. Nakamura, T. Moriya, S. Inoue, et al., "Estrogen differentially regulates expression of Per1 and Per2 genes between central and peripheral clocks and between reproductive and nonreproductive tissues in female rats," Journal of Neuroscience Research, vol. 82, no. 5, pp. 622–630, 2005.

68. P.-J. He, M. Hirata, N. Yamauchi, and M.-A. Hattori, "Up-regulation of Per1 expression by estradiol and progesterone in the rat uterus," Journal of Endocrinology, vol. 194, no. 3, pp. 511–519, 2007.

69. D. J. Kennaway, T. J. Varcoe, and V. J. Mau, "Rhythmic expression of clock and clock-controlled genes in the rat oviduct," Molecular Human Reproduction, vol. 9, no. 9, pp. 503–507, 2003.

70. P. E. Chappell, R. S. White, and P. L. Mellon, "Circadian gene expression regulates pulsatile gonadotropin-releasing hormone (GnRH) secretory patterns in the hypothalamic GnRH-secreting GT1-7 cell line," Journal of Neuroscience, vol. 23, no. 35, pp. 11202–11213, 2003.

71. J. M. A. Gillespie, B. P. K. Chan, D. Roy, F. Cai, and D. D. Belsham, "Expression of circadian rhythm genes in gonadotropin-releasing hormone-secreting GT1-7 neurons," Endocrinology, vol. 144, no. 12, pp. 5285–5292, 2003.

72. P. E. Chappell, C. P. Goodall, K. J. Tonsfeldt, R. S. White, E. Bredeweg, and K. L. Latham, "Modulation of gonadotrophin-releasing hormone secretion by an endog-

enous circadian clock," Journal of Neuroendocrinology, vol. 21, no. 4, pp. 339–345, 2009.

73. H. Dolatshad, E. A. Campbell, L. O'Hara, E. S. Maywood, M. H. Hastings, and M. H. Johnson, "Developmental and reproductive performance in circadian mutant mice," Human Reproduction, vol. 21, no. 1, pp. 68–79, 2006.

74. V. Pilorz and S. Steinlechner, "Low reproductive success in Per1 and Per2 mutant mouse females due to accelerated ageing?" Reproduction, vol. 135, no. 4, pp. 559–568, 2008.

75. J. D. Alvarez, A. Hansen, T. Ord, et al., "The circadian clock protein BMAL1 is necessary for fertility and proper testosterone production in mice," Journal of Biological Rhythms, vol. 23, no. 1, pp. 26–36, 2008.

76. B. H. Miller, S. L. Olson, F. W. Turek, J. E. Levine, T. H. Horton, and J. S. Takahashi, "Circadian Clock mutation disrupts estrous cyclicity and maintenance of pregnancy," Current Biology, vol. 14, no. 15, pp. 1367–1373, 2004.

77. S. Yamazaki, R. Numano, M. Abe, et al., "Resetting central and peripheral circadian oscillators in transgenic rats," Science, vol. 288, no. 5466, pp. 682–685, 2000.

78. A. B. Reddy, M. D. Field, E. S. Maywood, and M. H. Hastings, "Differential resynchronisation of circadian clock gene expression within the suprachiasmatic nuclei of mice subjected to experimental jet lag," Journal of Neuroscience, vol. 22, no. 17, pp. 7326–7330, 2002.

79. Y. Zhu, H. N. Brown, Y. Zhang, R. G. Stevens, and T. Zheng, "Period3 structural variation: a circadian biomarker associated with breast cancer in young women," Cancer Epidemiology Biomarkers and Prevention, vol. 14, no. 1, pp. 268–270, 2005.

80. J. L. Marino, V. L. Holt, C. Chen, and S. Davis, "Shift work, hCLOCK T3111C polymorphism, and endometriosis risk," Epidemiology, vol. 19, no. 3, pp. 477–484, 2008.

81. L. J. Kriegsfeld and R. Silver, "The regulation of neuroendocrine function: timing is everything," Hormones and Behavior, vol. 49, no. 5, pp. 557–574, 2006.

82. I. N. Karatsoreos and R. Silver, "Minireview: the neuroendocrinology of the suprachiasmatic nucleus as a conductor of body time in mammals," Endocrinology, vol. 148, no. 12, pp. 5640–5647, 2007.

83. L. P. Morin, K. M. Fitzgerald, B. Rusak, and I. Zucker, "Circadian organization and neural mediation of hamster reproductive rhythms," Psychoneuroendocrinology, vol. 2, no. 1, pp. 73–98, 1977.

84. H. E. Albers, A. A. Gerall, and J. F. Axelson, "Effect of reproductive state on circadian periodicity in the rat," Physiology and Behavior, vol. 26, no. 1, pp. 21–25, 1981.

85. S. E. Labyak and T. M. Lee, "Estrus- and steroid-induced changes in circadian rhythms in a diurnal rodent, Octodon degus," Physiology and Behavior, vol. 58, no. 3, pp. 573–585, 1995.

86. L. P. Morin, K. M. Fitzgerald, and I. Zucker, "Estradiol shortens the period of hamster circadian rhythms," Science, vol. 196, no. 4287, pp. 305–307, 1977.

87. H. E. Albers, N. Minamitani, E. Stopa, and C. F. Ferris, "Light selectively alters vasoactive intestinal peptide and peptide histidine isoleucine immunoreactivity within the rat suprachiasmatic nucleus," Brain Research, vol. 437, no. 1, pp. 189–192, 1987.

88. E. Leibenluft, "Do gonadal steroids regulate circadian rhythms in humans?" Journal of Affective Disorders, vol. 29, no. 2-3, pp. 175–181, 1993.

89. B. L. Parry, S. L. Berga, N. Mostofi, M. R. Klauber, and A. Resnick, "Plasma melatonin circadian rhythms during the menstrual cycle and after light therapy in premenstrual dysphoric disorder and normal control subjects," Journal of Biological Rhythms, vol. 12, no. 1, pp. 47–64, 1997.

90. K. Shibui, M. Uchiyama, M. Okawa, et al., "Diurnal fluctuation of sleep propensity and hormonal secretion across the menstrual cycle," Biological Psychiatry, vol. 48, no. 11, pp. 1062–1068, 2000.

91. F. C. Baker and H. S. Driver, "Circadian rhythms, sleep, and the menstrual cycle," Sleep Medicine, vol. 8, no. 6, pp. 613–622, 2007.

92. T. J. Nakamura, K. Shinohara, T. Funabashi, and F. Kimura, "Effect of estrogen on the expression of Cry1 and Cry2 mRNAs in the suprachiasmatic nucleus of female rats," Neuroscience Research, vol. 41, no. 3, pp. 251–255, 2001.

93. T. J. Nakamura, M. T. Sellix, M. Menaker, and G. D. Block, "Estrogen directly modulates circadian rhythms of PER2 expression in the uterus," American Journal of Physiology, vol. 295, no. 5, pp. E1025–E1031, 2008.

94. S. Gery, R. K. Virk, K. Chumakov, A. Yu, and H. P. Koeffler, "The clock gene Per2 links the circadian system to the estrogen receptor," Oncogene, vol. 26, no. 57, pp. 7916–7920, 2007.

95. S. L. Winter, L. Bosnoyan-Collins, D. Pinnaduwagez, and I. L. Andrulis, "Expression of the circadian clock genes Per1 and Per2 in sporadic and familial breast tumors," Neoplasia, vol. 9, no. 10, pp. 797–800, 2007.

96. F. P. M. Kruijver and D. F. Swaab, "Sex hormone receptors are present in the human suprachiasmatic nucleus," Neuroendocrinology, vol. 75, no. 5, pp. 296–305, 2002.

97. G. P. Chrousos, D. J. Torpy, and P. W. Gold, "Interactions between the hypothalamic-pituitary-adrenal axis and the female reproductive system: clinical implications," Annals of Internal Medicine, vol. 129, no. 3, pp. 229–240, 1998.

# CHAPTER 12

# A NEW APPROACH TO UNDERSTANDING THE IMPACT OF CIRCADIAN DISRUPTION ON HUMAN HEALTH

MARK S. REA, ANDREW BIERMAN, MARIANA G. FIGUEIRO, AND JOHN D. BULLOUGH

## 12.1 BACKGROUND

As the earth rotates, all species on the surface of the planet are exposed to 24-hour patterns of light and darkness. In response to these regular, daily oscillations to the natural light-dark cycle, these species have evolved endogenous circadian rhythms that repeat approximately every 24 hours [1,2]. Examples of circadian rhythms include oscillations in core body temperature [3], hormone secretion [4], sleep [5], and alertness [6]. Circadian oscillations also exist at a cellular level, including cell mitosis and DNA damage response [7,8]. These oscillations are a result of a small group of clock genes inside the cell nuclei creating interlocked transcriptional and post-translational feedback loops. The timing of these circadian clock genes is generally orchestrated by a master biological clock located in the suprachiasmatic nuclei (SCN) [9] of the hypothalamus of the brain

*This chapter was originally published under the Creative Commons Attribution License. Rea MS, Bierman A, Figueiro MG, and Bullough JD. A New Approach to Understanding the Impact of Circadian Disruption on Human Health.* Journal of Circadian Rhythms *6,7 (2008). doi:10.1186/1740-3391-6-7.*

[10]. The master clock in the SCN provides precise time cues throughout the body to regulate these diverse physiological, hormonal, and behavioral circadian patterns. However, in total darkness the timing of the SCN will become asynchronous with the solar day because in humans the period of the master clock is slightly longer than 24 hours [1]. To maintain synchrony with the external world, the light-dark pattern incident on the retina resets the timing of the SCN, so that as we travel across time zones, we can entrain our biological functions to the local environment. If the period of the light-dark pattern is too long or too short, or if the light and dark exposures become aperiodic, the master clock can lose control of the timing of peripheral circadian clocks.

Maintaining the phase-relation ordering of the various circadian rhythms from molecular to behavioral levels appears to be crucial for coordinated functions throughout the human body. Lack of synchrony between the master clock and the peripheral clocks can lead to asynchronies within cells (e.g., cell cycle) and between organ systems (e.g., liver and pancreas). This breakdown in synchrony, as demonstrated most profoundly with jet lag, disrupts sleep [11], digestion [12], and alertness [13]. Chronic disruptions can contribute to cardiovascular anomalies [14] and accelerated cancerous tumour growth [15] in animal models. In humans, epidemiological studies have shown that rotating-shift nurses, who experience a marked lack of synchrony between activity-rest patterns and light-dark cycles (as shown in this report), are at higher risk of having breast cancer compared to day-shift nurses [16]. In fact, the World Health Organization has identified rotating-shift work as a probable cause of cancer [17]. In addition to heightened cancer risks, other disorders have been associated with rotating-shift work, such as diabetes and obesity, suggesting again a role for circadian disruption in the development and progression of diseases [18].

Despite the growing evidence that circadian disruption negatively affects human health [18,19], the logical chain linking light-induced circadian disruption to morbidity and mortality still has not been forged. If the impact of circadian disruption is to be studied with any degree of accuracy, it is important to quantitatively characterize light and dark as it affects the human circadian system because the light-dark pattern is the primary synchronizing stimulus for our circadian system [1]. It is also necessary to quantify the temporal characteristics of circadian light and dark exposures actually experienced by people [20]. Without quantification of the actual circadian light and dark exposures experienced by people, it will be difficult to relate the findings from controlled laboratory studies of light-induced circadian disruption in humans to the expected health of any human sub-population, including rotating-shift workers. These actual circadian light and dark exposures in human populations must also be incorporated into parametric studies using animal models as surrogates for particular human diseases or maladies if we are to gain any detailed insight into the role of circadian disruption on human health. Since nocturnal species are used almost exclusively as animal models in this research, a method needs to be established to relate actual circadian light and dark exposures in humans to parametrically controlled exposures of light and dark using these animal models [21].

This paper is concerned with patterns of circadian light and dark as they affect behavioral entrainment and how more sophisticated studies of the relationship between light-induced circadian disruption and human health might be conducted. Here we present original data from the Daysimeter [20], a device for simultaneously recording light-dark and activity-rest data in humans. Significantly, these data reveal relationships between circadian light-dark patterns actually experienced by day-shift and rotating-shift nurses and their own activity-rest patterns. Original data are also presented for two groups of rats, one placed on a 12L:12D pattern of light and dark and the other placed on a 12L:12D pattern of light and dark regularly reversing every 48 hours. We present a novel methodology to quantify circadian entrainment/disruption in both diurnal and nocturnal species, so as to allow researchers to make direct comparisons of circadian entrainment/disruption across species. Attention to circadian entrainment/disruption, rather than to activity alone or to light and dark, per se, makes it possible to circumvent the diurnal-nocturnal conundrum plaguing many comparative studies of light-induced circadian entrainment/disruption using animal models. We found that the circadian entrainment/disruption patterns for day-shift and rotating-shift nurses were remarkably different, but they were remarkably similar to the patterns for two parallel groups of nocturnal rodents. The marked differences in circadian entrainment/disruption patterns within species together with the marked similarities in circadian entrainment/disruption across species, in addition to the new method for quantifying circadian entrainment/disruption, suggest that health-related problems associated with circadian disruption in humans can be parametrically studied using animal models.

## 12.2 METHODS

### 12.2.1 MEASURING AND CHARACTERIZING CIRCADIAN ENTRAINMENT PATTERNS ACTUALLY EXPERIENCED BY HUMANS

#### 12.2.1.1 DAYSIMETER

The Daysimeter was developed as a head-worn light-dosimeter and activity monitor to address measurements of the spectral and spatial response of the human circadian system (Figure 1) [20]. Two detectors are used to characterize the spectral-opponent, subadditive response of the circadian system to polychromatic light and thereby provide measurements of the circadian light stimulus (CS) for humans (Figure 2) [22]. A transfer function relating CS to nocturnal melatonin suppression was also developed [22] to characterize the effective stimulus for nonvisual responses associated with optical radiation on the retina (Figure 3). Entrainment to the circadian light-dark pattern is not directly related to nocturnal melatonin suppression, but as demonstrated by Zeitzer et al. [23], both light-induced phase shifting and nocturnal melatonin suppression in humans appear to have similar, if not identical, functional relationships to optical radiation of the same spectral power distribution.

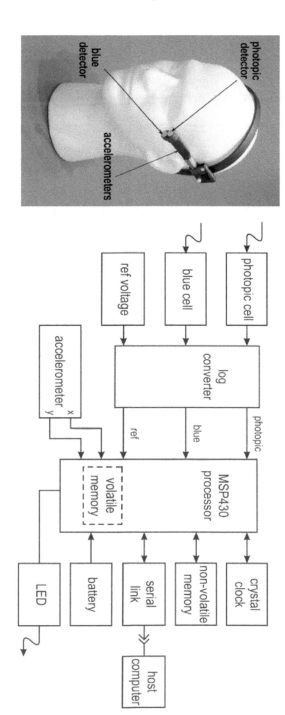

**FIGURE 1:** Daysimeter and functional block diagram.

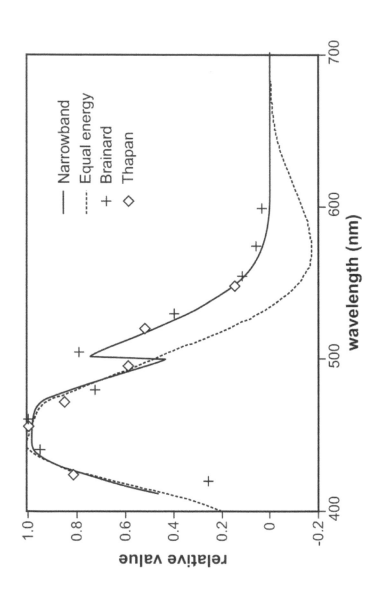

**FIGURE 2:** Spectral response graph. Spectral response functions generated from the model of human circadian phototransduction by Rea et al. [22]. The dashed line represents the predicted spectral response function for an equal energy spectrum light source. The continuous line represents the predicted spectral responses to individual, narrow-band light sources. The two sets of symbols represent empirical spectral response data from two independent laboratories [34, 35].

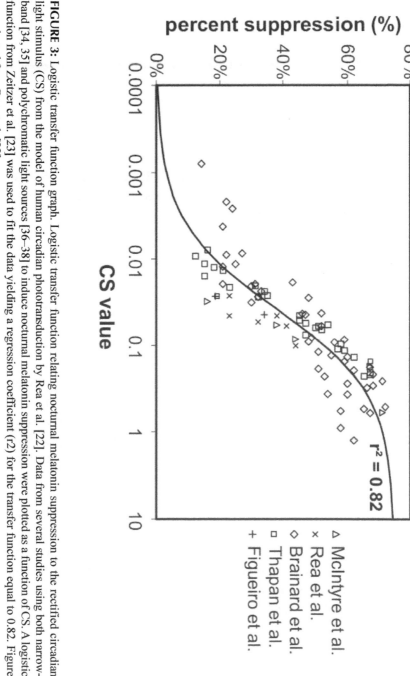

**FIGURE 3:** Logistic transfer function graph. Logistic transfer function relating nocturnal melatonin suppression to the rectified circadian light stimulus (CS) from the model of human circadian phototransduction by Rea et al. [22]. Data from several studies using both narrow-band [34, 35] and polychromatic light sources [36–38] to induce nocturnal melatonin suppression were plotted as a function of CS. A logistic function from Zeitzer et al. [23] was used to fit the data yielding a regression coefficient (r2) for the transfer function equal to 0.82. Figure was adapted from Rea et al. [22].

The Daysimeter also measures head movements with solid-state acceler-ometers to characterize behavioral activity. Detailed information about the Daysimeter is available elsewhere [20].

It should be emphasized that activity as measured by the Daysimeter is not a direct measure of the endogenous clock in the SCN. Like every downstream measure of circadian function, behavior can only yield partial insight into circadian entrainment. It is presently impossible to directly measure SCN activity in vivo, and thus it is impossible to measure en-trainment in the purest sense in living and active humans; the term "be-havioral entrainment" is used in this paper to describe the observed levels of synchrony between light-dark exposures and activity-rest responses as measured by the Daysimeter.

## 12.2.1.2 DATA COLLECTION

The Daysimeter was sent to nurses throughout the United States to mea-sure their actual CS exposures and activity for seven consecutive days. Forty-three pre-menopausal female nurses, both day-shift (n = 32) and rotating-shift nurses (n = 11), participated in the study. They wore the Daysimeter for seven consecutive days and were scheduled to work at least two and no more than three consecutive days during that period. The Daysimeter was worn while nurses were awake. The nurses were in-structed to place the Daysimeter next to them when they slept or bathed. After the seven-day recording session, they returned the device for data analyses. In addition to wearing the Daysimeter, participating nurses provided urine samples, obtained every four hours, for subsequent mela-tonin assay and filled out a chronotype questionnaire [Horne-Östberg Morningness-Eveningness Questionnaire (MEQ)] and a lighting survey. The nurses were also asked to keep a sleep log, writing down the times they went to bed and any other information about their sleep schedules. These sleep logs were used to match the exact time nurses started wear-ing the device. Presented here are only the Daysimeter data.

## 12.2.2 MEASURING AND CHARACTERIZING CIRCADIAN BEHAVIORAL ENTRAINMENT PATTERNS IN NOCTURNAL RODENTS

### 12.2.2.1 DATA COLLECTION

Forty albino female Sprague-Dawley rats (*Rattus norvegicus*) were housed in individual cages illuminated by a lighting system previously developed by Bullough et al. [24] to determine the spectral and absolute sensitivities of another nocturnal rodent (*murine*). Based upon the mouse phase response curve (PRC) obtained in that study, a spectral power distribution (nearly monochromatic green light; $\lambda_{max}$ = 525 nm, half-bandwidth = 35 nm) and irradiance (approximately 5 $\mu$W/cm$^2$ on the cage floor) were selected to provide the light stimulus to the Sprague-Dawley rats. This particular light stimulus for nocturnal rodents was estimated to be above threshold and below saturation for stimulation of the rat circadian system. The light stimulus for the rats was precisely controlled using a light-emitting diode (LED) light-delivery system fabricated and installed in every cage. The light-delivery system provided better controlled and more biologically meaningful circadian light stimulation to the rats than the fluorescent ceiling lighting traditionally used to provide bright, ambient illumination throughout an animal colony [21].

As with the nurse data, the rat data were obtained from two experimental groups: 20 rats were exposed to a consistently repeating pattern of 12 hours of light (12L) followed by 12 hours of darkness (12D), and another 20 rats (the "jet-lagged" group) were exposed to a 12L:12D pattern where the phase of the light-dark cycle was reversed every 48 hours (as if this group of rats instantly travelled back and forth from Asia to the Americas every other day). Animals were housed individually and allowed to eat and drink ad libidum.

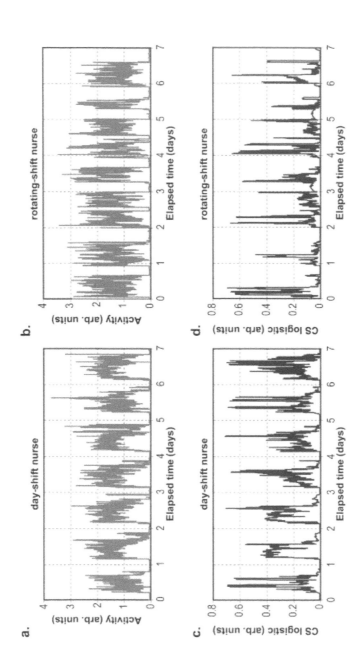

**FIGURE 4:** Activity and light exposure graphs: Nurses. Activity and light exposure data plotted as a function of elapsed number of days for a day-shift nurse (4a, 4c) and for a rotating-shift nurse (4b, 4d). Data collection started at a different clock time for each subject, so each "day" is a different 24-hour period of time for each subject. Circadian light stimulus (CS) exposures were measured with the Daysimeter [20], and transformed to range between the limits of human melatonin suppression (CS Logistic) shown in Figure 3.

Wheel running was measured continuously throughout the experimental session and used as the measure of activity-rest in these animals. The accumulated number of wheel revolutions was recorded at 10-minute time intervals. At the start of the experiment, the photoperiods for both groups were in phase with each other, and the animals exhibited typical nocturnal behavior (active during the dark phase, inactive during the light phase). To allow for acclimation to the cages and to the lighting by the rats, wheel-running data were not collected until the third day of the study, by which time the photoperiod for the "jet-lagged" group had reversed. Most of the activity in the "jet-lagged" group on that day occurred during the light phase. As shown below, the animals in this group were unable to entrain to the regularly reversing photoperiod and exhibited behavior similar to free-running, with similar amounts of activity in the light and in the dark throughout the eight-day observation period.

## 12.3 RESULTS

Figure 4 shows activity and CS exposure data for two representative nurses (one day-shift and one night-shift) and Figure 5 shows the wheel-running data and relative light level for two representative animals (one in the 12L:12D group and one in the "jet-lagged" group).

### 12.3.1 HUMANS

Figures 4a and 4b show activity for two representative nurses, one day-shift nurse (4a) and one rotating-shift nurse (4b), for seven consecutive days. Figures 4c and 4d illustrate the measured CS exposure values obtained directly from the Daysimeter and subsequently transformed using a logistic stimulus-response function representing the entire response range of the circadian system, from threshold to saturation (Figure 3). The transformation was employed to estimate the functional input to the human circadian system, which appears to apply to both light-induced nocturnal melatonin suppression and phase shifting [23].

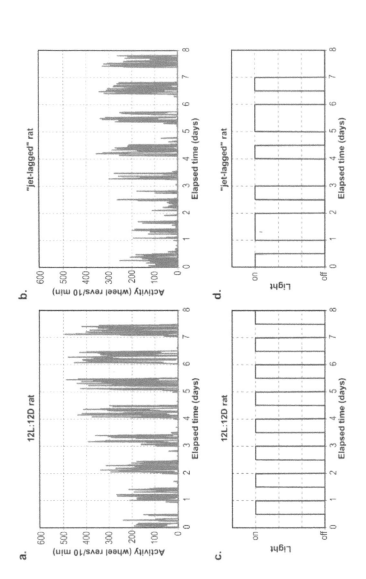

**FIGURE 5:** Activity and light exposure graphs: Rats. Activity and light exposure data plotted as a function of elapsed time (days) for a 12L:12D rat (5a, 5c) and for a "jet lagged" rat (5b, 5d). At the start of the experiment, the photoperiods were in phase. In the first two days of the experiment, the photoperiods for both groups were the same. Wheel-running data were not collected until the third day of the study, by which time the photoperiod for the "jet-lagged" group had reversed. Most of the activity in the "jet-lagged" group on that day occurred during the light phase.

Examination of Figure 4 reveals subtle but important differences in the activity and transformed CS data for these two nurses. In the case of the day-shift nurse (Figures 4a and 4c), there appears to be a consistent relationship between the activity and transformed CS values over the course of the seven-day measurement session. For the rotating-shift nurse (Figures 4b and 4d), however, this synchrony is much less pronounced. Qualitatively then, and as might be expected, these two example sets of data suggest that the day-shift nurse's behavior is much more synchronized to the light-dark cycle than that of the rotating-shift nurse. Parenthetically, Figure 4 also reveals "flat" periods for both nurses over the course of the seven-day measurement period, which indicate prolonged times of rest and, usually, darkness.

Although many analyses of the activity and of the transformed CS data are possible, the data in Figure 4 were used to develop a quantitative measure of circadian behavioral entrainment/disruption for day-shift and for rotating-shift nurses. The behavioral entrainment analyses were based on the circular cross-correlations of activity and light exposure data. Circular cross-correlation, an analysis technique commonly used in the field of signal processing, involves the concept of time-shifting one signal relative to another to determine relationships between signals that might otherwise be obscured due to relative timing differences. The activity and the transformed CS data can be considered as two time-varying signals whose time-matched values can be multiplied together and then the products at every time of data acquisition integrated into a single value. This value is proportional to the covariance of the two signals. When normalized by dividing by the number of data samples, subtracting the product of the individual signal means, and dividing by the product of the standard deviations of each signal, the result will always be limited to values between -1 and 1 (i.e., a correlation coefficient). The multiply-and-integrate operation can be repeated following a small shift in time by one of the signals (e.g., the activity trace, Figure 4a) with respect to the other (e.g., the transformed CS trace, Figure 4c) and a new correlation coefficient computed. Continuously repeating this process for the entire recording period yields a new time-varying function, the circular cross-correlation, bounded by -1 and 1, that reveals the degree to which the two signals are systematically related to one another for all possible alignments of phase between the two signals. This operation is adapted from standard signal processing techniques [25], and when performed on the periodic light and activity data, yields what are termed, for the purposes of this paper, behavioral entrainment-correlation functions.

Figure 6 shows two behavioral entrainment-correlation functions relating the transformed CS data to the activity data: one for the day-shift nurse (Figure 6a) and one for the rotating-shift nurse (Figure 6b) in Figure 4. As can be readily appreciated from Figure 6a, the activity of the day-shift nurse is highly entrained to her light-dark pattern throughout the seven days, as exhibited by the regularly oscillating, 24-hour period of her behavioral entrainment-correlation function. More specifically, this nurse, typical of almost all day-shift nurses, has a peak correlation near the zero-phase marker and again at every 24-hour multiple. This day-shift pattern is in marked contrast to the behavioral entrainment-correlation pattern for the rotating-shift nurse (Figure 6b). Her pattern is aperiodic, exhibiting minor correlation peaks at times other than at the 24-hour phase markers. The pattern of the rotating-shift nurse is of much lower amplitude and very distorted compared to the smoothly varying and periodic behavioral entrainment-correlation pattern of the day-shift nurse.

### 12.3.2 NOCTURNAL RODENTS

The wheel running data from the 12L:12D (e.g., see Figure 5a) rats were typical of those collected in innumerable studies, with more active periods associated with darkness and less active periods in the light. The "jet-lagged" group differed considerably from the 12L:12D group, however, in the apparent degree of association between the light-dark and the rest-activity data (e.g., see Figure 5b). For those rats in the 12L:12D group, almost all of their wheel running occurred in darkness; although, as is usually the case, there was some activity in the light, particularly near the transition times from light to dark, and there were intervals of quiescence sporadically occurring during the dark periods. In the "jet-lagged" group of rats, the association between wheel running and darkness was markedly less pronounced. Indeed, after several reversals of the light-dark cycle, the wheel running appeared to be disassociated with either light or dark.

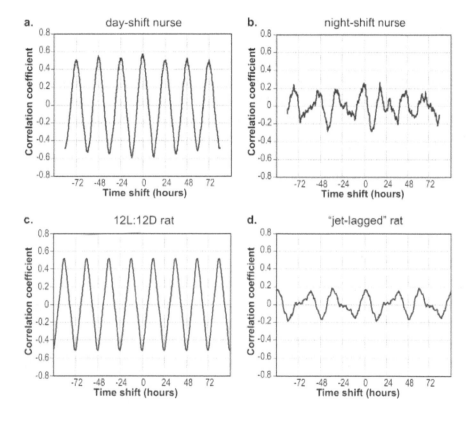

**FIGURE 6:** Behavioral entrainment-correlation functions. Behavioral entrainment-correlation functions relating activity and light exposures for two example nurses, one day-shift nurse (Figure 6a) and one rotating-shift nurse (6b) and two example rats, a rat exposed to a regular 12L:12D pattern of light and dark (6c) and a "jet-lagged" rat exposed to a 12:12 light-dark cycle that was phase-reversed every 48 hours (6d).

The same analyses performed on the data from the nurses were also applied to the data from the two groups of nocturnal rodents. The light exposure values were binary for the rats, zero when no cage lighting was present and a value of one when the cage lighting was administered. A behavioral entrainment-correlation function from one typical rat in the 12L:12D group is shown in Figure 6c. The similarity between the entrainment-correlation function for the sample day-shift nurse and the 12L:12D rat are remarkable; the only apparent difference is that the latter function is shifted approximately 12 hours with respect to the former. This shift reflects the expected difference between a diurnal and a nocturnal species; diurnal nurses are active during the day and inactive at night, whereas nocturnal rats are inactive during the light phase and active in the dark. Figure 6d shows a typical behavioral entrainment-correlation function for one rat in the "jet-lagged" group. Again, there is a marked similarity between the entrainment-correlation functions for the rotating-shift nurse in Figure 6b and for the "jet-lagged" rat in Figure 6d.

## 12.3.3 PHASOR REPRESENTATIONS OF CIRCADIAN BEHAVIORAL ENTRAINMENT

Plots of the behavioral entrainment-correlation functions for the day-shift nurses generally exhibit smooth, oscillating curves whereas those of the rotating-shift nurses exhibit much more irregular patterns. Estimates of the relationship between activity-rest and light-dark in terms of magnitude and phase can be determined for both groups of nurses through Fourier decomposition and spectral analysis of the behavioral entrainment-correlation functions. Phasors represent the magnitude and phase relationship between the activity-rest data and the light-dark data that underlie the entrainment-correlation functions for a particular spectral component obtained from the Fourier decomposition [26]. Since the 24-hour spectral component is of special interest in studies of circadian entrainment, the activity and light data for every nurse were first parsed into seven equal 24-hour periods. The behavioral entrainment-correlation functions were then calculated for each of these seven periods after which the seven corresponding phasors representing the frequency component corresponding to a 24-hour periodicity, f(24) for every one of the 43 nurses were determined. It should be noted that a systematic investigation of periods ranging from 22 to 26 hours in 10-minute increments was conducted for the day-shift nurse data. While the range of peak phasor amplitudes occurred for periods ranging from 23.7 to 24.56 hours as determined from quadratic curve-fits to the phasor magnitude versus period data, the mean was 24.035 hours, supporting the significance of the 24-hour period for this analysis.

Complex arithmetic [27] was then used to determine the average (n = 7) phasor for a given nurse and these average phasors for all the nurses are plotted in Figure 7a in polar coordinates. The length of each phasor is the magnitude of the average f(24) and reveals how well light and activity are correlated over the seven-day recording session. As a group, the day-shift nurses have larger phasor lengths than the rotating-shift nurses, implying that they have a much higher degree of behavioral entrainment.

Consistent with a diurnal species, all the phasor directions for the nurses are to the right, meaning that activity and light exposure occur at nearly the same time. The angular direction of a phasor indicates the phase relationship between light and activity for an individual. Greater amounts of activity near the onset of circadian light exposure than near the offset of circadian light exposure produces a phasor extending below the zero-phase polar axis line (labeled 0 hour). Conversely, greater amounts of activity near the offset of circadian light exposure than near the onset of circadian light exposure produces a phasor extending above the zero-phase line. Researchers [28] have used the terms "larks" and "owls" to refer to people with diurnal activity patterns biased toward morning or evening hours, respectively. These times, however, are not explicitly linked to actual light exposures. The phasor analysis does reveal similar behavioral characteristics, but ones referenced to actual light-dark exposures rather than to an arbitrary exogenous time reference (watch or wall-clock time). Borrowing the lark and owl terminology for describing the behavioral characteristics revealed by the phasor analyses, it is interesting to note that there are more owls than larks, particularly among the rotating-shift nurses, indicating that these people tend to be more active after the onset and subsidence of daily light exposure than before. Although it was true that for day-shift nurses the natural solar cycle was largely coincident with

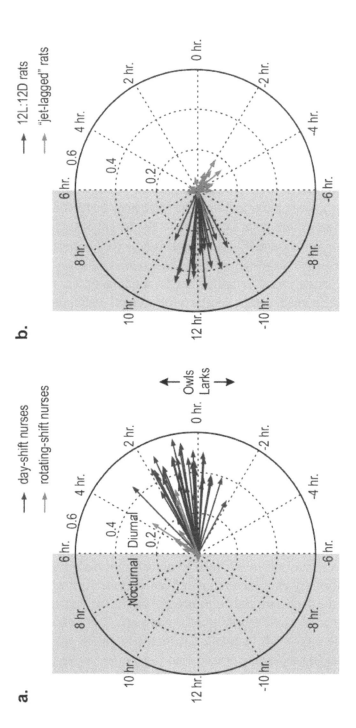

**FIGURE 7:** Phasor diagrams for day-shift and rotating-shift nurses and for 12L:12D and "jet-lagged" nocturnal rats.

the measured light-dark pattern, the phasor analyses are, again, performed without respect to any exogenous time reference. Theoretically then, a person exhibiting lark or owl behavior with respect to actual light and dark pattern could, in fact, be completely out of phase with the local solar day, as indeed would happen with a "true" night-shift worker.

The rats exposed to the consistent 12L:12D light-dark cycle produced average (n = 8) phasors with magnitudes similar to the day-shift nurses, but with directions to the left, clustered around a 12-hour phase shift between light and activity, as would be expected for an entrained nocturnal animal (Figure 7b). The "jet-lagged" rats experiencing the continually changing light-dark exposures have short, low magnitude average (n = 8) phasors with no consistent direction across individuals. (Two very different scenarios can result in the same low magnitude average phasors. One is that every phasor comprising the average is low in magnitude, which indicates that there is no systematic relationship between activity-rest and light-dark. The second, as exhibited by the "jet-lagged" rats, is that individual phasors representing 24-hour periods have significant magnitudes, but their phase varies widely in many directions resulting in a small magnitude average phasor. Either scenario, however, indicates low entrainment to the light-dark pattern when measured across multiple days.)

Figure 8 shows the average [27] phasor magnitudes and phase angles for the two groups of nurses and the two groups of rats. The common use of binary light-dark exposure levels and of wheel running as a measure of activity in caged animals can potentially affect the comparison of their phasor magnitudes to those obtained by humans using the Daysimeter. In a natural environment human activity varies continuously as does a person's light exposure. The phasor analysis based upon the Daysimeter data captures the association between the natural and continuously varying stimuli and responses. Conversely, caged animals have many fewer options with regard to self-regulated light exposures and with regard to running behavior. This situational difference between species may, in fact, have contributed to the relatively shorter phasor magnitudes in the 12L:12D group of rats than in the day-shift nurses. Clearly if cross-species comparisons are to be made, additional investigations need to be undertaken of actual light exposures and of alternative behavioral measures for both human and animal models.

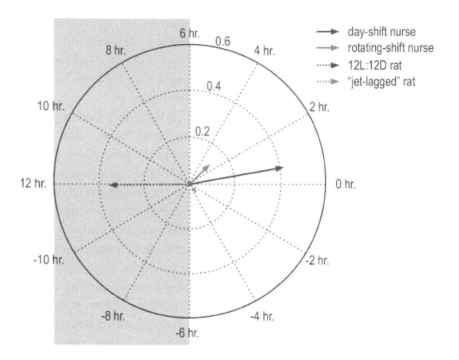

**FIGURE 8:** Mean phasors for nurses and for rats.


### 12.3.4 PHASORS COMPARED TO OTHER MEASURES OF CIRCADIAN BEHAVIORAL ENTRAINMENT

Considering only the degree of behavioral entrainment, Figure 9 shows the distribution of the f(24) phasor magnitudes for the two groups of nurses (Figure 9a) and for the two groups of rats (Figure 9b). Figure 9a shows a clear and statistically significant difference between the day-shift and rotating-shift nurse groups with widely separated group means and medians. Nevertheless, there is some overlap of the distributions, perhaps reflecting a true continuum of the degree of circadian behavioral-entrainment among individuals. The data from the rats in Figure 9b also show a clear and statistically significant separation, but undoubtedly because of the two radically different light-dark patterns, there is no overlap in the phasor amplitudes for these two groups of rats.

The interdaily stability (IS) and the intradaily variability (IV) statistics [29] have been used in numerous studies as measures of behavioral entrainment, or more precisely the coupling between rest-activity rhythms and assumed exogenous zeitgebers, or time givers [30-32]. Unlike the phasor analysis, these two statistics are computed based solely on activity and cannot be used to assess the phase relationship between measured activity and the actual light zeitgeber.

It is possible, however, to compare phasor magnitudes (Figure 9) and IS values by using the same sets of activity data as estimates of circadian entrainment. The distribution of the IS statistic was calculated from the activity data from nurses (Figure 10a) and from rats (Figure 10b). The two groups of nurses and the two groups of rats were significantly different in terms of their IS values. The ratio of the mean IS values for the two groups of nurses (2.6) and the ratio of the mean IS values for the two groups of rats (2.0) are similar to, but smaller than the ratios of the mean phasor magnitudes for the comparable groups shown in Figure 9 (3.2 for nurses and 4.9 for rats). This comparison between phasor magnitude ratios and IS value ratios suggests that a better assessment of behavioral entrainment can be made by relating measured activity-rest to actual light-dark exposures than to an exogenous time reference, such as local solar time, that may or may not be correlated with the actual zeitgeber for entrainment, that is, light.

The IV statistic was also calculated from the activity data from nurses and rats, but the values showed no significant difference between the two groups of nurses nor between the two groups of rats; the mean IV values for day-shift and rotating-shift nurses were 0.50 and 0.54 respectively with standard deviations of 0.20 and 0.16 respectively, and the mean values for the entrained and "jet-lagged" rats were 1.10 and 1.21 with standard deviations of 0.28 and 0.27 respectively. This lack of separation in IV values for the two groups of nurses and for the two groups of rats suggests that consolidation of activity patterns is not systematically related to the degree of circadian behavioral entrainment as measured either with IS values or with phasor magnitudes.

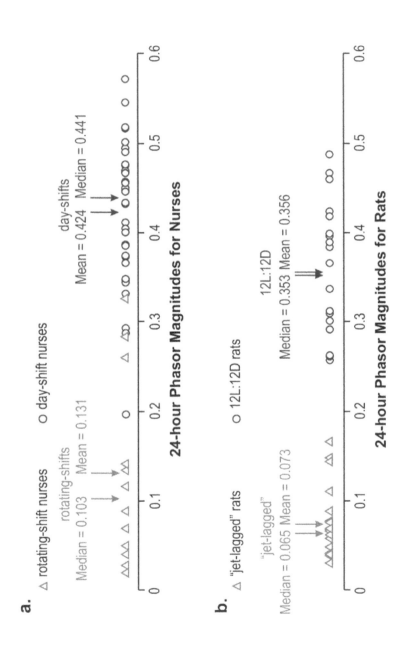

**FIGURE 9:** Phasor magnitudes for the day-shift, and rotating-shift nurses (a) and for the two groups of rats (b).

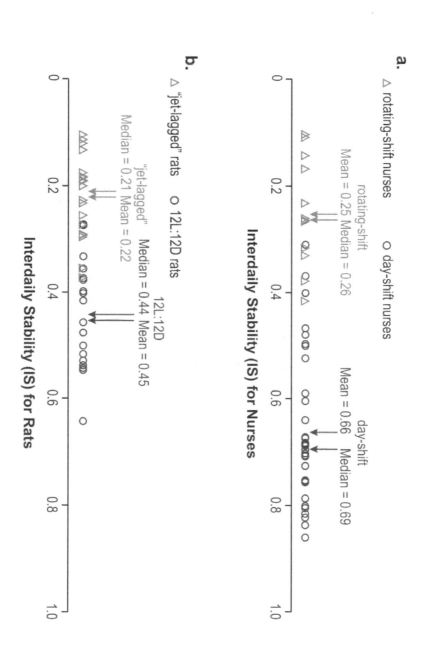

**FIGURE 10:** Interdaily stability (IS) statistics for the day-shift and rotating-shift nurses (a) and for the two groups of rats (b).

## 12.4 DISCUSSION

This paper provides a new framework for the study of the effects of circadian entrainment/disruption on human health, emphasizing three important links in the logical chain relating circadian disruption to maladies such as breast cancer, obesity, and sleep disorders [18].

First, circadian light (and dark) for humans and for animal models can now be quantitatively defined to such a degree that meaningful studies of light as a stimulus for circadian disruption can be undertaken, not only in humans but in nocturnal rodents as well. Without quantitative definitions of the light stimuli, it would simply be impossible to understand the results of any ecological study of circadian disruption on human health or how laboratory studies using animal models relate to the human condition. Second, with an understanding of circadian light, it is now possible to measure the synchrony between light-dark and activity-rest patterns in actual human living environments using tools like the Daysimeter [20]. These ecological light and activity data are necessary to develop the essential insights into circadian disruption actually experienced by modern people. Third, it is now possible to simply and quantitatively characterize degrees of circadian entrainment/disruption; that is, the levels of synchrony between light-dark exposures and activity-rest, in both humans and animal models. A focus on entrainment, rather than light per se or activity alone, makes it possible to relate ecological studies of diurnal humans to parametric studies of diseases using nocturnal animal models. In other words, parametric studies of circadian disruption employing animal models for human diseases can now be designed and conducted so as to more accurately reflect their relevance to the actual living conditions in humans.

It should be emphasized, too, that the methods presented here are not limited to the study of behavioral entrainment. Rather, this analysis provides the basis for assessing entrainment of other outcome measures from the circadian system, such as core body temperature or melatonin synthesis, to light-dark patterns. From these envisioned studies, modern maladies like diabetes, obesity, and poor sleep, as well as breast cancer and cardiovascular disease, can be meaningfully and systematically investigated. More important perhaps, forging the links identified in this paper will significantly accelerate a deeper understanding of the role of circadian disruption on human health [17] and thereby may accelerate medical treatment of these maladies with light and with drugs [33]. The techniques identified here also imply that, in the future, it will be possible to examine circadian entrainment/disruption on an individual basis so that each person can be treated with the appropriate light-dark exposure and/or with the appropriate pharmaceutical interventions.

## REFERENCES

1.  Moore-Ede MC Sulzman, F. M., Fuller, C. A.: The Clocks That Time Us. Cambridge, Harvard University Press; 1982.
2.  Refinetti R: Circadian Physiology. 2nd edition. Boca Raton, London, New York , CRC Taylor & Francis; 2006.
3.  Wever R: The Circadian System of Man: Results of Experiments Under Temporal Isolation. New York, Springer-Verlag; 1979.
4.  Aschoff J: Endocrine Rhythms. Edited by Krieger DTE. New York , Raven; 1979.
5.  Czeisler CA, Weitzman E, Moore-Ede MC, Zimmerman JC, Knauer RS: Human sleep: its duration and organization depend on its circadian phase. Science 1980, 210(4475):1264-1267.
6.  Conroy RTWL Mills, J. N.: Human Circadian Rhythms. London , Churchill; 1970.
7.  Collis SJ, Boulton SJ: Emerging links between the biological clock and the DNA damage response. Chromosoma 2007, 116(4):331-339.
8.  Zamborszky J, Hong CI, Csikasz Nagy A: Computational analysis of mammalian cell division gated by a circadian clock: quantized cell cycles and cell size control. J Biol Rhythms 2007, 22(6):542-553.
9.  Kalsbeek A, Palm IF, La Fleur SE, Scheer FA, Perreau-Lenz S, Ruiter M, Kreier F, Cailotto C, Buijs RM: SCN outputs and the hypothalamic balance of life. J Biol Rhythms 2006, 21(6):458-469.
10. Klein DC, Moore RY, Reppert SM: Suprachiasmatic nucleus: The mind's clock. New York, NY , Oxford University Press; 1991.
11. Sack RL, Auckley D, Auger RR, Carskadon MA, Wright KP Jr., Vitiello MV, Zhdanova IV: Circadian rhythm sleep disorders: part II, advanced sleep phase disorder, delayed sleep phase disorder, free-running disorder, and irregular sleep-wake rhythm. An American Academy of Sleep Medicine review. Sleep 2007, 30(11):1484-1501.
12. Kohsaka A, Bass J: A sense of time: how molecular clocks organize metabolism. Trends Endocrinol Metab 2007, 18(1):4-11.
13. Mallis MM, DeRoshia CW: Circadian rhythms, sleep, and performance in space. Aviat Space Environ Med 2005, 76(6 Suppl):B94-107.
14. Lemmer B: Importance of circadian rhythms for regulation of the cardiovascular system--studies in animal and man. Conf Proc IEEE Eng Med Biol Soc 2006, 1:168-170.
15. Filipski E, Li XM, Levi F: Disruption of circadian coordination and malignant growth. Cancer Causes Control 2006, 17(4):509-514.

16. Schernhammer ES, Laden F, Speizer FE, Willett WC, Hunter DJ, Kawachi I: Rotating night shifts and risk of breast cancer in women participating in the Nurses' Health Study. J Natl Cancer Inst 2001, 93:1563-1568.

17. Straif K, Baan R, Grosse Y, Secretan B, Ghissassi FE, Bouvard V, Altieri A, Benbrahim-Tallaa L, Cogliano V: Carcinogenicity of shift-work, painting, and fire-fighting. The Lancet Oncology 2007, 8(12):1065.

18. Stevens RG, Blask DE, Brainard GC, Hansen J, Lockley SW, Provencio I, Rea MS, Reinlib L: Meeting report: the role of environmental lighting and circadian disruption in cancer and other diseases. Environ Health Perspect 2007, 115(9):1357-1362.

19. Stevens RG, Rea MS: Light in the built environment: potential role of circadian disruption in endocrine disruption and breast cancer. Cancer Causes Control 2001, 12(3):279-287.

20. Bierman A, Klein TR, Rea MS: The Daysimeter: A device for measuring optical radiation as a stimulus for the human circadian system. Measurement Science and Technology 2005, 16:2292-2299.

21. Bullough JD, Rea MS, Figueiro MG: Of mice and women: light as a circadian stimulus in breast cancer research. Cancer Causes Control 2006, 17(4):375-383.

22. Rea MS, Figueiro MG, Bullough JD, Bierman A: A model of phototransduction by the human circadian system. Brain Res Rev 2005, 50(2):213-228.

23. Zeitzer JM, Dijk DJ, Kronauer R, Brown E, Czeisler C: Sensitivity of the human circadian pacemaker to nocturnal light: melatonin phase resetting and suppression. J Physiol 2000, 526(Pt. 3):695-702.

24. Bullough JD, Figueiro MG, Possidente BP, Parsons RH, Rea MS: Additivity in murine circadian phototransduction. Zoolog Sci 2005, 22(2):223-227.

25. Oppenheim AV Schafer, R. W.: Discrete-Time Signal Processing. Englewood Cliffs, NJ , Prentice-Hall; 1989.

26. Wikipedia contributors: Phasor (sine waves) . [http:/ / en.wikipedia.org/ w/ index. php?title=Phasor_%28sine_wave s%29&oldid=197396343]

27. Weisstein EW: Complex Number. From MathWorld-A Wolfram Web Resource. [http://mathworld.wolfram.com/ComplexNumber.html]

28. Roenneberg T, Wirz-Justice A, Merrow M: Life between clocks: daily temporal patterns of human chronotypes. J Biol Rhythms 2003, 18(1):80-90.

29. Witting W, Kwa IH, Eikelenboom P, Mirmiran M, Swaab DF: Alterations in the circadian rest-activity rhythm in aging and Alzheimer's disease. Biol Psychiatry 1990, 27(6):563-572.

30. Hatfield CF, Herbert J, van Someren EJ, Hodges JR, Hastings MH: Disrupted daily activity/rest cycles in relation to daily cortisol rhythms of home-dwelling patients with early Alzheimer's dementia. Brain 2004, 127(Pt 5):1061-1074.

31. Scherder EJ, Van Someren EJ, Swaab DF: Transcutaneous electrical nerve stimulation (TENS) improves the rest-activity rhythm in midstage Alzheimer's disease. Behav Brain Res 1999, 101(1):105-107.

32. Van Someren EJW, Hagebeuk EE, Lijzenga C, Scheltens P, de Rooij SE, Jonker C, Pot AM, Mirmiran M, Swaab DF: Circadian rest-activity rhythm disturbances in Alzheimer's disease. Biol Psychiatry 1996, 40:259-270.

33. Hrushesky WJ: Circadian timing of cancer chemotherapy. Science 1985, 228(4695):73-75.

34. Brainard GC, Hanifin JP, Greeson JM, Byrne B, Glickman G, Gerner E, Rollag MD: Action spectrum for melatonin regulation in humans: evidence for a novel circadian photoreceptor. J Neurosci 2001, 21(16):6405-6412.

35. Thapan K, Arendt J, Skene DJ: An action spectrum for melatonin suppression: evidence for a novel non-rod, non-cone photoreceptor system in humans. J Physiol 2001, 535(Pt 1):261-267.

36. Figueiro MG, Bullough JD, Parsons RH, Rea MS: Preliminary evidence for spectral opponency in the suppression of melatonin by light in humans. NeuroReport 2004, 15(2):313-316.

37. McIntyre IM, Norman TR, Burrows GD, Armstrong SM: Human melatonin suppression by light is intensity dependent. J Pineal Res 1989, 6(2):149-156.

38. Rea MS, Bullough JD, Figueiro MG: Phototransduction for human melatonin suppression. J Pineal Res 2002, 32(4):209-213.

# CHAPTER 13

# WAKING AND SLEEPING IN THE RAT MADE OBESE THROUGH A HIGH-FAT HYPERCALORIC DIET

MARCO LUPPI, MATTEO CERRI, DAVIDE MARTELLI, DOMENICO TUPONE, FLAVIA DEL VECCHIO, ALESSIA DI CRISTOFORO, EMANUELE PEREZ, GIOVANNI ZAMBONI, AND ROBERTO AMICI

## 13.1 INTRODUCTION

A possible link between insufficient sleep and metabolism dysregulation has been suggested by studies showing that a prolonged sleep curtailment may act as a key co-factor for the development of obesity and/or metabolic syndrome [1]. Sleep restriction protocols have been shown to reduce glucose tolerance and insulin sensitivity and to reduce the leptin/ghrelin ratio, possibly leading subjects to eat more than needed [1]. These data have been partly confirmed by the results of a recent study, showing that sleep restriction induced an increase in energy expenditure which was overcompensated by an increase in energy intake leading to weight gain, in spite of a concomitant increase in the leptin/ghrelin ratio [2].

*Reproduced with permission by Elsevier Publishing. Luppi M, Cerri M, Martelli D, Tupone D, Del Vecchio F, Di Cristoforo A, Perez E, Zamboni G, and Amici R. Waking and Sleeping in the Rat Made Obese Through a High-Fat Hypercaloric Diet.* Behavioural Brain Research *258,1 (2014), 145–152.* http://dx.doi.org/10.1016/j.bbr.2013.10.014.

However, it is worth noting that although the aforementioned effects appear to be very consistent on a short-term basis, the epidemiological evidence which is available so far does not appear strong enough to support the existence of a causal link between sleep curtailment and the development of obesity [3]. On the other hand, it has been shown in both humans [4] and mice [5] and [6] that obesity induced by an excess of food intake is per se associated with a decrease in the time spent in wakefulness (Wake) and an increase in the time spent in sleep. Similar changes to the wake–sleep pattern have also been observed in animals in which overfeeding was associated with a lack of either leptin peptide [7] and [8] or leptin receptors [9], [10] and [11].

Both long-term sleep curtailment and overfeeding, leading to obesity, may functionally interact at a hypothalamic level, where circuits involved in WS and body metabolism regulation have been described [12] and [13]. Within the hypothalamic region, a possible site of interaction is the preoptic area (POA), which is crucially involved in the regulation of body temperature and, hence, of basal metabolism [14]. In particular, data from our laboratory have shown that a depression of cellular activity at the POA level is associated with a profound REMS dysregulation [15] and [16].

Since no consistent data on the wake–sleep (WS) pattern in diet-induced obesity rats are available, in the present study we have investigated the fine architecture of the WS cycle during the development of obesity induced by the administration of a high-fat hypercaloric (HC) diet in animals kept under a standard 12 h:12 h LD cycle.

The effects of the development of obesity on REMS regulation have been investigated in more detail by exposing the animals to 12 h of continuous darkness (DD), a condition obtained by extending the D period of the light–dark cycle to the following L period, which is known to enhance REMS occurrence in the albino rat [17] through an increase in the frequency of REMS episodes [15]. The practicality of this behavioral tool in the assessment of the intervention of POA circuits in shaping the interaction between weight gain and REMS occurrence has been suggested by the finding that REMS enhancement under DD is depressed when the cellular activity at POA level is impaired [15].

## 13.2 MATERIALS AND METHODS

### 13.2.1 ANIMALS

Eighty adult male Sprague-Dawley rats (Charles River) were used. Animals were housed under normal laboratory conditions (nLab): free access to food and water, ambient temperature (Ta) $24.0 \pm 0.5$ °C, 12-h:12-h LD cycle (L: 09:00–21:00; 100 lux at cage level). The experiments were carried out according to the European Union Directive (86/609/EEC) and were under the supervision of the Central Veterinary Service of the University of Bologna and the National Health Authority.

### 13.2.2 EXPERIMENTAL PROTOCOL

After their arrival at the laboratory, all animals were fed a standard normocaloric (NC) laboratory diet (4RF21, Mucedola). Starting from the end of the sixth week of life, which was considered to be time = 0 of the experiment, animals were separated into two groups: the first group (n = 32) continued to be fed the standard NC diet, while the second group (n = 48) was fed a high-fat hypercaloric diet (PF4215, Mucedola: 35% fat). Both groups underwent EEG recordings after either 4 weeks (time = 4) or 8 weeks (time = 8) after diet differentiation. A group of animals was also studied at time 0. According to this protocol, five experimental groups were studied:

1.  Normocaloric diet at time = 0, NC0 (n = 8)
2.  Normocaloric diet at time = 4, NC4 (n = 7)
3.  High-fat hypercaloric diet at time = 4, HC4 (n = 7)
4.  Normocaloric diet at time = 8, NC8 (n = 8)
5.  High-fat hypercaloric diet at time = 8, HC8 (n = 6)

Animals were selected randomly for the NC (NC0, NC4, NC8) and HC (HC4, HC8) diet protocols from each of 4 consecutive litters. The population of HC candidates was kept larger than its NC equivalent since about 50% of Sprague-Dawley rats fed a HC diet appear to be obesity resistant (OR) [18]. In order to study the WS pattern, animals assigned to each diet protocol had to undergo surgery by seven to ten days before the EEG recordings were carried out. Regarding the EEG recordings, the selection of the NC experimental groups was identical to that for the diet protocol, while that of the HC experimental groups was the result of a further random choice performed on animals whose weight was over the median value of the population (obesity prone, OP, animals).

For all groups, the EEG recordings were carried out under nLAB for two consecutive days (LD1, LD2). A third day of recording was added to both the NC8 and the HC8 groups, during which animals were kept under a DD condition. Under the DD protocol the environmental light was switched off during the normal 12-h L period of the LD cycle (DD-L) and kept off for the following 12-h D period (DD-D).

### 13.2.3 SURGERY

While under deep general anesthesia (diazepam, Valium Roche, 5 mg/kg intramuscular; ketamine-HCl, Ketalar, Parke-Davis, 100 mg/kg intraperitoneal), 36 animals were implanted epidurally with two stainless-steel electrodes for frontal-parietal EEG recording. Furthermore, a thermistor mounted inside the tip of a stainless-steel needle (21G) was positioned above the left anterior hypothalamus to measure hypothalamic temperature (Thy). Plugs to connect EEG electrodes and the thermistor to the recording apparatus were embedded in acrylic dental resin (Res-Pal) anchored to the skull by small epidural stainless-steel screws implanted at the outer limit of the surgical field. Motor activity (MA) was monitored by means of a passive infrared detector (Siemens, PID11, Munich, FRG) placed on top of the recording cage.

### 13.2.4 EEG RECORDINGS

Animals were allowed to recover from surgery for at least one week, while adapting to the recording apparatus in individual Plexiglas cages kept in a thermoregulated and sound-attenuated box. After recovery from surgery, each rat was recorded continuously for 48 h, starting at the onset of the L period. The only exception was a brief time window from 09:00 to 09:15, during which bedding, food and water were changed.

Data were handled by software (QuickBASIC, Microsoft, CA, USA) developed in our laboratory. The EEG signal was amplified (amplification factor: approximately 7000), filtered (high-pass filter: −40 dB at 0.35 Hz; low-pass filter: −6 dB at 60.0 Hz) and, after analog-digital conversion (sampling rate: 128 Hz), was stored on a PC (486/100 DX-4). The EEG signal was subjected to online fast Fourier transform, and EEG power values were obtained for 4-s epochs in the Delta (DPW: 0.75–4.0 Hz), Theta (TPW: 5.5–9.0 Hz) and Sigma (SPW 11–16 Hz) bands. Thy signal was amplified (1 °C/1 V) before AD conversion (sampling rate: 8 Hz). MA signal was amplified and integrated before analog-digital conversion (sampling rate: 8 Hz) in order to make the output proportional to the amplitude and duration of movement (MA intensity). This system detected most of the movements related to the normal behavior of the rat, such as exploring, grooming, feeding and small movements during muscle twitching or brief awakenings in either non-REM sleep (NREMS) or REMS.

The method for the determination of the WS stages and their parameters has been described previously [19]. Briefly, the analysis comprised two steps. The first consisted in the visual scoring of the REMS episodes for the definition of the number and duration of REMS episodes and the duration of the time interval between REMS episodes (REMS interval). The time length for the minimal duration of a REMS episode, as well as that of a REMS interval was fixed at 8 s [20]. In the rat, the duration of the REMS intervals shows a bimodal frequency distribution with a minimum between the two modes at the 3-min class [21]. On this basis, two types of REMS were identified: single REMS, consisting of episodes preceded and followed by long REM sleep intervals (>3 min) and sequential REMS, consisting of episodes separated by short REM sleep intervals (≤3 min) and occurring in clusters. In the rat, the rate of occurrence of sequential REMS episodes represents the main factor in the modulation of REMS occurrence [15], [19], [20], [21] and [22]. The second step of the analysis consisted in the recognition of Wake and NREMS episodes by means of an automatic procedure developed and validated in our laboratory [19].

## 13.2.5 *BLOOD METABOLITES*

Glycemia, triglyceridemia, and total cholesterolemia were determined for the NC8 and HC8 experimental groups. At the end of the recording sessions, the rats were anaesthetized and a 5-ml blood sample was taken by cardiac puncture. Blood parameters were determined by means of standard kits used for human blood parameter determination.

## 13.2.6 *STATISTICAL ANALYSIS*

Statistical analysis was carried out using ANOVA (SPSS 20.0). A number of pre-planned orthogonal and non-orthogonal contrasts were made by means of the modified t-test (t*). For the non-orthogonal contrast the alpha level was adjusted by the "sequential" Bonferroni correction [23]. A separate analysis was carried out for data collected from all experimental groups during exposure to the normal LD cycle and for those related to the effects of DD exposure in the NC8 and HC8 groups.

Data collected during exposure to the normal LD cycle were analyzed using one-way ANOVA with either a 24-h or 12-h resolution. For the 24-h resolution analysis, the following orthogonal contrasts were carried out: (i) [NC4; NC8] vs. [HC4; HC8]; (ii) NC4 vs. NC8; (iii) HC4 vs. HC8; and the following non-orthogonal contrasts were also carried out: (i) NC0 vs. each experimental condition; (ii) HC4 vs. NC4; (iii) HC8 vs. NC8. For the 12-h resolution analysis, the following orthogonal contrasts were carried out: (i) [NC4-L; NC4-D; NC8-L; NC8-D] vs. [HC4-L; HC4-D; HC8-L; HC8-D]; (ii) [NC4-L; NC4-D] vs. [NC8-L; NC8-D]; (iii) [HC4-L; HC4-D] vs. [HC8-L; HC8-D]; (iv) L vs. D for all experimental conditions; as were the following non-orthogonal contrasts: (i) NC0, L or D vs. each of the other corresponding L or D experimental conditions; (ii) [HC4-L vs. NC4-L]; (iii) [HC4-D vs. NC4-D]; (iv) [HC8-L vs. NC8-L] (v) [HC8-D vs. NC8-D].

Data concerning the Continuous Darkness protocol were analyzed using two-way ANOVA for repeated measures on one factor, with either a 24-h or a 12-h resolution. In particular, for the 24-h resolution analysis, the following were considered as Main Factors: (i) Factor "Time", which was considered for the repeated measures, with three levels (LD1, LD2, DD), and (ii) Factor "Diet" with two levels (NC, HC). The following orthogonal contrasts were carried out: (i) [NC8-LD; HC8-LD] vs. [NC8-DD; HC8-DD]; (ii) [NC8-DD vs.HC8-DD], as were the following non- orthogonal contrasts: (i) NC8-DD vs. NC8-LD; (ii) HC8-DD vs. HC8-LD. For the 12-h resolution analysis, the following were considered as Main Factors: (i) Factor "Time", which was considered for the repeated measures, with six levels (LD1-L, LD1-D, LD2-L, LD2-D, DD-L, DD-D, and (ii) Factor "Diet" with two levels (NC, HC). The following orthogonal contrasts were carried out: (i) [NC8-LD-L; NC8-LD-D; HC8-LD-L; HC8-LD-D] vs. [NC8-DD-L; NC8-DD-D; HC8-DD-L; HC8-DD-D]; (ii) [NC8-DD-L; NC8-DD-D] vs. [HC8-DD-L; HC8-DD-D]; (iii) NC8-DD-L vs. NC8-DD-D; (iv) HC8-DD-L vs. HC8-DD-D, while several non-orthogonal contrasts were carried out to compare each NC8-LD or HC8-LD L or D value with the corresponding DD-L or DD-D value.

The weights of the animals were statistically analyzed using two-way ANOVA, considering the following as main factors: (i) Factor "Time", with three levels (0, 4, 8 weeks), and (ii) Factor "Diet", with two levels (NC, HC). The following orthogonal contrasts: (i) NC4 vs. HC4; (ii) NC8 vs. HC8; and the following non-orthogonal contrasts: (i) NC4 vs. NC0; (ii) NC8 vs. NC0; were carried out. Blood metabolite values were compared between HC8 and NC8 by means of a t-Student statistic.

Throughout all analyses, differences were considered statistically significant when $P < 0.05$.

## 13.3 RESULTS

### 13.3.1 EFFECTS OF HIGH-FAT HYPERCALORIC DIET DELIVERY ON BODY WEIGHT AND BLOOD METABOLITES

At time 0 (NC0), the weight of the animals was $176 \pm 3$ g. The delivery of the HC diet led to the development of a diet-induced obesity in the animals selected for the study, after either four (NC4 = $361 \pm 6$ g; HC4 = $405 \pm 7$

g; P < 0.05) or eight (NC8 = 459 ± 9 g; HC8 = 593 ± 15 g; P < 0.05) weeks of treatment. Also, an increase in blood concentration of glucose (+25.4 ± 16.4%; n.s.), triglycerides (+139.3 ± 29.1%; P < 0.05), and total cholesterol (+59.0 ± 15.5%; P < 0.05) was observed in the HC8 group when compared to the NC8 group.

## 13.3.2 EFFECTS OF HIGH-FAT HYPERCALORIC DIET DELIVERY ON TIME SPENT IN THE DIFFERENT WAKE–SLEEP STATES

As shown in Fig. 1, the time spent in the different WS states was affected by the development of obesity. In particular, obese animals, overall, spent less time in Wake (P < 0.05), and therefore, more time sleeping when compared to those that were lean. While the apparent increase in time spent in NREMS did not reach statistical significance, a significant increase in time spent in REMS was found in obese animals compared to lean ones (P < 0.05) and, in particular, when the HC8 group was individually compared to the NC8 group (P < 0.05). Interestingly, the latter effect can be explained by the apparent lack in the HC8 group of the slight decrease in REMS occurrence, which was observed in the NC8 group when compared to either the NC4 or the NC0 groups (P < 0.05, for both comparisons). The analysis of the partition between single and sequential REMS showed that the increase in REMS occurrence in obese animals was apparently mostly due to an increased occurrence of sequential REMS in HC4 and single REMS in HC8, although neither effect was statistically significant.

In the NC8 and HC8 groups, REMS occurrence was, on the whole, significantly enhanced by the exposure to the DD protocol (P < 0.05, DD vs. LD conditions). However, the effect was larger in lean than in obese animals, as also supported by the presence of a significant interaction (P < 0.05) between the two treatments (DD and Diet) and by the finding that the difference between the time spent in REMS in DD compared to the corresponding LD condition was significant for the NC8 group (P < 0.05) but not for the HC8 group. However, no significant differences in time spent in REMS under DD were observed between the NC8 and the HC8 groups. Also, no significant effects of DD were observed on time spent in either

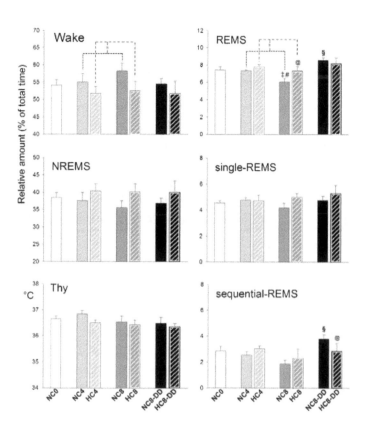

**FIGURE 1:** Time spent in the different wake–sleep states and hypothalamic temperature in obese and lean rats. The time rats spent in Wake, non-REM sleep (NREMS), and REM sleep (REMS) while kept under a normal 12 h:12 h Light–Dark (LD) cycle or under a Continuous Darkness (DD) protocol is shown. The amount of REMS occurring under the form of either single REMS or sequential REMS and hypothalamic temperature (Thy) levels are also shown. Animals underwent EEG recording after being fed either a standard normocaloric (NC, solid bar) or a high-fat hypercaloric (HC, dashed bar) diet for either 4 (light gray bar) or 8 (dark gray bar) weeks. A group of animals was also studied at time 0 (NC0, white bar). Following baseline recordings, animals from both NC8 and HC8 groups were also exposed to a DD condition (black bar), in which the environmental light was switched off during the normal 12-h L period of the LD cycle and kept off for the following 12-h D period. Values (means ± S.E.M.) are expressed as the percentage of each 24-h period. Data represent the average of two consecutive days of recording. Statistically significant differences are indicated: [NC4, NC8] vs. [HC4, HC8] (*P < 0.05); NC8 vs. NC4 (#P < 0.05); NC8 vs. NC0 (‡P < 0.05); HC8 vs. NC8 (@P < 0.05). [NC8, HC8] vs. [NC8-DD, HC8-DD] (*P < 0.05); NC8-DD vs. NC8 (§P < 0.05); HC8-DD vs. NC8-DD (@P < 0.05).

Wake (in spite of an apparent depression in Wake occurrence) or NREMS. The analysis of the partition between single and sequential REMS showed that the increase in REMS occurrence induced by DD was substantially due to an increase in the amount of sequential REMS (P < 0.05). As observed for total REMS, the enhancement was larger in lean than in obese animals, as supported by the finding of a statistically significant interaction (P < 0.05) between the two treatments (DD and Diet). Furthermore, the 24-h amount of sequential REMS under DD was significantly larger when compared to the corresponding LD values, in lean animals (P < 0.05) but not in obese ones and, differently from what was observed for total REMS, it was significantly larger in the NC8 group compared to the HC8 group.

Finally, the average 24-h levels of Thy were apparently lower in the obese animals than in the lean ones, but the difference still failed to reach statistical significance. Differences in Thy between obese and lean animals were not significant even when a wake–sleep state-dependent analysis of this parameter was carried out (data not shown).

In Table 1, the 12 h:12 h LD distribution of the time spent in the different WS states and Thy levels are shown. Data analysis confirmed the presence of a statistically significant decrease in overall Wake occurrence in obese animals compared to lean ones when L and D data were taken as a whole (P < 0.05). However, neither the observed changes in time spent in the different WS states nor those in Thy levels induced by the administration of the HC diet reached statistical significance when the 12-h levels observed in obese animals were individually compared to those seen in lean animals. Interestingly, the normal L vs. D distribution within the different WS parameters and within Thy, which was maintained throughout the five experimental conditions, was lost in the HC8 group regarding time spent in REMS and the amount of single REMS. In animals exposed to the DD protocol, the analysis showed an overall significant depression in Wake occurrence (P < 0.05) and confirmed the presence of a significant enhancing effect of DD on both the time spent in REMS (P < 0.05) and the amount of sequential REMS (P < 0.05). For both parameters, the increase was statistically significant in both the NC8 and the HC8 groups when the 12-h DD-L levels were compared to the 12-h LD-L levels (P < 0.05, for both comparisons), while no significant differences were observed when 12-h DD-D values were compared to those in 12-h LD-D, although REMS occurrence appeared to be slightly dampened under DD in HC8. No significant differences were found between the NC8 and the HC8 groups in either DD-L or DD-D.

### 13.3.3 EFFECTS OF HIGH-FAT HYPERCALORIC DIET DELIVERY ON THE FREQUENCY AND DURATION OF WAKE–SLEEP EPISODES

The main outcomes of the analysis of the number and duration of WS episodes (Table 2 and Table 3) were the tendency in obese animals toward a Wake fragmentation, accompanied by an overall increase in the number of single REMS episodes, as well as in that of REMS clusters, which were relatively shorter compared to those seen in lean animals. The effects on Wake and single REMS episodes were at their largest during the D period in HC8. More specifically, the number of Wake episodes, which was larger in obese animals in both L and D (although the overall effect did not reach statistical significance), was significantly higher in the HC8 group than in the HC4 group ($P < 0.05$). These effects were accompanied by a consistent decrease in the average duration of the Wake bout in obese animals, which reached statistical significance when the comparison between obese and lean animals was carried out taking L and D data as a whole ($P < 0.05$). Furthermore, the average duration of the Wake episode was significantly lower in the HC8 group during the D period when compared with either the NC8 ($P < 0.05$) or the HC4 ($P < 0.05$) groups. Taking into account the analysis of the partition between single and sequential REMS, a statistically significant increase in the number of single REMS episodes was observed in obese animals when the L and D data were taken as a whole ($P < 0.05$), and in HC8, during the D period, when compared to the NC8 group ($P < 0.05$). Moreover, when L and D data were taken as a whole, a significant increase in the number of REM sleep clusters ($P < 0.05$), which was apparently more marked in the L period, was observed in obese animals compared to lean ones. This effect was paralleled by a significant decrease in the average duration of the REM sleep cluster ($P < 0.05$).

**TABLE 1:** The time diet-induced obese rats spent in the different Wake–Sleep states and their hypothalamic temperature levels while they were kept under a 12 h:12 h Light–Dark cycle or under a Continuous Darkness protocol.

| | NC0 | NC4 | HC4 | NC8 | HC8 | NC8-DD | HC8-DD |
|---|---|---|---|---|---|---|---|
| | n = 8 | n = 7 | n = 8 | n = 7 | n = 6 | n = 8 | n = 6 |
| **Wake** | | | | | | | |
| L | 38.9 ± 2.8 | 41.1 ± 2.6 | 36.4 ± 3.0 | 43.2 ± 2.6 | 41.4 ± 3.3 | 37.9 ± 1.9 | 37.5 ± 5.3 |
| D | 68.7 ± 1.6§ | 68.4 ± 2.6§ | 66.5 ± 3.1§ | 72.8 ± 1.9§ | 63.3 ± 2.9§ | 70.5 ± 1.5§ | 65.4 ± 2.2§ |
| **NREMS** | | | | | | | |
| L | 52.3 ± 3.0 | 49.8 ± 2.9 | 53.1 ± 3.1 | 49.4 ± 2.4 | 50.2 ± 3.0 | 48.8 ± 1.5 | 50.2 ± 4.5 |
| D | 25.2 ± 1.3§ | 26.0 ± 2.3§ | 28.3 ± 2.5§ | 22.4 ± 1.8§ | 30.4 ± 2.5§ | 25.5 ± 1.5§ | 30.3 ± 2.2§ |
| **REMS** | | | | | | | |
| L | 8.8 ± 0.5 | 9.1 ± 0.6 | 10.5 ± 1.1 | 7.3 ± 0.7 | 8.4 ± 0.8 | 13.3 ± 0.5# | 12.3 ± 1.2# |
| D | 6.1 ± 0.8§ | 5.7 ± 0.5§ | 5.2 ± 0.7§ | 4.8 ± 0.5§ | 6.3 ± 0.8 | 4.0 ± 0.4§ | 4.2 ± 0.3§ |
| **Single REMS** | | | | | | | |
| L | 5.7 ± 0.4 | 5.9 ± 0.4 | 6.1 ± 0.9 | 5.3 ± 0.7 | 5.6 ± 0.8 | 6.8 ± 0.5 | 7.2 ± 1.0 |
| D | 3.5 ± 0.4§ | 3.6 ± 0.2§ | 3.4 ± 0.4§ | 3.1 ± 0.2§ | 4.4 ± 0.4 | 2.8 ± 0.3§ | 3.4 ± 0.3§ |
| **Sequential REMS** | | | | | | | |
| L | 3.1 ± 0.4 | 3.1 ± 0.5 | 4.4 ± 0.4 | 2.1 ± 0.4 | 2.8 ± 1.0 | 6.5 ± 0.6# | 5.0 ± 1.2# |
| D | 2.6 ± 0.5 | 2.0 ± 0.5 | 1.8 ± 0.4§ | 1.7 ± 0.3 | 1.9 ± 0.6 | 1.2 ± 0.2§ | 0.8 ± 0.1§ |
| **Thy (°C)** | | | | | | | |
| L | 36.3 ± 0.1 | 36.4 ± 0.1 | 36.1 ± 0.1 | 36.1 ± 0.3 | 36.1 ± 0.2 | 36.1 ± 0.2 | 36.1 ± 0.1 |
| D | 37.0 ± 0.1§ | 37.3 ± 0.2§ | 36.9 ± 0.1§ | 37.0 ± 0.2§ | 36.7 ± 0.2§ | 36.9 ± 0.2§ | 36.6 ± 0.1§ |

*The time rats spent in Wake, non-REM sleep (NREMS), and REM sleep (REMS) while kept under a normal 12 h:12 h Light–Dark (LD) cycle or under a Continuous Darkness (DD) protocol is shown. The amount of REMS occurring under the form of either single REMS or sequential REMS and hypothalamic temperature (Thy) levels are also shown. Animals underwent EEG recording after being fed either a standard normocaloric (NC4, NC8) or a high-fat hypercaloric (HC4, HC8) diet for either 4 or 8 weeks. A group of animals was also studied at time 0 (NC0). Following baseline recordings, animals from both NC8 and HC8 groups were exposed to a DD condition, in which the environmental light was switched off during the expected L period of the LD cycle and kept off for the following D period. Values (means ± S.E.M.) are expressed as the percentage of each 12-h L or D period. For animals kept under LD conditions average data from two consecutive days of recording are shown. The number of animals (n) is shown for each experimental condition. Only statistically significant differences between individual cells are indicated: LD vs. DD (#P < 0.05); D vs. L (§P < 0.05).*

**TABLE 2:** Number and duration of Wake and NREM sleep episodes in diet-induced obese rats kept under a 12 h:12 h Light–Dark cycle or under a Continuous Darkness protocol.

| | | NC0 | NC4 | HC4 | NC8 | HC8 | NC8-DD | HC8-DD |
|---|---|---|---|---|---|---|---|---|
| | | n = 8 | n = 7 | n = 8 | n = 7 | n = 6 | n = 8 | n = 6 |
| **Wake** | | | | | | | | |
| No. | L | 404.3 ± 17.3 | 465.9 ± 37.3 | 485.6 ± 26.6 | 502.3 ± 29.0 | 545.1 ± 25.5 | 378.1 ± 19.3 | 421.3 ± 46.0 |
| | D | 301.8 ± 53.0§ | 311.9 ± 37.1§ | 317.0 ± 35.4§ | 293.9 ± 17.6§ | 403.8 ± 45.7§ | 350.8 ± 24.7 | 509.8 ± 132.2 |
| Dur | L | 41 ± 3 | 38 ± 4 | 32 ± 3 | 37 ± 2 | 33 ± 4 | 42 ± 2 | 39 ± 6 |
| | D | 115 ± 15§ | 103 ± 10§ | 99 ± 14§ | 110 ± 8§ | 72 ± 7 *†§ | 90 ± 8#§ | 66 ± 9§ |
| **NREMS** | | | | | | | | |
| No. | L | 457.7 ± 68.3 | 491.9 ± 23.7 | 518.5 ± 38.6 | 504.9 ± 28.7 | 531.1 ± 28.0 | 373.9 ± 17.9# | 430.3 ± 43.9# |
| | D | 282.6 ± 36.1§ | 284.9 ± 13.4§ | 318.5 ± 43.5§ | 286.8 ± 17.6§ | 364.0 ± 25.8§ | 326.5 ± 19.0 | 384.5 ± 8.7 |
| Dur | L | 53 ± 6 | 43 ± 4 | 46 ± 5 | 42 ± 4 | 40 ± 3 | 56 ± 4# | 53 ± 9# |
| | D | 42 ± 4§ | 40 ± 4 | 41 ± 3 | 35 ± 3 | 36 ± 3 | 34 ± 3§ | 34 ± 2§ |

*The number and duration of episodes of Wake and non-REM sleep (NREMS) in rats kept under a normal 12 h:12 h Light–Dark (LD) cycle or under a Continuous Darkness (DD) protocol are shown. Animals underwent EEG recording after being fed either a standard normocaloric (NC4, NC8) or a high-fat hypercaloric (HC4, HC8) diet for either 4 or 8 weeks. A group of animals was also studied at time 0 (NC0). Following baseline recordings, animals of both NC8 and HC8 groups were exposed to a DD condition, in which the environmental light was switched off during the expected L period of the LD cycle and kept off for the following D period. Values (means ± S.E.M.) for the 12-h L and the 12-h D periods are shown. For animals kept under LD conditions average data from two consecutive days of recording are shown. The number of animals (n) is shown for each experimental condition. Only statistically significant differences between individual cells are indicated: vs. NC0 (\*P < 0.05); NC vs. HC (†P < 0.05); LD vs. DD (#P < 0.05); D vs. L (§P < 0.05).*

**TABLE 3:** Number and duration of REM sleep episodes in diet-induced obese rats kept under a 12 h:12 h Light–Dark cycle or under a Continuous Darkness protocol.

|               |   | NC0 | NC4 | HC4 | NC8 | HC8 | NC8-DD | HC8-DD |
|---------------|---|-----|-----|-----|-----|-----|--------|--------|
|               |   | n = 8 | n = 7 | n = 8 | n = 7 | n = 6 | n = 8 | n = 6 |
| **Single REMS** | | | | | | | | |
| No. | L | 28.2 ± 1.5 | 27.2 ± 1.3 | 26.4 ± 1.2 | 25.3 ± 1.8 | 26.3 ± 1.7 | 27.3 ± 1.4 | 29.0 ± 3.0 |
|     | D | 13.9 ± 1.2§ | 16.6 ± 1.8§ | 18.0 ± 1.6§ | 15.0 ± 1.0§ | 22.9 ± 2.2*† | 15.4 ± 2.0§ | 19.0 ± 2.1§ |
| Dur | L | 84 ± 6 | 93 ± 7 | 94 ± 11 | 86 ± 7 | 87 ± 10 | 102 ± 5 | 105 ± 11 |
|     | D | 106 ± 7§ | 95 ± 5 | 83 ± 9 | 90 ± 5 | 85 ± 7 | 83 ± 6§ | 79 ± 6§ |
| **Sequential REMS** | | | | | | | | |
| No. | L | 24.4 ± 3.1 | 22.6 ± 4.0 | 31.9 ± 5.3 | 14.2 ± 2.7 | 21.7 ± 8.2 | 36.8 ± 4.3# | 26.3 ± 5.1 |
|     | D | 14.0 ± 2.3§ | 11.8 ± 3.0 | 11.7 ± 2.7§ | 10.8 ± 2.7 | 13.4 ± 4.2 | 9.1 ± 1.6§ | 6.2 ± 1.2§ |
| Dur | L | 55 ± 4 | 61 ± 4 | 64 ± 7 | 63 ± 3 | 58 ± 4 | 75 ± 3 | 77 ± 8 |
|     | D | 82 ± 8§ | 83 ± 7§ | 66 ± 8 | 69 ± 7 | 62 ± 7 | 56 ± 4§ | 62 ± 8 |
| **REMS cluster** | | | | | | | | |
| No. | L | 10.3 ± 1.1 | 9.6 ± 1.4 | 13.7 ± 2.2 | 6.3 ± 1.1 | 9.1 ± 2.8 | 15.1 ± 1.6# | 11.8 ± 2.2 |
|     | D | 5.8 ± 0.9§ | 4.8 ± 1.0§ | 4.9 ± 0.9§ | 4.3 ± 0.7 | 5.6 ± 1.5 | 4.4 ± 0.8§ | 2.7 ± 0.5§ |
| Dur | L | 132 ± 7 | 138 ± 6 | 149 ± 14 | 146 ± 8 | 131 ± 9 | 181 ± 7 | 172 ± 17 |
|     | D | 188 ± 17§ | 185 ± 10§ | 146 ± 18 | 158 ± 13 | 136 ± 14 | 116 ±8#§ | 142 ± 16 |

*The number and duration of episodes of REM sleep (REMS) episodes in rats kept under a normal 12 h:12 h Light–Dark (LD) cycle or under a Continuous Darkness (DD) protocol are shown. Data concerning REMS episodes are shown according to the partition in single and sequential REMS and REMS clusters. Animals underwent EEG recording after being fed either a standard normocaloric (NC4, NC8) or a high-fat hypercaloric (HC4, HC8) diet for either 4 or 8 weeks. A group of animals was also studied at time 0 (NC0). Following baseline recordings, animals of both NC8 and HC8 groups were exposed to a DD condition, in which the environmental light was switched off during the expected L period of the LD cycle and kept off for the following D period. Values (means ± S.E.M.) for the 12-h L and the 12-h D periods are shown. For animals kept under LD conditions average data from two consecutive days of recording are shown. The number of animals (n) is shown for each experimental condition. Only statistically significant differences between individual cells are indicated: vs. NC0 (\*P < 0.05); NC vs. HC (†P < 0.05); D vs. L (§P < 0.05); LD vs. DD (#P < 0.05).*

The analysis of the number and duration of WS episodes in animals exposed to the DD protocol suggests that the depression of Wake occurrence under DD during the first 12-h period (DD-L) was apparently associated with a decrease in the number of Wake episodes, although this decrease was not statistically significant. On the whole, under DD, Wake was maintained significantly more fragmented in obese than in lean animals, as shown by the significantly higher number and lower duration of Wake episodes in obese animals ($P < 0.05$ for both parameters). The number of NREMS episodes was significantly reduced ($P < 0.05$) and their duration was significantly increased ($P < 0.05$) by DD. This effect was much larger during the first 12-h period of exposure (DD-L), since both the decrease in the number and the increase in the duration of the episodes were statistically significant when either the NC8 or the HC8 levels under DD-L were compared with the respective LD-L values ($P < 0.05$ for the 4 comparisons). Still, the overall number of NREMS episodes under DD was significantly larger in the HC8 group than in the NC8 group ($P < 0.05$). The analysis of the partition in single and sequential REMS episodes confirmed the presence of an overall significant enhancing effect of DD on the number of sequential REMS episodes and REMS clusters ($P < 0.05$) that was more evident during the first 12-h period of exposure (DD-L). These effects reached individual statistical significance ($P < 0.05$) in the NC8 group, but not in the HC8 group ($P < 0.05$, for both comparisons) during DD-L. During DD exposure, no significant differences were present regarding REMS parameters in obese animals compared to lean animals, in spite of the differences observed in Wake and NREMS parameters.

## 13.4 DISCUSSION

The results of the present study indicate that, in the rat, the long-term administration of a HC diet leading to the development of obesity, and to a concomitant alteration of related blood parameters, induced an overall decrease in the time spent in Wake and a reciprocal increase in the time spent in sleep. These results are both in accordance with what has previously been observed in mice made obese by HC diets [5] and [6] and in alignment with the presence of EDS in obese humans [4].

These WS effects caused by obesity are not immediately explainable by the hypothesized outcome of obesity induced by the enhancement of Wake and the curtailment of sleep [1]. However, the results on humans by Marckwald et al. [2] have shown that Wake enhancement induced an increase in energy expenditure which was overcompensated by an increase in food intake. This led to a significant weight gain concomitant with changes in the concentration of hormones promoting satiety and hormones reducing hunger. The hypothesis made by the Authors was that the increase of food intake associated with an enhancement of Wake is a behavioral over-adaptation which allows subjects to cope with an overall increase in energy needs. By taking obesity as a common end point of differently motivated overfeedings and sleep as a key role player in the regulation of energy metabolism, it may be hypothesized that the depression of Wake and the enhancement of sleep occurring in obese mammals is a behavioral over-adaptation aimed toward an overall reduction in energy intake.

Possible mechanisms leading to Wake depression and sleep enhancement in obese animals may lay in the ground of an alteration of the general molecular and hormonal asset due to the development of obesity. Obesity is associated with an increase in inflammatory cytokines [24], among which, tumor necrosis factor $\alpha$, interleukin-1 and interleukin-6 are known to have, to a differing extent, sleep promoting effects [25]. Also, metabolic signals coming from the energy deposits may operate at a hypothalamic level within the neural network in which the control of WS states and the regulation of food intake/metabolism overlap. Regarding this, a possible target could be the HCRT system, which is known to promote both the continuity of active Wake and food intake [13]. The tendency to Wake fragmentation observed in obese animals during the active period may be explained by the increase in leptin levels typically observed in obese subjects, since leptin has been shown to inhibit the activity of HCRT neurons [26].

In the present study, the development of a frank obesity led to a clear fragmentation of Wake, which was characterized by a significant decrease in the average duration of the Wake bouts, accompanied by a tendency toward an increase in their number. These data are in full agreement with what has been observed in mice fed a HC diet [5] and [6] and are consistent with the reported association between EDS and obesity in humans [4]. This intrusion of sleep into Wake during the active period was not the consequence of sleep disruption or shortening during the rest period, since no apparent signs of sleep fragmentation during the rest period were observed, but, possibly, the consequence of a modification in the Wake regulatory processes at a central level.

The relationship between a HC diet delivery and sleep in rats was also studied in a pioneering experiment in which animals were kept under a diet treatment for ten days only [27], showing the presence of an acute enhancing effect of the HC diet on both NREMS and REMS well before the development of obesity. In our study, the apparent overall presence of larger effects in the HC8 group than in the HC4 group suggests that the sleep changes were not a mere acute effect of diet delivery, but were, at least partially, associated with weight gain.

Studies carried out in genetically obese rodents [7], [8], [9], [10] and [11] have shown a tendency for the animals to spend more time in NREMS, while REMS resulted either unchanged or more evenly distributed between L and D periods [10] and [11].

The anatomico-functional substrate of the interaction between sleep curtailment and overfeeding, leading to obesity, may be found at the level of hypothalamic circuits involved in WS and body metabolism regulation. Among the hypothalamic structures which may share the function of regulating both sleep and body metabolism are the POA and the lateral hypothalamus (LH). POA, which is directly involved in the regulation of body temperature and, hence, of basal metabolism [14], has also been shown to be crucially involved in sleep regulation [12], while hypocretin-ergic (HCRT) neurons at LH level are known to be involved in both meal assumption and the central control of WS behavior [13]. Further support to the presence of a functional interaction between sleep and body metabolism regulation at POA level is given by the fact that the hypothalamic control of body temperature is specifically suspended during REMS [28] and that, consequently, thermoregulatory activation depresses REMS occurrence [19].

In our study, the most evident change in sleep pattern across the development of obesity was the increase in REMS occurrence, in particular when the HC8 group was compared to the NC8 group. Cues for the interpretation of this finding come from the analysis of the effects of the exposure of NC8 and HC8 animals to the DD condition. This condition, which is known to specifically enhance REMS occurrence in the albino rat [17], was shown to be less powerful in concomitance with a depression of cellular activity at preoptic-hypothalamic level [15]. The results show that both NC8 and HC8 animals were responsive to DD stimulation, since a large and significant increase in the amount of REMS was observed during either the whole 24-h period of DD or, more specifically, during the first 12 h period in which L was substituted by D. However, the increase seen in the HC8 group was smaller than that observed in the NC8 group, as shown by the presence of a significant interaction between the factors "time" and "diet" and by the presence of a significant difference between LD and DD conditions in the NC8 group, but not in the HC8 group, on a 24-h basis.

On these bases, on one hand the presence of a normal response to the stimulus in the NC8 group (i.e. a large increase in sequential REMS and REMS clusters: see [15]) indicates that the depression in REMS occurrence observed in the NC8 group in comparison to the NC0 group lies in the range of a possible physiological adaptive response to the 8-week stay under laboratory conditions and it was not due to a non-specific pathological incapacity of these animals to generate REMS. On the other hand, the dampening of the response to DD in the HC8 animals is not comparable to that previously observed in the presence of a preoptic-hypothalamic impairment, since, in the latter, a depression in REMS occurrence was observed even when animals were kept under a normal LD schedule [16]. However, the dampening of the response in term of an increase in sequential REMS observed in the HC animals, may be taken as the presence of an hypothalamic impairment in the regulation of REMS occurrence revealed by the specific challenge of DD. This may lead to a ceiling effect limiting the increase of REMS under DD.

In conclusion, our results confirm that processes underlying energy homeostasis strongly interact with those underlying WS behavior. Furthermore, they suggest that this interaction tends to induce a behavioral optimization of energy use and storage: briefly, it would appear that on one hand an excess of Wake promotes an excess of energy accumulation, while on the other side an excess of energy accumulation reduces the amount Wake. On this basis, diet-induced obese rats represent a very good experimental model with which to investigate the interaction between WS disturbances and the development of obesity in humans.

## REFERENCES

1.  K. Spiegel, E. Tasali, R. Leproult, E. Van Cauter Effects of poor and short sleep on glucose metabolism and obesity risk Nat Rev Endocrinol, 5 (2009), pp. 253–261
2.  R.R. Markwald, E.L. Melanson, M.R. Smith, J. Higgins, L. Perreault, R.H. Eckel Impact of insufficient sleep on total daily energy expenditure, food intake, and weight gain Proc Natl Acad Sci, 110 (2013), pp. 5695–5700
3.  N.S. Marshall, N. Glozier, R.R. Grunstein Is sleep duration related to obesity? A critical review of the epidemiological evidence Sleep Med Rev, 12 (2008), pp. 289–298
4.  A.N. Vgontzas, E.O. Bixler, T.L. Tan, D. Kantner, L.F. Martin, A. Kales Obesity without sleep apnea is associated with daytime sleepiness Arch Intern Med, 158 (1998), pp. 1333–1337
5.  J.B. Jenkins, O. Takenori, G. Zhiwei, A.N. Vgontzas, E.O. Bixle, J. Fang Sleep is increased in mice with obesity induced by high-fat food Physiol Behav, 87 (2006), pp. 255–262
6.  Z. Guan, A.N. Vgontzas, E.O. Bixler, J. Fang Sleep is increased by weight gain and decreased by weight loss in mice Sleep, 31 (2008), pp. 627–633
7.  A.D. Laposky, J. Shelton, J. Bass, C. Dugovic, N. Perrino, F.W. Turek Altered sleep regulation in leptin-deficient mice Am J Physiol, 290 (2006), pp. R894–R903
8.  A. Silvani, S. Bastianini, C. Berteotti, C. Franzini, P. Lenzi, V.L. Martire et al. Sleep modulates hypertension in leptin-deficient obese mice Hypertension, 53 (2009), pp. 251–255
9.  J. Danguir Sleep patterns in the genetically obese Zucker rat: effect of acarbose treatment Am J Physiol, 256 (1989), pp. R281–R283
10. D. Megirian, J. Dmochowski, G.A. Farkas Mechanism controlling sleep organization of the obese Zucker rats J Appl Physiol, 84 (1998), pp. 253–256
11. A.D. Laposky, M.A. Bradley, D.L. Williams, J. Bass, F.W. Turek Sleep–wake regulation is altered in leptin-resistant (db/db) genetically obese and diabetic mice Am J Physiol, 295 (2008), pp. R2059–R2066
12. R. Szymusiak, I. Gvilia, D. McGinty Hypothalamic control of sleep Sleep Med, 8 (2007), pp. 291–301
13. M. Mieda, T. Sakurai Overview of orexin/hypocretin system Prog Brain Res, 198 (2012), pp. 5–14
14. S.F. Morrison, C.J. Madden, D. Tupone Central control of brown adipose tissue thermogenesis Front Endocrinol, 3 (2012), p. 5
15. G. Zamboni, R. Amici, E. Perez, C.A. Jones, P.L. Parmeggiani Pattern of REM sleep occurrence in continuous darkness following the exposure to low ambient temperature in the rat Behav Brain Res, 122 (2001), pp. 25–32
16. G. Zamboni, C.A. Jones, R. Domeniconi, R. Amici, E. Perez, M. Luppi et al. Specific changes in cerebral second messenger accumulation underlie REM sleep inhi-

bition induced by the exposure to low ambient temperature Brain Res, 1022 (2004), pp. 62–70

17. R. Fishman, H.P. Roffwarg REM sleep inhibition by light in the albino rat Exp Neurol, 36 (1972), pp. 166–178
18. B.E. Levin, J. Trsicari, A.C. Sullivan Relationship between sympathetic activity and diet-induced obesity in two rat strains Am J Physiol, 245 (1983), pp. R367–R371
19. M. Cerri, A. Ocampo-Garces, R. Amici, F. Baracchi, P. Capitani, C.A. Jones et al. Cold exposure and sleep in the rat: effects on sleep architecture and the electroencephalogram Sleep, 28 (2005), pp. 694–705
20. R. Amici, G. Zamboni, E. Perez, C.A. Jones, I. Toni, F. Culin et al. Pattern of desynchronized sleep during deprivation and recovery induced in the rat by changes in ambient temperature J Sleep Res, 3 (1994), pp. 250–256
21. R. Amici, G. Zamboni, E. Perez, C.A. Jones, P.L. Parmeggiani The influence of a heavy thermal load on REM sleep in the rat Brain Res, 781 (1998), pp. 252–258
22. D. Martelli, M. Luppi, M. Cerri, D. Tupone, E. Perez, G. Zamboni et al. Waking and sleeping following water deprivation in the rat PLoS ONE, 7 (2012), p. e46116
23. S. Holm A simple sequentially rejective multiple test procedure Scand J Stat, 6 (1979), pp. 65–70
24. A.N. Vgontzas, D.A. Papanicolaou, E.O. Bixler, A. Kales, K. Tyson, G.P. Chrousos Elevation of plasma cytokines in disorders of excessive daytime sleepiness: role of sleep disturbance and obesity J Clin Endocr Metab, 82 (1997), pp. 1313–1316
25. M.R. Opp Cytokines and sleep Sleep Med Rev, 9 (2005), pp. 355–364
26. D. Burdakov, J. Antonio González Physiological functions of glucose-inhibited neurons Acta Physiol, 195 (2008), pp. 71–78
27. J. Danguir Cafeteria diet promotes sleep in rats Appetite, 8 (1987), pp. 49–53
28. P.L. Parmeggiani Thermoregulation and sleep Front Biosci, 8 (2003), pp. s557–s567

*There are several supplemental files that are not available in this version of the article. To view this additional information, please use the citation information cited on the first page of this chapter.*

# CHAPTER 14

# EFFECT OF SLEEP DEPRIVATION ON BRAIN METABOLISM OF DEPRESSED PATIENTS

JOSEPH C. WU, J. CHRISTIAN GILLIN, MONTE S. BUCHSBAUM, TAMARA HERSHEY, J. CHAD JOHNSON, AND WILLIAM E. BUNNEY, JR.

Sleep deprivation has been shown to have a rapid, nonpharmacologic antidepressant effect in studies involving over 1,500 patients (1–3). In normal subjects sleep deprivation is associated with diminished vigilance and decreased metabolism in the thalamus and midbrain, according to studies using positron emission tomography (PET) (4). Since normal and depressed subjects seem to have different responses to sleep deprivation (1), a different regional metabolic response to sleep deprivation might well occur in such patients, perhaps involving the cingulate and other limbic structures. The limbic system has been hypothesized to be involved in mood (5). In this report we present the results of what we believe to be the first study of sleep deprivation in depression using PET with [18F]deoxyglucose (FDG) to assess limbic system metabolic correlates of mood and the antidepressant effects of sleep deprivation.

*Reprinted with permission from the American Psychiatric Association and the* American Journal of Psychiatry. *Wu JC, Gillin JC, Buchsbaum MS, Hershey T, Johnson JC, and Bunney WE. Effect of Sleep Deprivation on Brain Metabolism of Depressed Patients.* American Journal of Psychiatry *49,4 (1992), 538-543.*

## 14.1 METHOD

### 14.1.1 SUBJECTS

The subjects in this study were 15 normal control subjects (nine women, six men; mean age=31.9 years, SD=9.1) and 15 depressed outpatients (12 women, three men; mean age=30.5 years, SD=10.2). They were studied with FDG PET scans after a night of normal sleep and again after all-night sleep deprivation. All depressed subjects met the DSM-III-R criteria for unipolar major depression and had scores on the Hamilton Rating Scale for Depression of 17 or greater at the time of screening. Neither the patients nor the normal subjects had taken psychoactive medications for at least 2 weeks before the study. Ten of the patients had never taken antidepressants. The other five had previously received amitriptyline, desipramine, or alprazolam. The mean time without medication for these five patients was 4.7 months (SD=4.0). They reported that they had achieved clinical response to these medications and had relapsed when the medications were discontinued.

All subjects were free of physical disorders. The control subjects and their first-degree relatives were determined to be without mental disorders. Eight of the 15 normal control subjects in this study were reported on in our previous study of normal subjects (4). The depressed and normal control subjects were recruited through newspaper advertisements. Informed consent was obtained after the procedure was fully explained.

### 14.1.2 EXPERIMENTAL PROTOCOL AND CLINICAL ASSESSMENT

The subjects were deprived of sleep and kept under continuous supervision from approximately 7:00 a.m. until after the scanning procedure the following afternoon at 1:00-5:00 p.m. Mood was measured with the 21-item

Hamilton questionnaire, from which questions 4-6 were deleted because they deal with how the subject sleeps and are not applicable when the subject is deliberately deprived of sleep. The questionnaire was administered between 9:00 a.m. and noon on the baseline PET scan day (after a night of normal sleep) and on the second PET scan day (after sleep deprivation). On the basis of our previous findings (6), patients were defined as responders to sleep deprivation if their Hamilton depression scores decreased by at least 40% after total sleep deprivation. The FDG PET procedure has been described previously (7). During the uptake of FDG the subjects did the continuous performance test, a visual vigilance task (8).

### 14.1.3 BRAIN IMAGING PROTOCOL

Approximately 45 minutes after the injection of FDG, nine slice images were obtained. The repositioning of the patients during the two studies was accurate to within 2 mm because for each patient we reused a custom-molded thermoplastic mask that was aligned with the anatomical landmarks of the lateral canthus and external auditory meatus. The scan was transformed to a glucose metabolic rate as described previously (7).

Cortical metabolic rates were measured by using our cortical peel technique (4). Subcortical structures were assessed by using stereotaxic coordinates derived from a standard neuroanatomical atlas (9), as we have previously described (7). We analyzed the absolute metabolic rate, which was expressed in micromoles of glucose per 100 g of tissue per minute.

The brain was divided into eight main systems: lateral cortex (average of frontal, temporal, parietal, and occipital lobes), medial cortex (precuneus, paracentral, medial frontal, rectal gyri, calcarine, and medial temporal), limbic system (average of amygdala, hippocampus, and cingulate), basal ganglia (average of caudate, putamen, and globus pallidus), thalamus, white matter (average of frontal white matter, corpus callosum, and optic radiation), midbrain, and cerebellum.

Statistical analysis comprised a four-way repeated measures multivariate analysis of variance (MANOVA) with BMDP 4V software (10), followed by post hoc t tests. The dimensions of the MANOVA were diagnostic group, brain system, hemisphere, and sleep condition. All significant interactions between group and sleep condition are reported. When significant interactions between brain regions and conditions were observed, we used simple effects analysis and t tests as post hoc contrasts.

## 14.2 RESULTS

### 14.2.1 CLINICAL RESPONSE

Of the 15 depressed patients, four were identified as responders (decrease in Hamilton depression score 40%). The responders and nonresponders did not differ significantly in mean age (responders: mean=29.8 years, SD=10.3; nonresponders: mean=30.8 years, SD= 10.6), sex distribution (responders: four women; nonresponders: eight women and three men), or mean baseline Hamilton depression score (responders: mean= 19.8, SD=5.9; nonresponders: mean=21.3, SD=7.3). The responders showed a significantly greater decrease in depression score; their mean Hamilton score after sleep deprivation was 6.0 (SD=2.1), compared to 19.9 (SD=9.4) for the nonresponders.

### 14.2.2 CHANGES IN REGIONAL METABOLIC RATES

At baseline the responders differed significantly from the nonresponders in their metabolic rate pattern (see table 1). Simple effects analysis and follow-up t tests revealed that the baseline glucose metabolic rate in the limbic system was significantly higher in the depressed responders than in either the depressed nonresponders or the normal control subjects (see table 1). Similar analyses indicated that the depressed responders had a significantly higher metabolic rate in the medial cortex than did the normal control subjects. No differences in whole brain metabolic rate were found, i.e., the main effect of subject group was not significant.

There was a significant difference in the patterns of change in absolute brain system metabolic rates after sleep deprivation among the responders, nonresponders, and normal control subjects (see table 1). The responders experienced a significant decrease in their initially high metabolic rate in the limbic system after sleep deprivation, whereas neither the normal control subjects nor the nonresponders showed a significant change as indicated by ANOVA. Again, no main effect across all structures was confirmed, indicating regional specificity for the effect.

**TABLE 1:** Brain Metabolism and Visual Vigilance Before and After Sleep Deprivation in Depressed Responders, Depressed Nonresponders, and Normal Subjects[a]

| Variable and Condition (before or after sleep deprivation) | Responders (N = 4) | | Nonresponders (N = 11) | | Normal Subjects (N = 15) | |
|---|---|---|---|---|---|---|
| | Mean | SD | Mean | SD | Mean | SD |
| Glucose metabolic rate (prnol/iOO g tissue/mm) | | | | | | |
| Cortical surface | | | | | | |
| Before | 31.5 | 6.3 | 26.2 | 6.5 | 24.0 | 6.6 |
| After | 27.4 | 6.9 | 26.0 | 9.9 | 23.7 | 7.1 |
| Medial cortex | | | | | | |
| Before | 38.3[b] | 7.4 | 31.1 | 7.4 | 28.3 | 7.4 |
| After | 33.2 | 8.3 | 31.2 | 11.0 | 28.3 | 8.0 |
| Limbic system | | | | | | |
| Before | 26.6[c] | 8.3 | 19.8 | 3.5 | 18.9 | 4.6 |
| After | 21.5 | 6.4 | 19.1 | 7.1 | 18.5 | 5.7 |
| Thalamus | | | | | | |
| Before | 31.0[d] | 5.1 | 25.1[e] | 6.0 | 26.6 | 6.8 |
| After | 28.1 | 9.3 | 26.1 | 10.7 | 23.6 | 7.9 |
| Basal ganglia | | | | | | |
| Before | 34.4 | 6.4 | 27.7 | 6.7 | 27.1 | 6.5 |
| After | 27.6 | 6.5 | 27.0 | 11.0 | 25.7 | 8.7 |
| White matter | | | | | | |
| Before | 21.1 | 5.6 | 17.5 | 4.6 | 16.2 | 4.3 |
| After | 20.1 | 5.4 | 18.1 | 6.3 | 17.9 | 5.3 |
| Midbrain | | | | | | |

**TABLE 1:** *Cont.*

| Variable and Condition (before or after sleep deprivation) | Responders (N =4) | | Nonresponders (N = 11) | | Normal Subjects (N = 15) | |
|---|---|---|---|---|---|---|
| | Mean | SD | Mean | SD | Mean | SD |
| Before | 21.9 | 8.9 | 17.1 | 4.1 | 17.1 | 4.4 |
| After | 17.6 | 5.9 | 16.5 | 7.6 | 15.6 | 4.7 |
| Cerebellum | | | | | | |
| Before | 22.0[f] | 8.4 | 18.9 | 4.5 | 19.2 | 5.4 |
| After | 18.0 | 7.2 | 20.4 | 11.0 | 16.6 | 5.6 |
| Score on continuous performance task (d') | | | | | | |
| Before | 4.1[g] | 0.0 | 3.4 | 0.8 | 3.3 | 1.0 |
| After | 35[h] | 0.5 | 2.9[i] | 0.9 | 2.8[j] | 0.9 |

[a]*Significant Condition by Brain System by Group interaction (F=2.41, df=14, 40, p=0.02) and System by Group interaction for baseline only (F=2.60, df=14, 40, p=O.OO9) (MANOVA).*
[b]*Siguificantly higher in responders than in normal subjects (t=2.41, df=17, p=0.03).*
[c]*Siguificantly higher in responders than in nonresponders (t=2.25, df=12, p=0.04) or normal subjects (t=2.54, df=17, p=0.02) (F=4.13, df=2,26, p=0.02; Bonferroni criterion: n.s.). Negative correlation with change in visual vigilance (r= –0.95, df=2, p<0.05).*
[d]*Negative correlation with change in visual vigilance (r= –0.96, df=2, p<0.05).*
[e]*Positive correlation with change in visual vigilance (r=0.71, df=9, p<0.05).*
[f]*Negative correlation with change in visual vigilance (r= –0.97, df=2, p<0.05).*
[g]*Significantty higher in responders than in nonresponders (t=2.68, df=12, p<0.0S) or normal subjects (t=3.19, df=17, p<0.05).*
[h]*Significantly lower than at baseline (t=2.32, df=3, p<0.05).*
[i]*Significantly lower than at baseline (t=3.58, df=9, p<0.05).*
[j]*Significantly lower than at baseline (t=4.01, df=14, p<0.05).*

The rates in the cingulate, amygdala, and hippocampus were measured to obtain the limbic system average (see figures 1 and 2). At baseline the depressed responders had significantly higher cingulate and amygdala glucose metabolic rates than either the nonresponders or the normal control subjects. In contrast, the glucose metabolic rates in the hippocampus did not significantly differ between the responders and either the nonresponders or the normal control subjects. The glucose metabolic rate in the cingulate decreased significantly after sleep deprivation for the responders, whereas the nonresponders and normal control subjects showed little change. The amygdala did not show a statistically significant decrease in the responders. These findings were confirmed by a three-way ANOVA interaction (Diagnostic Group by Brain System by Sleep Condition: $F=2.74$, $df=3.69$, $48.02$, $p<0.05$, Greenhouse-Geisser corrected) and exploratory post hoc t tests.

After sleep deprivation all of the responders showed a decrease in the cingulate of at least 2.0 μmol glucose/ 100 g tissue per minute. Of the 11 nonresponders, four showed similar decreases, two showed increases, and five showed no change.

Vigilance was assessed quantitatively by using the d' measure (4). Greater vigilance is associated with a higher d' value. Before sleep deprivation the mean d' vigilance score on the continuous performance test was higher for the depressed responders than for either the depressed nonresponders or the normal control subjects (see table 1). All three groups had lower d' values after sleep deprivation, and the change was significant for all three groups according to paired t tests, but the differences did not vary between groups.

Significant negative correlations between change in vigilance score and baseline metabolic values in the limbic system, thalamus, and cerebellum were found for the depressed responders (see table 1). A significant positive correlation was found between the baseline thalamus metabolic value and change in d' score for the depressed nonrespondenrs.

Hypofrontality values were calculated by taking the metabolic mates for the four frontal lobe segments in each hemisphere (superior, middle, inferior frontal gyri, and precentral gyrus) and dividing these by the occipital lobe metabolic rate. No significant group differences were found between the depressed responders and either the depressed nonresponders or normal control subjects according to ANOVAs on t tests.

## 14.3 DISCUSSION

The baseline metabolic rates for the cingulate cortex and amygdala were significantly higher in the depressed patients who responded to sleep deprivation than in the patients who did not respond or the normal control

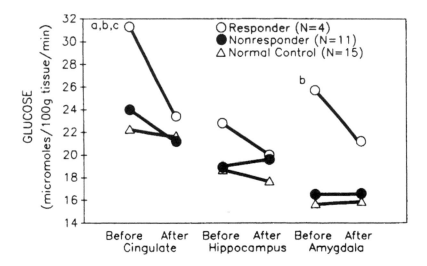

<sup>a</sup>Significant difference between responders and nonresponders at baseline (t=2.69, df=12, p=0.02).
<sup>b</sup>Significant difference between responders and normal subjects at baseline for cingulate (t=2.75, df=17, p=0.01) and for amygdala (t=3.09, df=17, p=0.01)..
<sup>c</sup>Significant difference between rates before and after sleep deprivation (t=2.42, df=17, p=0.03).

**FIGURE 1:** Mean Glucose Metabolic Rates for Limbic System Structures Before and After Sleep Deprivation in Depressed Responders, Depressed Nonresponders, and Normal Subjects

subjects. The metabolic mate for the cingulate fell significantly toward normal in the depressed responders after sleep deprivation, while that for the amygdala decreased nonsignificantly. These findings should be viewed as preliminary because of the relatively small number of responders and should be replicated in a larger cohort of depressed patients.

On the basis of our findings, we tentatively hypothesize that overactivation in the limbic system as measured by FDG PET scans is present in a subset of depressed patients before sleep deprivation. We suggest that in this subset sleep deprivation reduces depression by reducing the overactivity in these regions. These interpretations are consistent with earlier suggestions (11, 12) that some depressed patients are "overaroused" and that sleep deprivation acts by reversing this abnormality.

A subset of depressed patients have subnormal slow wave sleep (13, 14), and it may be this subset who respond best to sleep deprivation (15). Slow wave sleep has been hypothesized (16, 17) to slow down metabolic activity as a way of dissipating the heat load incurred during awake time. An impaired ability to activate slow wave sleep in a subset of depressed patients could result in an inability to slow down metabolism. Depressed patients have been shown to have abnormally high core body temperatures during the sleep period (18-20), and this finding is especially true in the subtype of patients who respond to sleep deprivation (21). Wehr (22) has hypothesized that prolonged awake time might reduce body metabolism. Prolonged awake time (i.e., sleep deprivation) might act like slow wave sleep to reduce body metabolism, whereas REM sleep may maintain high body temperature.

In addition to subnormal slow wave sleep and higher than normal nocturnal temperature, high levels of thynoid hormones differentiate the subset of depressed patients who respond to sleep deprivation (23). Higher than normal levels of thyroid hormones may be a neuroendocrine correlate of overarousal in this subset of depression.

We also observed higher baseline vigilance scones (as measured by the d' on the continuous performance test) in the depressed responders than in either the nonresponders or the normal control subjects. This observation is consistent with the theory of overarousal in depression, since vigilance is associated with arousal (11, 12). In a study of sleep deprivation in 16 depressed patients by Bouhuys et al. (24), self-reported arousal was cor-

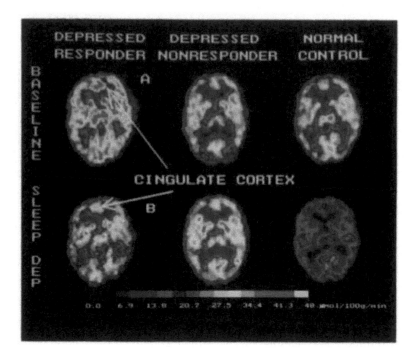

[a]All images are displayed with the same metabolic rate scale, shown as a bar at the bottom. Note the high cingulate activity (A) in the responders before sleep deprivation and the normalization of cingulate activity (B) after sleep deprivation.

**FIGURE 2:** PET Scans for Depressed Responders, Depressed Nonresponders, and Normal Subjects Before and After Sleep Deprivationa

related with mood response. The cingulate cortex has been implicated in maintenance of vigilance (25), which is also associated with arousal (26).

In a previous study (7), the cingulate gyrus was the only cortical structure with a significantly higher glucose metabolic rate during REM sleep than during the normal waking state. REM sleep is associated with an increase in cholinergic activity and a decrease in aminergic activity (27). Short REM latency in depressed patients may also be an indicator of hyperarousal. Further studies are needed to determine the causal chain of events.

The cingulate cortex is innervated by cholinergic input from cells in the basal forebrain (28, 29). Depressed patients have been hypothesized to have an overactive cholinergic system (30), in part because of a supersensitive responsiveness to the cholinergic REM induction test (31, 32). An overactive cingulate cortex might also be associated with an underactive aminergic system, which has also been hypothesized for depression (30). Depressed patients treated with sertraline, a serotonergic reuptake inhibitor, were found to have significantly decreased cingulate cortex metabolism, as assessed by PET scans (J.C. Wu, unpublished data). Enhancement of serotonergic function by lithium has been shown to prevent relapse with recovered sleep after total sleep deprivation (33) or after partial sleep deprivation (34). Decreasing serotonergic function through tryptophan depletion has been found to precipitate a depressogenic relapse in patients who have responded to antidepressants (35).

The large decrease seen in the cingulate cortex of the depressed responders after sleep deprivation was seen in only a few of the nonrespondenrs and normal control subjects. In our previous study of normal subjects (4), in which eight of the 15 normal control subjects in this study were also studied, the limbic system did not show a significant decrease in glucose metabolic rate after sleep deprivation. Our present analysis with the larger cohort of normal control subjects also shows no significant decrease in the cingulate cortex rate for normal subjects. The limbic system was the only one of eight brain systems (including the dorsolateral cortex, medial cortex, basal ganglia, thalamus, midbrain, white matter, cerebellum) that showed a significant difference between depressed responders and both the normal subjects and depressed nonresponders.

The method used to study the regions of interest relics on stereotaxic coordinates based on a neuroanatomical atlas (9). Using the Talairach atlas (36), we estimated the volume of the hippocampus to be 3000 mm². The approximate dimensions of the hippocampus are 12 mm thick by 25 mm long by 10 mm wide. The dimensions of the hippocampus can easily accommodate our stereotaxic boxes, which are 10 mm thick by 6 mm long by 6 mm wide. The approximate dimensions of the amygdala are 8 mm thick by 12 mm long by 10 mm wide, for a total volume of approximately 960 mm². Although it is smaller, this structure can also accommodate our 10 mm by 6 mm by 6 mm stereotaxic box. Talairach et al. (36) and Vanier et al. (37) have demonstrated that a proportional system for localizing structures in the brain is much more reliable than using distances from bony landmarks in millimeters. This is because a proportional-based system normalizes the brains of different individuals and permits individual cases to be reduced to a common scale. Random variation caused by individual differences in brain proportions, vertical position of the plane studied, and variation in head position and reposition would all tend to create random error and diminish group differences.

The higher right precentral gyrus metabolic rate in the depressed responders than in the depressed nonresponders is consistent with the hypofrontality in depressed unipolar patients previously reported by our group (38), but it is not consistent with the hypofrontality reported by Baxter et al. (39). This may be due to the differences in the cognitive task studied during the glucose-uptake period.

This study has some important clinical implications. It may be possible to better characterize subtypes of depression with different responses to treatment by using an objective biological measure (e.g., PET scans) as a basis for classification. This study provides evidence for a distinct subtype of depression with overactive limbic system metabolism that responds to sleep deprivation.

## 14.4 ADDENDUM

Since this manuscript was submitted, similar findings were presented by D. Ebert, H. Feistel, and A. Barocka at the 5th World Congress of the World Federation of Societies of Biological Psychiatry, Florence, Italy,

June 9-14, 1991. Using technetium $^{99m}$Tc HMPAO SPECT, they showed that responders to sleep deprivation, but not nonresponders, were more hyperperfused in the limbic system than normal control subjects.

## REFERENCES

1. Wu JC, Bunney WE: The biological basis of an antidepressant response to sleep deprivation and relapse: review and hypothesis. Am J Psychiatry 1990; 147:14-21
2. Gillin JC: The sleep therapies of depression. Prog Neuropsychopharmacot Biol Psychiatry 1983; 7:351-364
3. Hittman E, Kripke DF, Gillin JC: Sleep restriction, exercise, and bright lights: alternative therapies for depression, in American Psychiatric Press Review of Psychiatry, vol 9. Edited by Tasman A, Kaufman C, Gotdfinger S. Washington, DC, American Psychiatric Press, 1990
4. Wu JC, Gittin JC, Buchsbaum MS, Hershey T, Haztett E, Sicotte N, Bunney WE: The effect of sleep deprivation on cerebral glucose metabolic rate in normal humans assessed with positron emission tomography. Sleep 1991; 14:155-162
5. Papez JW: A proposed mechanism of emotion. Arch Neurol Psychiatry 1937; 38:725-743
6. Gillin JC, Janowsky DS, Risch SC, Kripke DF: Effects of brief naps on mood and sleep in sleep-deprived depressed patients. Psychiatry Res 1989; 27:253-265
7. Buchsbaum MS, Wu JC, Haier R, Haztett E, Ball R, Katz M, Sokolski K, Lagunas-Sotar M, Langer DH: Positron emission tomography assessment of effects of benzodiazepines on regional cerebral glucose metabolic rate of patients with anxiety disorder. Life Sci i987; 40:2393-2400
8. Nuechtertein KH, Parasuraman R, Jiang Q: Visual sustained attention image degradation produces rapid sensitivity decrement over time. Science 1983; 220:327-329
9. Matsui T, Hirano A: An Atlas of the Human Brain for Computerized Tomography. Tokyo, Igaku-Shoin, 1978
10. Dixon WJ (ed): BMDP Statistical Software Manual. Berkeley, University of California Press, 1981
11. van den Burg W, Van den Hoofdakker RH: Total sleep deprivation in endogenous deprivation. Arch Gen Psychiatry 1975; 32: 1121-1125
12. Gillin JC, Sitaram N, Wehr T, Duncan W, Post R, Murphy DL, Mendelson WB, Wyatt RJ, Bunney WE: Sleep and affective illness, in Neurobiology of Mood Disorders. Edited by Post RM, Ballenger JC. Baltimore, Williams & Wilkins, 1984
13. Reynolds CF, Gillin JC, Kupfer DF: Sleep and affective disorder, in Psychopharmacology: The Third Generation of Progress. Edited by Meltzer HY. New York, Raven Press, 1987
14. Borbety AA, Wirz-Justice A: Sleep, sleep deprivation and depression. Human Neurobiology 1982; 1:205-210

15. Duncan WC, Gitlin JC, Post RM, Gerner RH, Wehr TA: Relationship between EEG sleep patterns and clinical improvement in depressed patients treated with sleep deprivation. Biol Psychiatry 1980; 15:879-889

16. Berger RM, Phillips NH: Comparative aspects of energy metabolism, body temperature, and sleep. Acta Physiol Scand (Suppl) 1988; 574:21-27

17. McGinty D, Szymusiak R, Moriarty 5: Thermoregulatory controt of slow wave sleep. Sleep Res 1991; 20:5 1

18. Avery DH, Wildshiodt G, Rafaelson OJ: Nocturnal temperature in affective disorders. J Affective Disord 1982; 4:61-71

19. Beersma DGM, Van den Hoofdakker RH, van Berkestijn HWBM: Circadian rhythms in affective disorders: body temperature and sleep physiology in endogenous depressives. Adv Biol Psychiatry 1983; 11:114-127

20. Schulz H, Lund R: Sleep onset REM episodes are associated with circadian parameters of body temperature: a study in depressed patients and normal controls. Biol Psychiatry 1983; 18:1411-1426

21. Elsenga 5, Van den Hoofdakker RH: Body core temperature and depression during total sleep deprivation in depressives. Biol Psychiatry 1988; 24:53 1-540

22. Wehr TA: Manipulations of sleep and phototherapy: nonpharmacological alternatives in the treatment of depression. Clin Neuropharmacot 1990; 13(suppl 1):s54-s65

23. Baumgartner A, Riemann D, Berger M: Neuroendocrinological investigations during sleep deprivation in depression, II: longitudinat measurement of thyrotropin, TH, cortisol, prolactin, GH, and LH during sleep and sleep deprivation. Biol Psychiatry 1990; 28:569-587

24. Bouhuys AL, Ftentge F, Van den Hoofdakker RH: Effects of total sleep deprivation on urinary cortisol, self-rated arousal, and mood in depressed patients. Psychiatry Res 1991; 34:149-162

25. Posner MI, Petersen SE, Fox PT, Raichle ME: Localization of cognitive operations in the human brain. Science 1988; 240: 1627-1631.

26. Mirsky AF, Carson PV Jr: A comparison of the behavioral and physiological changes accompanying sleep deprivation and chlorpromazine administration in man. Electroencephalogr Clin Neurophysiol 1962; 14:1-10

27. Hobson JA, Lydic R, Baghdoyan HA: Evolving concepts of sleep cycle generation: from brain centers to neuronal populations. Behavioral and Brain Sciences 1986; 9:371-448

28. Saper CB: Organization of cerebral cortical afferent systems in the rat, II: magnocellular basal nucleus. J Comp Neurot I 984; 222:313-342

29. Borst JGG, Leung SWS, MacFabe DF: Electrical activity of the cingulate cortex, II: cholinergic modulation. Brain Res 1987; 407:81-93

30. Janowsky DL, El-Yousef MK, Davis JM: A cholmnergic-adrenergic hypothesis of mania and depression. Lancet I 972; 2:632-635

31. Gillin JC, Sutton L, Ruiz C, Kelsoe J, Dupont R, Darko D, Risch SC, Golshan F, Janowsky D: The cholinergic REM induction test with arecholine in depression. Arch Gen Psychiatry 1991; 48: 264-270

32. Berger M, Riemann D, Hochli D, Spiegel R: The cholinergic rapid eye movement sleep induction test with RS-86: state or trait marker of depression? Arch Gen Psychiatry 1989; 46:421-428

33. Grube M, Hartwich P: Maintenance of antidepressant effect of sleep deprivation with the help of lithium. Eur Arch Psychiatry Neurol Sci 1990; 240:60-61

34. Baxter LRJr, Liston EH, SchwartzJM, Altshuler LL, WilkinsJN, Richeimer 5, Guze BH: Prolongation of the antidepressant response to partial sleep deprivation by lithium. Psychiatry Res 1986; 19:17-23

35. Delgado PL, Charney DS, Price LH, Aghajanian GK, Landis H, Heninger GR: Serotonin function and the mechanism of antidepressant action: reversal of antidepressant-induced remission by rapid depletion of plasma tryptophan. Arch Gen Psychiatry 1990; 47:411-418

36. Talairach J, Szikla G, Tournoux P, Prossalentis A, Bordas-Ferrer M, Covello L, Jacob M, Mempet A, Buser P, Bancaud J: Atlas d'anatomie stereotaxique du telencephale. Paris, Masson, 1967

37. Vanier M, Roch Lecours A, Ethier R, Habib M, Poncet M, Milette PC, Salamon G: Proportional localization system for anatomical interpretation of cerebral computed tomograms. J Cornput Assist Tomogr 1985; 9:715-724

38. Buchsbaum MS, Wu J, DeLisi LE, Holcomb H, Kessler R, Johnson J, King AC, Hazlett E, Langston K, Post RM: Frontal cortex and basal ganglia metabolic rates assessed by positron emission tomography with ['8F]2-deoxyglucose in affective illness. J Affective Disord 1986; 10:137-152

39. Baxter LR Jr, SchwartzJM, Phelps ME, Mazziotta JC, Guze BH, 5dm CE, Gerner RH, Sumida RM: Reduction of prefrontal cortex glucose metabolism common to three types of depression. Arch Gen Psychiatry 1989; 46:243-250

# AUTHOR NOTES

## CHAPTER 1

### Author Contributions

ELB sampled the *Cry1-/-Cry2-/-* mice and performed behavior experiments on *Cry1-/-Cry2-/-* mice. SH sampled the melanopsin-deficient mice and triple knockout mice. MYC performed the tissue sectioning, in situ hybridizations and all quantitative analyses. MYC, ELB and QYZ drafted the manuscript. ELB, SH, MYC and QYZ designed the studies. All authors read and approved the final manuscript.

### Acknowledgments

We thank David R. Weaver and King-Wai Yau for providing helpful discussions, in situ probes and critical comments on the manuscript. We would also like to thank Aziz Sancar for providing access to *Cry1-/-Cry2-/-* mice, Frances Leslie for helpful discussions and equipment use, James Belluzzi for help with statistical analysis, Alex Lee for mice running-wheel setup and data analysis, Clayton Bullock and Jia-da Li for technical assistance and discussions. The research is partially supported by NIH grants (to QYZ and ELB). MYC was supported in part by a NIDA training grant and by a predoctoral fellowship from PhRMA Foundation.

## CHAPTER 2

### Author Contributions

MAO and SS performed the analysis. RRA, DCD and WJJ assisted in data interpretation. IPA supervised the study. All authors read and approved the final manuscript.

## Acknowledgments

Support for this work has been partially provided by USEPA-funded Environmental Bioinformatics and Computational Toxicology Center (ebCTC), under grant number GAD R 832721-010 and National Institutes of Health under grant number GM 24211. This work has not been reviewed by and does not represent the opinions of the funding agencies.

## CHAPTER 3

### Competing Interests

The authors declare that they have no competing interests.

### Author Contributions

MMZ wrote the manuscript and performed the literature review. MLCG revised the manuscript and made suggestions for intellectual content. MBM helped in literature background and revised the manuscript. SMFV supervised the project and revised the manuscript. All authors have read and approved the final version of the manuscript.

## CHAPTER 4

### Funding

This work was supported by a project grant (SFB 654) of the German Research Foundation (DFG) to HO and HL; HO is an Emmy Noether fellow of the DFG and a Lichtenberg fellow of the Volkswagen Foundation. The funders had no role in study design, data collection and analysis, decision to publish, or preparation of the manuscript.

### Competing Interests

The authors have declared that no competing interests exist.

### Acknowledgments

The authors would like to acknowledge Ms Christin Helbig for technical assistance.

## Author Contributions

Conceived and designed the experiments: HL HO. Performed the experiments: JLB BB JH JM-K NN HO. Analyzed the data: JLB SMS HO. Wrote the paper: JLB HO.

## CHAPTER 7

### Competing Interests

The authors declare that they have no competing interests.

### Author Contributions

This manuscript is based on doctoral research completed by OJM with additional analysis and interpretation by RHW. OJM, RHW, and RES did the immunohistochemistry and quantification of immunostaining, OJM and MMC analyzed the behavioral data, and NU advised and provided financial support for the study, while OJM and HDP performed the statistical tests. OJM, RHW, and HDP wrote the paper.

### Acknowledgments

Supported by project grants from the BBSRC to HDP and by an MRC-GSK Industrial Collaborative Studentship to OJM. We thank Johan Oldekopp for technical assistance.

## CHAPTER 8

### Funding

This work was supported by the Korea Research Foundation (KRF) grants funded by Korea government (MEST) (Nos. 331-2006-1-C00212, 313-2007-2-C00625, 2008-0062417, 2009-0088886). The funders had no role in study design, data collection and analysis, decision to publish, or preparation of the manuscript.

### Competing Interests

The authors have declared that no competing interests exist.

## Author Contributions

Conceived and designed the experiments: JAY GHS SC. Performed the experiments: JAY DHH JYN MHK SC. Analyzed the data: JYN DHH GHS KK CJK YKP SC. Contributed reagents/materials/analysis tools: KK YKP CJK SC. Wrote the paper: JYN DHH GHS SC.

## CHAPTER 9

### Acknowledgments

The author is supported by DARPA Young Faculty Award N66001-09-1-2117 and NINDS 1R15NS070734.

## CHAPTER 10

### Competing Interests

The authors declare that they have no competing interests.

### Author Contributions

AH wrote the manuscript and performed circadian phenotyping. SK and KM edited the manuscript. All authors read and approved the final manuscript.

### Acknowledgments

This study was supported by Grants-in-Aid for Scientific Research from the Ministry of Education, Culture, Sports, and Technology of Japan and from the Ministry of Health, Labour, and Welfare of Japan. A part of this study is the result of "Understanding of molecular and environmental bases for brain health" carried out under the Strategic Research Program for Brain Sciences by the Ministry of Education, Culture, Sports, Science and Technology of Japan.

## CHAPTER 11

### Acknowledgments

The author would like to thank J. Mohawk, M. Hagenauer, and J. Koch for reviews of earlier drafts of this manuscript.

## CHAPTER 12

### Competing Interests

The authors declare that they have no competing interests.

### Author Contributions

MSR conceived the study, lead the team in its execution and drafted major sections of the paper, AB formulated the analyses and drafted portions of the Results and Discussion sections, MGF was instrumental in acquiring the nurse data, drafted sections of the paper and provided expertise while preparing the manuscript, JDB was instrumental in acquiring the rat data and provided expertise while preparing the manuscript. All authors participated equally in discussions and the exchange of ideas during the study, and all reviewed and approved the final manuscript.

### Acknowledgments

The authors would like to thank Dr. Bernard Possidente at Skidmore College and Drs. Irma and Jose Russo at Fox Chase Cancer Research Institute for collaboration with the animal experiments. Thanks also to Mr. Terry Klein who helped develop and calibrate the Daysimeter, to Mr. Yutao Zhou for performing several analyses, Mr. Dennis Guyon for graphical support, as well as to Ms. Jennifer Taylor who provided editorial support, all of whom are at the Lighting Research Center at Rensselaer Polytechnic Institute. This work was supported in part by CDC Grant 1R01 OH008171 to Dr. Eva Schernhammer at Harvard Public Health and by the Trans-NIH Genes, Environment and Health Initiative Grant 1U01 DA023822-01 to the first author.

## CHAPTER 13

### Conflict of Interest

The authors declare no competing financial interests.

### Acknowledgments

This work has been supported by the Ministero dell'Università e della Ricerca Scientifica (MIUR), Italy, (PRIN 2009, Project 2009SPTHRK) and by the University of Bologna (University Strategic Project 2006). The authors wish to thank Dr. Silvia Laudadio for technical help and Ms Melissa Stott for reviewing the English.

# INDEX

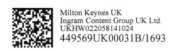